Register
Access

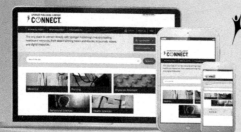

SPRINGER PUBLISHING COMPANY
CONNECT™

Your print purchase of *The Physician Assistant Student's Guide to the Clinical Year: Emergency Medicine* **includes online access to the contents of your book**—increasing accessibility, portability, and searchability!

Access today at:

http://connect.springerpub.com/content/book/ 978-0-8261-9537-1 or scan the QR code at the right with your smartphone and enter the access code below.

Scan here for quick access.

8P393CM1

M000205074

Titles in *The Physician Assistant Student's Guide to the Clinical Year* Series

Family Medicine

Gerald Kayingo
Deborah Opacic
Mary Carcella Allias

Internal Medicine

David Knechtel
Deborah Opacic

Emergency Medicine

Dipali Yeh
Erin Marthedal

Surgery

Brennan Bowker

OB/GYN

Elyse Watkins

Pediatrics

Tanya L. Fernandez
Amy Akerman

Behavioral Health

Jill Cavalet

THE PHYSICIAN ASSISTANT STUDENT'S GUIDE

to the Clinical Year

Dipali Yeh, MS, PA-C, CHSE, is an assistant professor at Rutgers University Physician Assistant Program in New Jersey and has been a faculty member for 10 years. She received her BS in biology in 1999 from Seton Hall University and then went on to complete her Master of Science in Physician Assistant degree in 2001 from the joint University of Medicine and Dentistry of New Jersey (UMDNJ)/Seton Hall University program. She has 18 years of experience in emergency medicine and continues to work clinically at Robert Wood Johnson University Hospital. Ms. Yeh is a certified healthcare simulation expert in the PA program. Her role includes coordinating all simulation activity for the program and is involved in interprofessional education for the School of Health Professions. She is also currently pursuing her PhD in Interdisciplinary Healthcare Studies at Rosalind Franklin University.

Erin Marthedal, MS, PA-C, holds a volunteer faculty appointment as a clinical instructor in the department of primary care at the Rutgers School of Health Professions, where she works with PA students and faculty. Ms. Marthedal also works in clinical practice at a private urgent care center in New Jersey. From 2010 to 2016 she was a cinical instructor in the emergency department at the Robert Wood Johnson School of Medicine. She has experience in emergency medicine, urgent care medicine, clinical preceptorship, and community-based primary care clinic work in the United States and abroad. Ms. Marthedal is a graduate of the Rutgers School of Health Professions, Master of Science Physician Assistant program. She works with the New Jersey State Society for Physician Assistants Foundation and was awarded the 2018 Rutgers School of Health-Related Professions Distinguished Service Award. She has previously been published in a peer-reviewed journal and has given academic presentations for the Robert Wood Johnson Emergency Medicine residency program and New Jersey State Society for Physician Assistants educational conference.

Maureen Knechtel, MPAS, PA-C (Series Editor), received a bachelor's degree in health science and a master's degree in physician assistant (PA) studies from Duquesne University in Pittsburgh, Pennsylvania. She is the author of the textbook *EKGs for the Nurse Practitioner and Physician Assistant*, first and second editions. Ms. Knechtel is a fellow member of the Physician Assistant Education Association, the American Academy of Physician Assistants, and the Tennessee Academy of Physician Assistants. She is the academic coordinator and an assistant professor with the Milligan College Physician Assistant Program in Johnson City, Tennessee, and practices as a cardiology PA with the Ballad Health Cardiovascular Associates Heart Institute. Ms. Knechtel has been a guest lecturer nationally and locally on topics including EKG interpretation, chronic angina, ischemic and hemorrhagic stroke, hypertension, and mixed hyperlipidemia.

THE PHYSICIAN ASSISTANT STUDENT'S GUIDE

to the Clinical Year

EMERGENCY MEDICINE

Dipali Yeh, MS, PA-C, CHSE
Erin Marthedal, MS, PA-C

SPRINGER PUBLISHING COMPANY

Copyright © 2020 Springer Publishing Company, LLC

Springer Publishing Company, LLC
11 West 42nd Street
New York, NY 10036
www.springerpub.com
http://connect.springerpub.com/home

Acquisitions Editor: Suzanne Toppy
Compositor: diacriTech

ISBN: 978-0-8261-9527-2
ebook ISBN: 978-0-8261-9537-1
DOI: 10.1891/9780826195371

19 20 21 22 23 / 5 4 3 2 1

The author and the publisher of this Work have made every effort to use sources believed to be reliable to provide information that is accurate and compatible with the standards generally accepted at the time of publication. Because medical science is continually advancing, our knowledge base continues to expand. Therefore, as new information becomes available, changes in procedures become necessary. We recommend that the reader always consult current research and specific institutional policies before performing any clinical procedure or delivering any medication. The author and publisher shall not be liable for any special, consequential, or exemplary damages resulting, in whole or in part, from the readers' use of, or reliance on, the information contained in this book. The publisher has no responsibility for the persistence or accuracy of URLs for external or third-party Internet websites referred to in this publication and does not guarantee that any content on such websites is, or will remain, accurate or appropriate.

CIP data is on file at the Library of Congress.
Library of Congress Control Number: 2019912917

Contact us to receive discount rates on bulk purchases.
We can also customize our books to meet your needs.
For more information please contact: sales@springerpub.com

Publisher's Note: New and used products purchased from third-party sellers are not guaranteed for quality, authenticity, or access to any included digital components.

Printed in the United States of America.

This book is dedicated to the faculty and staff of the Robert Wood Johnson Emergency Department. Thank you for raising me. And, of course, also to Sloane, Gavin, Logan, and Bella for climbing into my heart.

—DIPALI YEH

To the loved ones who supported me through the writing of this book; to the instructors, mentors, and patients who have taught me so much; and to the students and providers embarking on new career paths; I am forever grateful.

—ERIN MARTHEDAL

Contents

e-Chapter 8. Case Studies in Emergency Medicine
https://connect.springerpub.com/content/book/978-0-8261-9537
-1/chapter/ch08

e-Chapter 9. Review Questions in Emergency Medicine
https://connect.springerpub.com/content/book/978-0-8261-9537
-1/chapter/ch09

e-Chapter 10. Additional Resources to Enhance the Emergency
Medicine Rotation
https://connect.springerpub.com/content/book/978-0-8261-9537
-1/chapter/ch10

Contributor

John P. Bastin, MHS, PA-C, EM-CAQ, CPAAPA,   Assistant Professor, School of Physician Assistant Practice, Florida State University College of Medicine, Tallahassee, Florida

Peer Reviewers

Craig Hritz, MPAS, PA-C   Assistant Professor, Manchester–Worcester Physician Assistant Program, Manchester, New Hampshire and Massachusetts College of Pharmacy and Health Sciences, Worcester, Massachusetts

Justin Mizelle, MSPA-C   Emergency Medicine, Tri-Cities Regional Emergency Physicians, Johnson City, Tennessee

Melissa A. Witzigman, MPH, PA-C   Lead Physician Assistant, Tri-Cities Regional Emergency Physicians, Johnson City, Tennessee

Preface

For a physician assistant student, the clinical year marks a time of great excitement and anticipation. It is a time to hone the skills you have learned in your didactic training and work toward becoming a competent and confident healthcare provider. After many intense semesters in the classroom, you will have the privilege of participating in the practice of medicine. Each rotation will reinforce, refine, and enhance your knowledge and skills through exposure and repetition. When you look back on this time, you will likely relish the opportunities, experiences, and people involved along the way. You may find an affinity for a medical specialty you did not realize you enjoyed. You will meet lifelong professional mentors and friends. You may even be hired for your first job.

Although excitement is the overlying theme, some amount of uncertainty is bound to be present as you progress from rotation to rotation, moving through the various medical specialties. You have gained a vast knowledge base during your didactic training, but may be unsure of how to utilize it in a fast-paced clinical environment. As a clinical-year physician assistant student, you are not expected to know everything, but you are expected to seek out resources that can complement what you will learn through hands-on experience. Through an organized and predictable approach, this book series serves as a guide and companion to help you feel prepared for what you will encounter during the clinical year.

Each book was written by physician assistant educators, clinicians, and preceptors who are experts in their respective fields. Their knowledge from years of experience is laid out in the pages before you. Each book will answer questions such as, "What does my preceptor want me to know?" "What should I be familiar with prior to this rotation?" "What can I expect to encounter during this rotation?" This is followed by a guided approach to the clinical decision-making process for common presenting complaints, detailed explanations of common disease entities, and specialty-specific patient education.

Chapters are organized in a way that will allow you to quickly access vital information that can help you recognize, diagnose, and treat commonly seen conditions. You can easily review suggested labs and diagnostic imaging for a suspected diagnosis, find a step-by-step guide to frequently performed procedures, and review urgent management of conditions specific to each rotation. Electronic resources are available for each book. These include case studies with explanations to evaluate your clinical reasoning process, and review questions to assist in self-evaluation and preparation for your end-of-rotation examinations as well as the Physician Assistant National Certifying Exam.

As a future physician assistant, you have already committed to being a lifelong learner of medicine. It is my hope that this book series will outline expectations, enhance your medical knowledge base, and provide you with the confidence you need to be successful in your clinical year.

MAUREEN KNECHTEL, MPAS, PA-C
Series Editor
The Physician Assistant Student's Guide to the Clinical Year

Introduction

The Approach to the Patient in Emergency Medicine

According to the American Academy of Physician Assistants' (AAPA) 2016 statistical data set, 13.2% of physician assistants (PAs) went into emergency medicine (EM).[1] It is one of the few specialties that allows for intimate cross-collaboration with public health, law enforcement, pastoral care, and prehospital medicine. This requires competence in interprofessional teamwork and communication.

If you are a PA student who is not sure what specialty you wish to pursue, completing an EM rotation can help solidify that decision. Emergency medicine is a popular field for PAs, in part due to the variety of conditions you have an opportunity to evaluate and manage. It is important to understand that the EM rotation has a wide depth and breadth of information, requiring self-motivation and self-learning outside of your time spent in the ED.

WHAT TO EXPECT

In order to be successful on this rotation, you must be motivated to learn, and you must be confident in making decisions quickly. The ability to take a focused history, perform a physical examination, and use your clinical acumen are skills that will develop throughout your time in the ED. A focused history and physical examination can allow you to create and narrow a comprehensive differential diagnosis and determine an appropriate workup and treatment plan without ordering unnecessary diagnostic tests.

THE ENVIRONMENT

Many healthcare providers find the ED environment to be chaotic. The monitors at the nurses' station often produce a cacophony of beeps. There may be a dedicated behavioral health area with patients suffering from hallucinations.

You will hear simultaneous conversations happening between providers, in person and on the phone. It can be difficult to adjust to the constant commotion.

Students are required to simulate the schedule of a true ED provider. As a result, you should expect to work varied hours, including doing shift work and overnight shifts. Most ED rotations have shift lengths varying in time from 8 to 12 hours. This is also a procedure-heavy rotation with the potential to be exposed to bodily fluids. For these reasons, you will likely be allowed to wear scrubs.

THE OBJECTIVES

One of the primary objectives of an ED provider is to determine whether the patient is "sick versus not sick." In addition to acute management, correct evaluation of the patient's disposition is a clinical endeavor every ED provider hopes to accomplish. Just because a patient is triaged to a lower acuity area, does not guarantee there is not a more serious underlying problem. For example, a toothache can be an acute myocardial infarction (MI) presentation in a patient with diabetic neuropathy.

There are three main entities specific to establishing the disposition of the patient in EM:

1. Sick versus not sick: It is necessary to be able to determine whether a patient requires immediate intervention and/or admission to the hospital.
2. Often, EDs may be divided into zones based on patient acuity. Know that your approach to the patient will not only be based on complaint acuity but also the location of the unit you are working in.
   - Low-acuity patients, such as those with sore throat, ankle sprains, superficial lacerations, and uncomplicated musculoskeletal pain, are usually placed in a section known broadly as *fast track*.
   - Moderate-acuity patients, such as those with abdominal pain, chest pain, and patients who are stable but may have an infection, may be placed in a middle-acuity section.
   - The main ED is where the highest acuity patients are, such as those with acute congestive heart failure (CHF), unstable urosepsis, or cardiac arrest. This is the location of the ED with the most equipment, code carts, resuscitation bays, and trauma surgery equipment at the bedside.
3. Transfer of care: Care transfer occurs more frequently in the ED compared to any other setting. As a result, there is a greater potential for errors here. Medical errors are the third leading cause of death. The most common cause of errors is poor communication.[2,3] Further research shows the lack of communication may happen at the most integral time known as the *handoff*.[2] This refers to the point at which one provider signs patients out at the end of a shift for care by another provider. The information exchange must be brief, concise, relevant, and timely. As a result, the Agency for Healthcare Research and Quality (AHRQ) has developed a dedicated communication curriculum known as TeamSTEPPS (Team

Strategies and Tools to Enhance Performance and Patient Safety). The purpose of TeamSTEPPS is multifactorial. Components include identifying barriers to workplace success and team structure, identifying the factors that allow for a team to work well, and integrating a dedicated communication format to facilitate a collaborative, patient-centered culture. Several mnemonics exist to help the provider facilitate this communication, including IPASStheBATON and SBAR.[4] These are outlined in Tables I.1 and I.2.

TABLE I.1 IPASStheBATON Mnemonic

I	Introduce	Introduce yourself
P	Patient information	Name, identifiers, age, sex, location
A	Assessment	Relevant diagnoses and complaints, vital signs, symptoms
S	Situation	Current status (i.e., ADL, intake, elimination, behavior, cognition), circumstances, code status, level of uncertainly, recent changes, response to treatment
S	Safety	Critical lab values, reports, allergies, alerts, falls, isolation
The		
B	Background	Other diagnoses, previous episodes, current medications, history
A	Actions	What actions were taken or are required? Provide a brief rationale.
T	Timing	Level of urgency and explicit timing and prioritization of actions
O	Ownership	Who is taking responsibility (APRN, nurse, doctor, PA)?
N	Next	What will happen next? Anticipated changes? What is the plan?

ADL, activities of daily living; APRN, advanced practice registered nurse; PA, physician assistant.

Source: Agency for Healthcare Research and Quality. About TeamSTEPPS®. http://www.ahrq.gov/teamstepps/aboutteamstepps/ index.html. Published August 2015.

TABLE I.2 SBAR Mnemonic

S	Situation	What is going on with the patient?
B	Background	What is the clinical background or context?
A	Assessment	What do you think the problem is?
R	Recommendation/Request	What would you do to correct it?

Source: Agency for Healthcare Research and Quality. About TeamSTEPPS®. http://www.ahrq.gov/teamstepps/about-teamstepps/index.html. Published August 2015.

WHAT YOUR PRECEPTOR WANTS YOU TO KNOW

Although your main objective during your EM rotation is to learn, there are a few things that your preceptor will want you to know prior to your first shift. You will not be expected to be fully proficient in all of these areas at the start of your rotation, but if you have a firm grasp on the following concepts, you will be able to maximize your ED rotation experience:

COMMUNICATION

The ability to communicate with your preceptor and with the other members of the ED team is of paramount importance. You should introduce yourself to all members of the team that you will be working with for your shift. Maintain open lines of communication with nurses, medical technicians, consultant services, PAs, attending physicians, residents, and fellow students. This is particularly important to facilitate order input, testing, administration of treatment, and keep all team members aware of a patient's status at any given time. Your preceptor will want to know which patients you are preparing to examine prior to you examining them and should be made aware of any patient with unstable vital signs or a potentially life-threatening illness as soon as you recognize this.

TIME MANAGEMENT

Your preceptor will want you to know how to perform a focused history and physical exam in an efficient manner, and to present your findings succinctly. You will be expected to manage multiple patients at the same time, which entails following up on results, consultations, and dispositions of existing patients while continuing to evaluate new patients. Your preceptor will want you to know how to simultaneously balance patient evaluation, documentation, procedures, and consultations.

BASIC PATIENT EVALUATION AND MANAGEMENT

Learn how to present your patient in a concise way and include:

- Patient demographics (e.g., age, gender)
- Chief complaint
- Pertinent history of present illness (HPI)
- Pertinent past medical/surgical/family/social history
  - Generally limited only to information related to present complaint or illness
- Physical exam
  - Pertinent positive and negative findings only, including vital signs
    You should then be able to review your assessment and plan, including your differential diagnosis
- Differential diagnosis
  - Keep in mind life-threatening diagnoses that will need to be excluded
- Diagnostic studies you would like to order
  - Labs, radiologic imaging, EKG, and so forth
- Therapeutic measures you would like to order
  - Medications, intravenous (IV) fluids, procedures, and so forth

- Begin thinking about the disposition of the patient, which can change at any time based on results of diagnostic studies and response to therapies:
  - Potential consultation services
  - A general idea of whether or not your patient will require admission to the observation unit or the hospital

In continuing to manage your patient, be sure to:

- Follow-up results of diagnostic testing, patient status, and maintain communication about this information with your preceptor, other members of the ED team, and your patient
  - It is important to note any significant change in the status (e.g., decompensation, improvement) of your patient during the course of his or her ED evaluation.
- Efficiently present your patient to admission or consultant teams when necessary
  - Keep in mind, your presentation to an admission team or consultant will be even more abbreviated/succinct than your original presentation; a few brief sentences regarding demographics, chief complaint, HPI/patient history will suffice.
  - Include pertinent diagnostic testing findings and patient status updates during the patient's ED evaluation and, most important, the reason for the patient's admission/consultation.
- Provide ongoing communication with the patient regarding results, response to therapy, and disposition/plan
- Continue to participate in the patient's care until the patient is discharged or transfer of care has been completed

BASIC SKILLS

Being able to interpret diagnostic studies, familiarity with procedures, and having a basic understanding of certain procedural skills will help you to maximize your EM rotation and further hone your abilities. If you are familiar with these concepts at the start of your rotation, you will have the knowledge base and confidence needed to further improve your skills through firsthand experience. These skills include:

- Interpretation of lab results
- X-ray interpretation
  - Chest x-rays and x-rays corresponding to extremities involved in common orthopedic injuries (e.g., shoulder, wrist, hand, knee, ankle)
- EKG interpretation
  - Particularly life-threatening arrhythmias, atrial fibrillation, acute MI
- Basic suturing technique
- IV placement
- Phlebotomy
- Principles of splinting injured joints
- Basic incision and drainage technique

Preceptor Expectations for Successful Students

- Jump at every opportunity to learn.
  - Even if it is just through observation, watching fellow ED staff or consultants perform procedures provides a great educational opportunity.
  - Make yourself available to perform procedures.
  - Advocate for yourself—you will only be able to perform a procedure if you pursue the opportunity to do so.
- Take advantage of your resources.
  - Ask questions, participate in educational rounds, attend lectures, learn from admission teams/consultants.
- Know your limitations.
  - Never be afraid to ask for help or to notify any member of the ED staff if you are concerned about a patient or if you feel uncomfortable in a situation.
  - If you are uncertain about any aspect of evaluation and management of your patient (especially procedures), ask for further instruction or clarification.
  - Be able to assess your strengths and weaknesses in an objective way.
    - Learn from constructive criticism.
    - It can be helpful to set objectives with your preceptor at the beginning of a shift and to discuss at the end which objectives were met and where you might improve for your next shift.

What Previous PA Students Wish They Knew Before This Rotation

- The ED is an intense, fast-paced environment and can be physically, emotionally, and mentally demanding.
- If you want to learn how to perform a specific procedure or skill, make sure you are in the right place at the right time; do not be timid about volunteering to try something new.
- You are not expected to be proficient at everything. Do not be afraid to ask for help if you are uncertain about how to do something.
- The ED is full of learning opportunities; do not pass up the chance to learn from others (e.g., nurses, patient care technicians, consultants) by being too focused on "your patients."
- Make yourself available to help other staff members; clinicians, nurses, residents, and consultants are more likely to include you in a teaching opportunity if you demonstrate that you are a team player.
- Do not underestimate the breadth of knowledge you will need for the ED. Although there are some complaints that are more common than others, you will need a solid foundation in many areas of medicine in order to be successful in EM.

- The ED is a unique learning environment where you will encounter diverse patients and medical complaints; it is important to approach this rotation with an open mind and to avoid prejudgment.

Pertinent Specialty-Specific Physical Exams

Although there are no special physical exam tests unique to EM, it is important to keep the following things in mind when examining your patient in the ED:

- Always completely expose the area(s) of the body related to the chief complaint.
  - Full exposure of the affected area is necessary for adequate examination (affected limb—joints above and below; abdomen—surgical scars, distension; skin—rash in an area of pain).
  - Keep patient modesty in mind during your examination.
    - Be sure to have a chaperone present if you are exposing sensitive areas during your examination, particularly if the patient is of the opposite sex.
- The ability to do a rapid, comprehensive neurologic exam is an important skill to master.
- Concerning physical exam findings should be brought to the attention of your preceptor immediately and may include:
  - Abnormal vital signs or altered mental status
  - Pallor, diminished pulse, weakness of an extremity
  - Focal neurologic deficit
  - Signs of severe distress (e.g., tachypnea, severe pain)
  - Evidence of an acute abdomen
  - Open fracture

Use of Interprofessional Consultations

Pharmacist

- Many EDs have EM pharmacists available for consultation about medication administration (e.g., dosing, antidotes/reversal agents, medication interactions).
- EM pharmacists are also readily available to collaborate with clinicians for efficient dispensation and administration of complex or time-sensitive medications in cases of cardiac arrest, stroke, anaphylaxis, or other life-threatening emergencies.

Social Worker

- Can provide community resources to patients such as alcohol or substance abuse programs, homeless shelters, or welfare benefits

- Can aid in collecting collateral information from family members or household contacts for patients who might not be able to provide historical information, such as those with psychiatric emergencies

Case Manager

- Assisting in medication acquisition and follow-up care for patients with complex diagnoses, such as arranging anticoagulation therapy and monitoring for a patient with thromboembolism who is getting discharged home from the ED
- Aiding discharge planning for patients who require placement in long-term care facilities or patients with in-home care needs such as home health aides, home physical therapy, or medical equipment such as a nebulizer machine or a walker

Forensic Nurse

- Available to aid in evaluation of sexual assault patients who wish to file criminal charges and who require forensic examination for evidence collection

Law Enforcement

- Officers are needed for patients who wish to report a crime, such as assault victims, and providers who suspect abuse or neglect. This is typically done in conjunction with social work.

Poison Control

- Cases requiring toxicology consultation such as chemical exposure or ingestion of toxic substance

Respiratory Therapy

- Aid in management of ventilators for patients who require intubation/ventilator support
- Can perform specialized diagnostic testing, such as negative inspiratory force (NIF) testing in myasthenia gravis patients

Physical Therapy

- Can evaluate a patient's ability to ambulate safely and make recommendations about exercise programs, ambulation assistance devices, or need for inpatient or outpatient rehabilitation

Radiology Technician

- Can perform bedside imaging studies, including portable x-ray, and can assist in more complex radiographic tests such as contrast-enhanced studies

CONFIDENTIALITY PRACTICES AND ETHICS

Maintaining patient confidentiality is the legal and ethical responsibility of students and clinicians working in all areas of medicine, including the ED. Patients visiting the ED are commonly in emotional and physical distress; it is important to ensure that patient privacy is protected to facilitate evaluation and management of all medical conditions. Confidentiality practices in EM should aim to allow patients to disclose sensitive information to the provider in a private manner without fear of judgment, discrimination, or disclosure of that information to others without the permission of the patient. Maintaining the confidence of the patient is an important aspect of the patient–provider relationship. Students and clinicians should consider patient confidentiality in all interactions and communication with other medical providers and ancillary staff.

It is the ethical responsibility of a PA to use his or her best judgment at all times in clinical practice and to take into consideration each individual patient's preferences, autonomy, dignity, and right to make his or her own decisions regarding medical care. Providers should give patients unbiased information regarding potential risks, benefits, costs, and treatment options to allow them to make informed decisions about their care. In addition to acting in the patient's best interest, providers must also consider the preferences of the healthcare team, ethical principles, and legal obligations in caring for patients. PAs should strive to maintain the four bioethical principles outlined by the AAPA's *Guidelines for Ethical Conduct for the PA Profession* at all times. Respect the patient's autonomy, act in the patient's best interest, avoid harm, and provide similar care to all patients in similar circumstances.[5]

DOCUMENTATION

PROCEDURE NOTES DOCUMENTATION

EM requires distinct procedural documentation. A few things to keep in mind include patient consent with the appropriate documentation of risks versus benefits of the procedure, type of equipment used, the time it took, any additional interventions to be documented, and patient instruction given. See Exhibit I.1 for an example of an EM note.

Exhibit I.1 Sample Emergency Medicine Note

Patient Name: Jane Doe

DOB: 02/02/1977

Age: 42 years old

MR #: 8675308

Insurance: Horizon Blue Cross Blue Shield

Primary Care Doctor:

Dr. Ludwig

66 James Road, Suite 101

Anywhere, AS 10298

(686) 908-5438

Cc: Abdominal Pain × 3 days

HPI: This is a 42-year-old Caucasian female with a past medical history of laparoscopic appendectomy 4 years ago who presents with RUQ abdominal pain described as colicky with gradual onset 1 hour after eating dinner this evening, 5/10 in severity, and nonradiating. She reports associated nausea and one episode of nonbilious vomiting. She has not taken anything for pain and leaning forward relieves her pain slightly. LNMP was 1 week ago. Surgical history is significant for appendectomy 4 years ago with no complications. She denies heartburn symptoms, dysphagia, hematemesis, melena, hematochezia, dysuria, fever, chills. Last PO intake was 3 hours ago with dinner of pasta with meatballs. Her diet is fairly healthy with oatmeal for breakfast, salad for lunch, and she almost always has pasta for dinner. Her last BM was this morning and normal, with BM daily. She denies any previous history of similar pain.

Medications: Acetaminophen for knee pain prn, otherwise no medications

Allergies: PCN-rash, no seasonal or food allergies

Family Hx: mother had gallstones; dx age 48

Social hx: (-)tobacco use, (-)EtOH use, (-)illicit substance use

Occupation: works as a high school teacher

ROS: Ht: 5′2″ Weight: 134 lbs; (-)weakness, (-)fatigue, (-)fever, (-)chills, (-)night sweats

Skin: (-)color changes

EENT: (-)voice hoarseness

CV/RESP: (-)chest pain, (-)palpitations, (-)dyspnea

ABD: see HPI (-)appetite changes, (-)jaundice

Neuro: (-)altered mental status

Physical Exam General: This is a middle-aged female in mild painful distress with one episode of vomiting in the ED.

Vitals: Temp 98.8, HR 110 bpm, BP: 120/78 mmHg, Pulse ox 97% RA

SKIN: No jaundice

HEENT: No scleral icterus

CV/Resp: regular heart rate; S1, S2, lungs clear to auscultation bilaterally

(continued)

Exhibit I.1 Sample Emergency Medicine Note *(continued)*

ABD: Soft, bowel sounds active, mild RUQ tenderness, (-)Murphy's sign, (-)organomegaly

Neuro: Alert, awake, and oriented × 3

Laboratory/Diagnostics

Urine pregnancy test: negative

EKG: NSR, rate 72 bpm; no acute ST-T wave changes

CBC: WBC: 8, H/H: 13/30, Plt 360

BMP:

Na: 135 mg/dL

K: 4.2 mg/dL

Cl: 102 mg/dL

Glucose: 120 mg/dL

BUN: 29 mg/dL

Creat: 0.1 mg/dL

CO_2: 20 mmol/L

LFTs:

Bilirubin: 5 ʊmol

Alkaline phosphatase: 35 IU/L

AST: 5 IU/L

ALT: 5 IU/L

Albumin: 40 IU/L

Lipase: 0.2 U/L

RUQ ultrasound: (+)gallstones noted in gallbladder; no evidence of gallbladder wall thickening or pericholecystic fluid; liver and pancreas within normal limits

IMPRESSION: Biliary colic

ED Treatment/Course: Patient seen by PA student. Initiated IV line placement. Labs sent. Treated with ondansetron 4 mg IV, morphine 2 mg IV, hydrated with IVNS 1L WO. Repeat vital signs: Temp 98.6°F, HR 78, BP 118/70 mmHg, pulse ox 98% RA. On reexamination, patient has no abdominal tenderness and reports improved pain. PO fluid challenge given with apple sauce and tolerated.

DISCHARGE Instructions: Patient instructed to follow up with Dr. Ludwig for further evaluation in 2–3 days. Instructed to follow a low-fat/low- residue diet. Given discharge instructions regarding gallstones. Return to the ED for any worsening symptoms, persistent vomiting, high fever, or any other concern. ED workup and EHR sent to Dr. Ludwig's office.

Provider e-signature

ABD, abdomen; ALT, alanine aminotransferase; AST, aspartate aminotransferase; BM, bowel movement; BMP, basic metabolic panel; BP, blood pressure; BUN, blood urea nitrogen; CBC, complete blood count; CV, cardiovascular; DOB, date of birth; EENT, eye, ear, nose, and throat; EHR, electronic health record; EtOH, alcohol use; HEENT, head, ear, eye, nose, and throat; HPI, history of present illness; HR, heart rate; IV, intravenous; LFT, liver function test; LNMP, last known menstrual period; NSR, normal sinus rhythm; PA, physician assistant; PCN, penicillin; PO, per os; RA, room air; RESP, respiration; ROS, review of systems; RUQ, right upper quadrant; WBC, white blood cell.

REFERENCES

1. National Commission on Certification of Physician Assistants. *2016 statistical profile of certified physician assistants: an annual report of the National Commission on Certification of Physician Assistants.* Johns Creek, GA: Author; 2017. https://prodcmsstoragesa.blob.core.windows.net/uploads/files/2016StatisticalProfileofCertifiedPhysicianAssistants.pdf

2. Makary MA, Daniel M. Medical error—the third leading cause of death in the US. *BMJ.* 2016;353:i2139. doi:10.1136/bmj.i2139

3. World Health Organization. *Framework for Action on Interprofessional Education and Collaborative Practice* (No. WHO/HRH/HPN/10.3). Geneva, Switzerland: World Health Organization; 2010.

4. Agency for Healthcare Research and Quality. *About TeamSTEPPS®.* Rockville, MD: Agency for Healthcare Research and Quality; 2019. http://www.ahrq.gov/teamstepps/about-teamstepps/index.html.

5. American Academy of PhysicianAssistants. 2018–2019 policy manual: guidelines for ethical conduct for the PA profession. https://www.aapa.org/download/36739/. Accessed February 3, 2019.

Common Presentations in Emergency Medicine

INTRODUCTION

During your emergency medicine (EM) rotation, you will evaluate a variety of presentations and disease entities. Although not all inclusive, this chapter reviews some of the more commonly encountered chief complaints. These include

1. Abdominal pain
2. Altered mental status
3. Chest pain
4. Headache
5. Injury
6. Low-back pain

ABDOMINAL PAIN

Abdominal pain is a commonly encountered clinical problem, accounting for nearly 10% of all visits to the ED.[1] The etiology of abdominal pain in the acute setting is a difficult one as benign conditions can present with instability and, conversely, patients with acute pathology can present in a benign format. As a result, the key to diagnosis is an algorithmic approach that requires a comprehensive yet concise history and appropriate physical exam skills. Because the physician assistant (PA) curriculum requires competency in these skills, you are already prepared for this rotation.

The key to being a good provider is differentiating whether the presentation is one that may lead to decompensation quickly, as in the case of a dissecting aortic aneurysm, or one that may be fairly benign such as dyspepsia. The utility of physical exam findings and other objective measures, such as vital signs, is also relevant in determining the approach to the diagnosis. These simple tools should allow the emergency medicine provider to have a streamlined approach and prevent the use of unnecessary imaging.

> **CLINICAL PEARL:** Select populations with abdominal pain in whom to consider emergent processes include pediatric and geriatric patients, pregnant females, and postoperative patients.

Differential Diagnosis

The differential diagnosis of abdominal pain can be narrowed by the location of the pain, as seen in Table 1.1. Keep in mind that many processes can present in multiple locations, such as an ovarian cyst, torsion, ischemic bowel, and sickle cell crisis.

TABLE 1.1 Differential Diagnosis of Abdominal Pain by Location

Right Upper Quadrant	Subxiphoid	Left Upper Quadrant
Biliary colic (cholelithiasis)	PUD	Gastritis
Cholecystitis	Dyspepsia	Esophagitis
Hepatitis	Gastritis	DKA
Ascending cholangitis	Acute MI	Pulmonary infarct
Choledocolithiasis	Pancreatitis	
Pancreatitis	Aortic aneurysm	
Pulmonary infarct		
Sickle cell crisis		
Fitz-Hugh–Curtis syndrome		

Right Middle Quadrant	Periumbilical	Left Middle Quadrant
Same as RUQ	Early appendicitis	Ileus
Renal colic	Early gastroenteritis	Intestinal obstruction
Occult malignancy	Colitis	Occult malignancy
	Early small bowel obstruction	
	Celiac sprue	
	Intestinal ischemia	
	Porphyria	

Right Lower Quadrant	Suprapubic/Hypogastric	Left Lower Quadrant
Ovarian cyst	Cystitis	Diverticular disease
Adnexal torsion	Pregnancy	Colonic lesion
Tubo-ovarian abscess	Threatened abortion	Enteritis
Testicular torsion	Urethritis	Colitis
Diverticular disease	Pelvic inflammatory disease	Hernia (inguinal/femoral)
Hernia (inguinal/femoral)	Bladder distention	Crohn's disease
Ectopic pregnancy	Endometriosis	Ectopic pregnancy
Renal colic		Testicular torsion
		Renal colic

DKA, diabetic ketoacidosis; MI, myocardial infarction; PUD, peptic ulcer disease; RUQ, right upper quadrant.
Source: Henderson M, Tierney LM, Smetana GW. *The Patient History.* 2nd ed. New York, NY: McGraw-Hill; 2012; Bickley LS. *Bates' Guide to Physical Examination and History Taking.* 12th ed. Philadelphia, PA: Wolters Kluwer; 2017:449–508.

You can also frame the differential diagnosis based on age:

- Young female: Ectopic pregnancy, ruptured ectopic pregnancy, ovarian torsion
- Older male: Abdominal aortic aneurysm (AAA), ruptured viscous
- Alcohol use: Pancreatitis
- Anticoagulant use: Lower gastrointestinal (GI) bleed
- Young male: Testicular torsion

History

In determining the etiology of pain, recall human embryological development. Epigastric pain typically derives from the foregut structures, including the stomach, pancreas, and proximal duodenum. Any pain deriving from the periumbilical region can be attributed to the midgut structures, including appendix and small bowel. Suprapubic pain can develop from hindgut organs such as the genitourinary (GU) system, bladder, or terminal colon. Location of the pain can facilitate diagnosis due to the anatomical structures within the abdominal cavity.

In taking the history of present illness, use the OPQRST format to further narrow the differential diagnosis:

O: Onset: When was the onset of the pain? Was it sudden or more gradual?
P: Provocation/palliative components: Any provocating or palliating components? Postprandial? Previous history of similar pain?
Q: Quality: What is the quality of the pain? Is it sharp, dull, achy, burning?
R: Radiation: Does the pain have any radiation?
S: Severity: On a scale of 1–10, how severe is the abdominal pain?
T: Timing: How long does the pain last? Is it constant or does it wax and wane?

Determine the onset of pain and its quality. If the patient had acute onset, consider diagnoses related to acute visceral injury such as perforated ulcer, renal colic, or ruptured ovarian cyst. Pain with a more gradual onset presents with inflammatory etiologies, such as biliary colic, diverticulitis, and hepatitis.

- Pain: Visceral fibers are attached to organs and do not localize pain very well. As a result, the pain is usually dull and secondary to other reasons such as ischemia or stretching. The somatic fibers innervate the peritoneum. When activated by inflammation or blood, the pain is more localized and patients complain of the pain being sharp. Asking about the quality of pain will facilitate your decision-making process.
- Radiation: The concept of pain radiation is also key to determining the etiology of abdominal pain in the adult. Pain, such as biliary colic, may radiate to the right shoulder, to the midepigastrium or even to the right flank. Renal colic radiates to the flank of the ipsilateral side and patients may describe it as radiating to the scrotum for males and to the labia for females.

○ The pain from appendicitis is dynamic due to the evolving nature of the disease. The pain from appendicitis typically begins in the umbilicus and then radiates to the right lower quadrant.

○ Pain secondary to renal colic may start in the flank but may travel to a testicle for male patients. This is relevant because if the patient has a testicular torsion that is causing pain instead, it can be a missed diagnosis with heavy consequences such as lifetime infertility. Testicular torsion is an emergent condition requiring rapid diagnosis and intervention.

• Timing: Timing will vary depending on the etiology of the patient's pain. Visceral conditions, such as biliary colic, tend to progress over time. The same goes for diverticulitis, in which left lower quadrant (LLQ) pain is felt for several days.

○ When the pain started and the quality of the pain are relevant to diagnosis. Visceral pain tends to be more insidious. It also tends to present in a location other than where the actual disease process is.

Past Medical History Specific to Complaint

Past medical history contributing to a patient's abdominal pain can be brief, but there are a few distinct questions that stand out when obtaining this information. The preceding description of the OPQRST format allows for the history of present illness. When following the standard format for outlining past medical history, the following additional considerations should be discussed:

• Medications: All current medications should be documented along with prescription, those sold over the counter, home remedies, vitamins, minerals, and supplemental herbs. There are certain medications that can lead to abdominal pain. Opiates can lead to constipation and abdominal pain. Pain secondary to a peptic ulcer disease can present if related to heavy nonsteroidal anti-inflammatory drug (NSAID) use. Certain medications, such as bisphosphonates and antibiotics, have been implicated in the development of pill esophagitis.

• Allergies: Patients with allergies or intolerances can present with GI symptoms. Consider not only medications but certain food, seasonal, environmental, and animal allergies. Some more common etiologies of foods include shellfish, which can lead to crampy abdominal pain and vomiting. Consider dairy leading to abdominal pain and diarrhea due to lactose intolerance. Patients on the spectrum of celiac conditions may develop abdominal pain and weight loss with ingestion of wheat products.

• Past medical history: Some medical conditions, such as inflammatory colitis or irritable bowel syndrome, have a more insidious development over time, so it is relevant to ask patients whether they have had similar symptoms in the past and with the equivalent severity. Specifically inquire about renal disease, endocrine conditions such as thyroid or diabetes, cancer, liver disease, and autoimmune conditions.

- Surgery: Noting the date and type of abdominal intervention is relevant. This not only goes for surgical intervention but upper or lower endoscopies as well. Some patients often do not think having a dilation and curettage or ovarian intervention is considered "abdominal surgery" but in a fertile female, these should be documented.

- Injuries: Ask about any potential injuries to the abdomen. Blunt abdominal trauma is discussed in another section.

- Immunizations: This is particularly important for patients with recent travel. There are certain countries where hepatitis A is quite prevalent, particularly in regions where questionable sanitation is reported.

- Screening: With reference to abdominal pain, questions about screening apply to patients with risk factors of family history of cancer or age over 50. For example, all patients above the age of 50 should be screened for colorectal cancer via fetal occult bloiod test (FOBT)/sigmoidoscopy/colonoscopy in the United States.[2]

- Family history should be obtained, in particular, history of malignancy.

- Social history: Certain habits, when followed in excess, can predispose patients to abdominal conditions. Ask about tobacco and alcohol use in particular. Patients with excessive alcohol use are predisposed to pancreatitis and gastritis. Patients with tobacco use are at risk for carcinoma of the structures of the upper abdomen, including the pancreas and esophagus, and the bladder in the lower abdomen. For patients with blunt trauma, asking about seatbelt use is relevant as patients may present with abdominal pain and no obvious signs of injury. In addition, ask about occupation to ensure the abdominal pain is not a trauma related to a job requiring physical strain. One example is the development of hernias in patients who work in a factory or who move furniture, where heavy lifting is required.

- Sexual history: For patients who present with abdominal pain and/or pelvic pain with or without urethral or vaginal discharge, asking a detailed sexual history determines risk factors for the development of urethritis in males and pelvic inflammatory disease (PID) in females. It is also relevant to rule out scrotal pain so as not to miss a potentially infertility-inducing diagnosis of testicular torsion in males. Male patients with renal colic sometimes complain of flank pain radiating into the testicles, so it is relevant to ask about radiation of pain as well.

- In the review of systems (ROS), the symptoms and events associated with a presentation of abdominal pain refer to symptoms that may have been present in the past 6 months. Inflammatory colitis, for example, may present severely during a patient's arrival but further historical questioning may reveal the patient has had similar symptoms in the past without realizing it. The past medical history components of ROS to note and their implications related to abdominal complaints are seen in Table 1.2.

Physical Examination

The abdominal examination involves employing skills in a particular sequence in order to appropriately form a differential diagnosis. The sequence is inspection, auscultation, percussion, and palpation.[2] Before initiating the physical exam, have the patient empty his or her bladder. A full bladder can be not only distracting to the patient but also prevent you from being able to palpate appropriately.

TABLE 1.2 Past Medical History and Review of Systems Specific to Abdominal Pain

System	Pertinent Past Medical History
General	Document present height and weight (patients with unintentional weight loss/who complain their clothes do not fit may have developed a neoplasm) Weakness, fatigue, malaise, night sweats: these may be associated findings with conditions such as hepatitis
Skin	Tendency to bruise can manifest in patients with underlying hepatic pathology or carcinoma Development of clubbing of the nails may occur in patients with chronic pancreatitis Jaundice may manifest in patients with diseases involving organs of the RUQ, including the liver, gallbladder, and pancreas
Eyes	Scleral icterus is concerning for liver or advanced biliary conditions
Nose/Sinus/Oral cavity	Patients with low platelets secondary to liver disease may present with coagulopathy manifested as epistaxis or bleeding gums Patients with inflammatory bowel conditions, such as Crohn's colitis, may present with frequent aphthous ulcer development in the mouth
Breast	Gynecomastia may occur in male patients with alcoholic cirrhosis
Cardiopulmonary	Respiratory and cardiac conditions should be considered in patients with upper abdominal pain as part of the differential diagnosis
GI	Inquire about Appetite changes Heartburn symptoms Dysphagia Odynophagia Obstipation, constipation, bloating, flatulence Stool consistency (color of stool and melena/bleeding, floating) Diarrhea Rectal conditions such as hernias, hemorrhoids, and fissures/fistulas Hernia
GU	Male: Testicular pain or swelling, dysuria or urethral discharge Female: LNMP, home pregnancy test results; obstetrical history, including gravida/parity and elective/spontaneous abortions and gynecologic history such as PID; vaginal discharge, fibroids, and ovarian cysts

(continued)

TABLE **1.2** Past Medical History and Review of Systems Specific to Abdominal Pain (*continued*)

System	Pertinent Past Medical History
CNS	Speech and memory disorders may be associated with Wernicke–Korsakoff syndrome, secondary to thiamine deficiency from alcoholism
	Tremors, such as asterixis, may be noted in patients with metabolic encephalopathy for patients with liver disease[3]

CNS, central nervous system; GI, gastrointestinal; GU, genitourinary; LNMP, last known menstrual periods; PID, pelvic inflammatory disease; RUQ, right upper quadrant.

INSPECTION

- Have the patient's abdomen fully exposed from the subxiphoid region to the pubic symphysis. If your patient is in a hospital gown but is wearing jeans or pants, they should be removed so as to appropriately view the entire abdomen.
- Have the patient lie supine with arms at the sides, not over the head or across the chest, in order to allow for full evaluation of the upper quadrants. Positioning the arms over the head can also cause abdominal muscle contractions, making it more difficult to do a physical exam. Have the patient's knees bent in order to ensure further relaxation of the abdominal wall.

Prior to palpation, consider the cough test. Have the patient cough and point to where he or she feels the pain. This motion causes movement of the peritoneum and may indicate the etiology of the pain along with indicating early signs of peritonitis. Patients may report abdominal pain during a bumpy ride to the ED, or pain may be elicited by tapping the bottom of a foot or jumping up and down.

AUSCULTATION

- When auscultating the abdomen, always begin away from the site of pain. The purpose is to assess for bowel sounds. Hypoactive bowel sounds are an indication of developing ileus or obstruction. In addition to bowel sounds, it is important to auscultate specific regions for vascular bruits, particularly in patients with advanced age and hypertension. Table 1.3 outlines the anatomical quadrant and corresponding vascular bruits.

TABLE **1.3** Anatomical Quadrant and Corresponding Bruit

Anatomical Quadrant	Associated Vascular Bruit
LUQ and RUQ	Renal artery
LLQ and RLQ	Iliac artery
Midline subxiphoid/just left to subxiphoid	Aorta

LLQ, left lower quadrant; LUQ, left upper quadrant; RLQ, right lower quadrant; RUQ, right upper quadrant.

PERCUSSION

- When percussing the abdomen, begin with light percussion of all four quadrants.

PALPATION

- Move from light to deep palpation. This allows for differentiation of superficial masses, such as a ventral hernia or lipoma, versus deep masses such as carcinomatosis, a liver lesion, or colonic mass. Be sure to palpate all four quadrants.
- Some abdominal conditions are associated with constitutional symptoms such as hepatitis, neoplasms, or chronic infections. In these patients, organomegaly may be present. If this is suspected, palpate the margins of both the liver and the spleen. Physical exam findings with correlating pathologic conditions are outlined in Table 1.4.
- Physical exam special tests can be performed to help determine the severity of illness and the presence of peritonitis. These include Rovsing's, psoas, and obturator signs.

Associated GU Exam

No abdominal exam in the acute care setting is complete without an appropriate GU exam. Asking a patient about abdominal pain radiation helps narrow down the differential diagnosis and guides the physical exam. For example, if a patient presents with flank pain radiating into the testicle for males or labia for females, consider renal colic and perform a hernia exam.

In order to rule out GU pathology, a concomitant pelvic and/or rectal exam may be necessary. Utilizing the digital rectal exam (DRE) in the setting of abdominal pain can help determine whether there is blood in the stool. These exams allow for a visual inspection of the external genitalia and can help rule out perirectal hemorrhoids, abscess development, or even evidence of sexually transmitted infections. There is data to suggest the utility of DREs is questionable, especially considering some of these exams are time intensive, may require a chaperone, and most patients with abdominal pain are lined up in a busy hallway with limited privacy.[4]

The utility of a pelvic exam for the female patient does help narrow the differential diagnosis, which includes reproductive pathology. As a result, a comprehensive, private, and chaperoned bimanual pelvic exam should be performed to allow for palpation of both ovaries and the uterus.

TABLE 1.4 Correlating Physical Exam Findings With Pathologic Conditions

Body System	Physical Exam Finding	Associated Clinical Condition
Skin	Pink–purple striae	Cushing syndrome
	Dilated veins (caput medusa)	Cirrhosis or IVC obstruction
	Abdominal wall/flank ecchymosis	Intraperitoneal or retroperitoneal hemorrhage

(continued)

TABLE 1.4 Correlating Physical Exam Findings With Pathologic Conditions (*continued*)

Body System	Physical Exam Finding	Associated Clinical Condition
GI	Abdominal distention or bulges	Ascites/distended bladder/pregnant uterus; ventral, femoral, or inguinal hernia; enlarged organ or mass; constipation
	Altered bowel sounds	Diarrhea, obstruction, paralytic ileus
	Hepatic friction rub	Hepatoma, gonococcal infection, splenic infarction, and pancreatic carcinoma
	Involuntary rigidity, Rovsing's sign, obturator sign, psoas sign	These indicate peritoneal inflammation and provider should suspect appendicitis, cholecystitis, or perforation
	Decreased liver span on percussion	Free air below the diaphragm indicates hollow viscus or perforated bowel
	Tenderness over the liver	Hepatitis, congestion from heart failure, cholecystitis
	(+)splenic percussion sign	Indicates splenomegaly; consider portal HTN, heme malignancies, HIV, splenic infarct, or hematoma in the setting of blunt trauma
	(+)test for shifting dullness or a (+)fluid wave shift	Ascites
	(+)point tenderness at McBurney's point or localized tenderness to the RLQ	Appendicitis
	(+)Murphy's sign	Acute cholecystitis
PV	Increased pulsations	AAA
	Bruits	Over vascular site (iliac, renal, or femoral) indicates vasoocclusive or stenotic disease
	Hypertension + bruit	Renal artery stenosis
GU	CVA tenderness on percussion of the kidneys	Pyelonephritis/hydronephrosis secondary to renal colic
	Lower quadrant unilateral pain	Tubo-ovarian abscess, ectopic pregnancy, ovarian torsion, endometriosis, STI, PID, nephrolithiasis

AAA, abdominal aortic aneurysm; CVA, cerebrovascular accident; GI, gastrointestinal; GU, genitourinary; HTN, hypertension; IVC, inferior vena cava; PID, pelvic inflammatory disease; PV, peripheral vascular; STI, sexually transmitted infection; RLQ, right lower quadrant.

Source: Bhuiya FA, Pitts SR, McCaig LF. Emergency department visits for chest pain and abdominal pain: United States, 1999–2008. NCHS data brief no. 43. Washington, DC: U.S. Department of Health and Human Services; 2010. https://www.cdc.gov/nchs/data/databriefs/db43.pdf

Diagnostic Plan

The primary purpose of a diagnostic plan in assessing abdominal pain is to expose the patient to the lowest amount of radiation while simultaneously determining the etiology. First, note whether the patient is stable. Upon receiving the triage sheet/patient chart, evaluate the vital signs after noting the patient's correct identifying factors. If the vitals are unstable with evidence of hypotension, tachycardia, or fever, order tests based on the most urgent diagnoses with the potential for decompensation/necrosis. As with everything in emergency medicine, the diagnostic approach to abdominal pain should follow an algorithmic strategy as noted in Table 1.5.

Determining which tests to order next is based on the patient's history and presentation.

LABS
- Urine studies
  - Evaluate for pregnancy with point-of-care approach.
  - Quick urine dipstick allows for detection of blood and leukocytes to rule out urethritis, renal colic, or cystitis.
  - Hematuria may be present in patients with nephrolithiasis but can be a false positive if the patient is menstruating.
- Complete blood count (CBC)
  - CBC is often useful in the evaluation of patients with abdominal pain. White blood cell (WBC) elevation may occur with acute infections such as gastroenteritis, appendicitis, or diverticulitis.
  - A low hematocrit may be noted in GI bleeding or in a patient with dysfunctional uterine bleeding.
- Lipase
  - If pancreatitis is suspected, the most useful diagnostic test is a serum lipase elevated to at least double the normal value. Serum amylase is no longer used for the diagnosis of acute pancreatitis.[5]
- Basic metabolic panel (BMP)
  - The BMP can give clues to severity of disease in patients presenting with abdominal pain. Excess electrolyte losses in vomiting and diarrhea from a variety of conditions, such as pancreatitis, cholecystitis, gastroenteritis, and colitis, can lead to excess chloride and potassium loss, warranting the need for repletion. Elevated blood urea nitrogen (BUN) cansignify dehydration or early GI bleed.
- Serum ketone can help determine the severity of acidosis, such as in patients with possible diabetic ketoacidosis (DKA). Keep in mind that acidosis can occur in many metabolic conditions.
- The role of serum lactate in the setting of acute abdominal pain is becoming more prevalent. Serum lactate is usually elevated in states leading to decreased tissue perfusion such as pancreatic necrosis due to chronic pancreatitis, sepsis in the setting of a perforated viscous or spontaneous bacterial peritonitis, or bowel ischemia.[5]

TABLE 1.5 Diagnostic and Management Plan Based on Suspected Diagnosis

Suspected Diagnoses	Diagnostics to Order	ED Management
Peritonitis, sepsis, organ failure, perforation of ulcer, appendix, or gallbladder	Stabilize the patient and order initial tests; call surgery immediately if patient appears hypotensive, tachycardic, or toxic	Aggressive fluid resuscitation Send off lab work (including type and screen) Keep NPO Immediate consultation with surgery
Cholecystitis Cholelithiasis Cholangitis Hepatic pathology	CBC with diff BMP Liver function test Coagulation profile Lipase RUQ ultrasound Possible HIDA versus ERCP/MRCP Urinalysis Urine pregnancy test Serum lactate level	IV fluids Antiemetics for vomiting Consider type and screen for blood products Pain control PPIs if upper GI bleed/varices (parenteral) Gastroenterology referral Surgery versus IR consult depending on findings
Gastritis PUD, duodenal ulcer GERD	CBC with differential (check for H/H for ulcer-related blood loss with type and screen)	IV fluids and antiemetics if vomiting PPI
Dyspepsia Pancreatitis (gallstone or alcohol)	EKG, troponin (rule out acute MI/ACS) Urine pregnancy (one of the more common symptoms is heartburn) Lactate (elevated in developing organ failure such as pancreatitis) Alcohol level if history indicates Urine drug screen if cocaine ingestion	GI cocktail: Bentyl, Mylanta, and lidocaine PO Thiamine 100 mg IV if alcoholic history, folate Consider type and screen for blood products Replace electrolytes as needed Admit for patients who are unable to tolerate PO intake, have low H/H, EKG findings consistent with heart disease or evidence of sepsis due to pancreatitis If symptoms improve and patient can tolerate PO intake, discharge home on PPI with low-residue diet and follow up with GI
Appendicitis Diverticulitis, colon neoplasm, colitis (infectious, antibiotic-associated, travel-related), enteritis, lower GI bleed, SBO	CBC with diff (WBC elevated in infectious etiology) CMP (low K and low Cl if vomiting or diarrhea) Lactate (evidence of acidosis, sepsis)	IV line placement with fluid resuscitation, administer pain medication, keep NPO during evaluation; order CT scan with PO and IV contrast (if IV contrast is contraindicated, PO alone is ok)

(continued)

TABLE 1.5 Diagnostic and Management Plan Based on Suspected Diagnosis (*continued*)

Suspected Diagnoses	Diagnostics to Order	ED Management
		If uncomplicated diverticulitis with appropriate follow-up and patient demonstrates tolerating PO intake, discharge home If uncomplicated infectious colitis, can be managed as outpatient with antibiotics and bowel rest
Urinary symptoms, if involving flank or back pain, consider pyelonephritis; in female patients, consider pelvic etiology such as ovarian, pregnancy, uterine	Urine pregnancy test in females of fertile status Urinalysis (No need for blood work if hx is clear that this is simple UTI or cystitis) Only send blood work if H&P is unequivocal to a diagnosis or patient appears toxic/has persistent vomiting Pelvic exam should be done if history indicates it is required	Outpatient antibiotics Pyridium if patient has severe urinary symptoms Anti-inflammatory medications for pain management PO fluid hydration If there is evidence of toxicity, patient unable to tolerate PO intake, lack of follow-up, admit for management to medicine with GI consult Discharge instructions about UTI prevention Complete antibiotic course even if symptoms improve
		PO fluid hydration encouraged Follow up with primary care team if outpatient For pregnancy-related management, see OB/GYN clinical rotation guide If patient has suspected ovarian cyst without evidence of torsion or rupture, call OB/GYN for follow-up arrangement If patient is unable to tolerate PO intake, has pain that cannot be managed, patient should be admitted

ACS, acute coronary syndrome; BMP, basic metabolic panel; CBC, complete blood count; CMP, comprehensive metabolic panel; ERCP, endoscopic retrograde cholangiopancreatography; GERD, gastroesophageal reflux disease; GI, gastrointestinal; H/H, hemoglobin and hematocrit; HIDA, hepatoiminodiacetic acid; IR, interventional radiology; IV, intravenous; MI, myocardial infarction; MRCP, magnetic resonance cholangiopancreatography; NPO, nothing by mouth; PO, by mouth; PPI, proton pump inhibitor; PUD, peptic ulcer disease; RUQ, right upper quadrant; SBO, small bowel obstruction; UTI, urinary tract infection; WBC, white blood cell.

DIAGNOSTIC IMAGING

- Plain radiography of the abdomen has very limited use except to evaluate for free air under the diaphragm in the setting of a perforated viscous or to check air fluid levels and dilated bowel loops for patients with small bowel obstruction (SBO). For the perforated hollow viscous, an upright film is recommended.

- CT scan of the abdomen is the imaging modality of choice when imaging is urgently needed. It has a reliable degree of accuracy and allows for discernment of various organs and structures, including the appendix, the reproductive organs of the abdomen, and the liver and spleen. It also allows for visualization of the retroperitoneal structures. If you are assessing for nephrolithiasis, a CT scan of the abdomen/pelvis should be ordered without contrast in order to visualize the ureters and renal parenchyma. If you are assessing other structures, ordering a CT scan with both by mouth (PO) and intravenous (IV) contrast is best. However, IV contrast should not be administered until the patient's allergies, serum creatinine, and medication list have been reviewed. In order to clear contrast out of the system, patients should be adequately hydrated following the CT scan study.

> **CLINICAL PEARL:** Patients on metformin are at risk for lactic acidosis with IV contrast administration and should hold this medication for 2 to 3 days post IV contrast administration.

- For more emergent use, bedside ultrasound is recommended if available. This is especially relevant for those conditions that can lead to rapid hemodynamic instability. These include dissecting abdominal aortic aneurism (AAA), ectopic pregnancy, blunt abdominal trauma with hypotension, and assessment of the structures in the right upper quadrant (RUQ) if cholecystitis or pancreatitis is suspected. Because the ultrasound is operator dependent, it does require availability of an individual who can perform it well. Ultrasound has limited capability for small or large bowel disorders but is the preferred method of choice for biliary tree disease.[6]

INVASIVE TESTING

- Nasogastric tube insertion should be performed for any upper GI bleed suspicion such as in a patient with hematochezia or melena. It is not only diagnostic but also therapeutic as well since blood is cathartic.

Initial Management

- In addressing treatment for various abdominal pain conditions, initial management is often symptom dependent. If a patient is suspected of having vomiting due to an SBO, he or she should receive IV antiemetics in the form of promethazine, metoclopramide, ondansetron, or prochlorperazine.
- For patients with vomiting due to gastroenteritis, we generally avoid giving multiple doses of antiemetics. These patients respond well to

aggressive parenteral fluid hydration. Typically after 2 to 3 L of IV normal saline (IVNS), patients are able to tolerate PO clear liquids. Once that is accomplished, they can be discharged with instructions for a BRAT diet (banana, rice, apple sauce, toast). Hydration should also be aggressive for patients with severe sepsis and evidence of lactic acidosis, severe diarrhea with volume loss, and GI bleed.

- For patients with evidence of GI infection, such as cholecystitis, diverticulitis, or colitis with underlying inflammatory bowel disease, antibiotic treatment should be initiated with appropriate Gram-negative coverage. This includes metronidazole and a quinolone. If there is suspicion of sepsis, consider parenteral piperacillin–tazobactam.[6]
- Patients with GU symptoms from uncomplicated urethritis or cystitis should receive appropriate oral antibiotics.

Key Points...

- Vitals
  - o Any patient with abnormal vital signs and a rigid abdomen is considered to have a suspected viscous perforation for which a surgical consult should be obtained immediately.
- CV/peripheral vascular (PV)
  - o Any patient with coronary artery disease (CAD) risk factors or age greater than 50 years should have an EKG done to rule out cardiac etiology for epigastric or upper quadrant abdominal pain.
  - o Because patients over the age of 50 with our without hypertension (HTN) are at risk for AAA, an abdominal ultrasound should be done to rule out AAA as it is a medical emergency.
- GI
  - o If a patient presents with severe unilateral pain with negative results of all other diagnostics studies, suspect varicella zoster as the pain typically precedes onset of rash.
  - o Do not perform a rectal exam on a neutropenic cancer patient on chemotherapy.
- GU
  - o All female patients who are of fertile age should have a pregnancy test as ectopic pregnancy should be assumed until proven otherwise.
  - o Ovarian torsion is a medical emergency. If a female patient presents with pelvic pain and a negative pregnancy test, suspect and rule out ovarian torsion urgently.

References

1. Henderson M, Tierney LM, Smetana GW. *The Patient History*. 2nd ed. New York, NY: McGraw-Hill; 2012.
2. Bickley LS. *Bates' Guide to Physical Examination and History Taking*. 12th ed. Philadelphia, PA: Wolters Kluwer; 2017:449–508.
3. Bhuiya FA, Pitts SR, McCaig LF. Emergency department visits for chest pain and abdominal pain: United States, 1999–2008. NCHS data brief no. 43. Washington, DC: U.S. Department of Health and Human Services; 2010. https://www.cdc.gov/nchs/data/databriefs/db43.pdf
4. Ball J, Dains JE, Flynn JA, et al. *Seidel's Guide to Physical Examination: An Interprofessional Approach*. 9th ed. St. Louis, MO: Mosby; 2018.
5. Quaas J, Lanigan M, Newman D, et al. Utility of the digital rectal examination in the evaluation of undifferentiated abdominal pain. *Am J Emerg Med*. 2009;27(9):1125–1129. doi:10.1016/j.ajem.2008.08.027
6. Walls R, Hockberger R, Gausche-Hill M, eds. *Rosen's Emergency Medicine: Concepts and Clinical Practice*. 9th ed. Philadelphia, PA: Elsevier; 2018.

ALTERED MENTAL STATUS

Altered mental status (AMS) is one of the most common entities in EM. The approach to the evaluation of AMS requires the provider to first ensure the patient has a patent airway, is breathing, and has measurable vital signs. The most relevant component in the acute approach to AMS is obtaining a thorough history. If this cannot be reliably obtained from the patient, begin with whomever brought the patient to the ED.

- Ask emergency medical services (EMS) about the scene prior to their arrival. Were they called to the patient's home? Did they find the patient at the bottom of the stairs (indicating head injury)? Were they called to a park where a patient was found lying on a bench next to drug paraphernalia? Perhaps they were called to a nursing home for an elderly patient with the complaint of AMS but the last set of vitals reported a high fever (indicating sepsis).
- If EMS are unable to provide any further history and your ED has electronic health records (EHRs), you may be able to look up the patient's history to see whether he or she has been there before. A history of alcohol ingestion can lead you to consider alcohol intoxication with delirium tremens.
- Inquire about past medical history. A history of diabetes mellitus can be relevant in a presentation of diabetic ketoacidosis (DKA).
- If there are family or friends who bring the patient to the ED, use the same approach in obtaining a history.

Differential Diagnosis

Due to the complexity of how AMS presents, the differential diagnosis is very broad, but can be narrowed (Table 1.6).

TABLE **1.6** Differential Diagnosis of Altered Mental Status

Neurological	Adverse reaction to a new medication/dosage
	Ischemic stroke
	Intracranial bleeding
	Traumatic brain injury
	Concussive syndrome
	Seizure disorder
	Encephalitis, meningitis (viral, bacterial, fungal)
	Neoplasm/mass
Toxicology	Ethylene glycol ingestion (antifreeze)
	Methamphetamine ingestion
	Cocaine use
	PCP use
	Marijuana use
	Opioid use
	Acute alcohol intoxication
	Benzodiazepine use
Endocrine	Hypoglycemia
	Diabetic ketoacidosis
	Thyroid storm
	Myxedema coma
Electrolytes	Uremic syndrome
	Hyponatremia
	Hypercalcemia
Cardiac/pulmonary	Hypoxia-induced AMS
	Sepsis from infected valve
	Pneumonia
	Hypercarbia
Geriatric	Dementia/depression
	Urosepsis
	Hyponatremia
Sports medicine	Rhabdomyolysis
	Heat stroke
	Hypothermia
GI disease	Hepatic encephalopathy
	Hypovolemia from acute GI bleed
	Delirium tremens secondary to alcoholic cirrhosis
Behavioral health	Acute decompensation from mental illness
	Dementia
	Delirium
	Schizophrenia
	Schizoaffective disorder
	Depression
	Bipolar syndromes
	Personality disorders
	Adverse reactions to medication

AMS, altered mental status; GI, gastrointestinal; PCP, phencyclidine.

History

- Onset, duration, timing: Onset is crucial. Conditions in which the behavior changes *suddenly* include acute brain injury, hypoglycemia, and those of toxicological etiologies such as ethylene glycol ingestion, alcohol, or opioid use. Conditions associated with *gradual* behavior change are those of more organic etiologies such as sepsis, hepatic encephalopathy, and DKA. The same applies to conditions with electrolyte imbalance such as hyponatremia.

- Provoking/alleviating factors: Mental illness is another disease entity in which onset and historical components may facilitate diagnosis. This is an especially important example as it may be a diagnosis of exclusion. If a patient presents with AMS and has normal vitals and labs with no organic etiology, ask family/friends about behavior changes. Patients with schizophrenia or schizoaffective disorder may present with paranoid behavior over several months. In bipolar conditions, patients present after manic episodes occur over several months, including spending money in excess or losing sleep over that time period.

- Having a list of the patient's medications is vital in determining the etiology of mental illness. As a student in EM, you have the luxury of time. Consider calling the patient's pharmacy to determine not only the types of medication he or he is taking but also whether there has recently been a change in dosage, lack of adherence to medication regimen, or discontinuation. Medications that can be implicated in AMS include opioids, benzodiazepines, tricyclic antidepressants (TCAs), gabapentin, cold medications such as those containing pseudoephedrine, antiseizure medications, diphenhydramine, and allergy medications.

- Quality: Determining the quality of AMS will facilitate the differential diagnosis by ruling out organic versus nonorganic etiologies. Acute altered behavior is typically induced with an exogenous source such as ingestion of medications and substances. Those with a more insidious and slow-presenting quality are secondary to organic etiologies such as sepsis, meningitis, or DKA.

- Severity: The severity of AMS can range from changes in behavior to comatose.

- Timing: Inquire as to whether the AMS is intermittent or progressively constant. Delirium takes place over a few days, whereas dementia is more insidious in onset. Delirium can be fluctuating but dementia is stable in that it persists over a long period of time. Delirium may be associated with movement disorders, whereas dementia is not.

Past Medical History Specific to Complaint

- Head and neck: Traumatic brain injury (TBI), head injury
- CV: Cardiac tamponade, pneumonia in the elderly, hypoxia- nduced AMS from heart failure/infectious pericarditis

- Abdomen: Sepsis secondary to spontaneous bacterial peritonitis in a renal-failure patient, patient with rigid abdomen, hepatic encephalopathy
- Musculoskeletal system (MSS): Heat stroke, rhabdomyolysis
- Neurology: Meningitis, seizure disorder, epilepsy
- Endocrinopathies: Low blood sugar, DKA
- Renal disease: hyperkalemia /hypokalemia; hyperkalemia/hypochloremia, hypermagnesemia/hypomagnesemia; hypernatremia/hyponatremia

Physical Examination

The physical exam for patients with AMS must be comprehensive and should include a Mini-Mental State Exam. Monitoring of vital signs allows for recognition of hemodynamic compromise and more urgent disease states. Clues, such as hypotension and/or fever, may indicate sepsis in an elderly patient. Tachycardia may be a result of cocaine ingestion if a young patient presents with agitation. Next, check finger-stick glucose. If a patient has a history of diabetes, hypoglycemia from a lack of oral intake or too much insulin can lead to AMS.

- Head, eye, ear, nose, and throat (HEENT) exam: Look for signs of head trauma, bleeding, hemotympanium, evidence of Battle's sign. Check the pupils for reactivity. Pinpoint pupils may indicate substance ingestion. Ethanol (ETOH) intoxication tends to dilate pupils. If a patient exhibits AMS with one blown pupil that is fixed and irregularly shaped, this may indicate a substantial head injury.
- CV/lung exam: Auscultate the lungs for airway patency. If a patient was in a motor vehicle accident, there may be hypoxia from a tension pneumothorax leading to AMS.
- ABD: Assess the liver for tenderness and size. Patients with chronic alcohol abuse may have evidence of epigastric tenderness due to pancreatitis with no hepatomegaly. Cirrhotic patients may present with AMS due to encephalopathy. Ascites may also be present.
- Neuro: Because AMS may be a presentation of cerebrovascular accident (CVA), doing a bedside focused assessment with sonography in trauma (FAST) exam is crucial, which can then be followed up as needed with additional testing. The acronym FAST components include having the patient perform **facial** movement, holding the **arms** out, assessing **speech** by asking the patient to say a common phrase, and **time**, or, asking when the symptoms started. This is a public health endeavor by the National Stroke Association. Doing a quick Mini-Mental State Exam will also help narrow down the differential diagnosis. Ask the patient the following questions to get a sense of her or his state of mind: What is your name? Do you know where you are? Who is the president? A summary of pertinent physical exam findings and their associated condition is seen in Table 1.7.

> **CLINICAL PEARL:** Consider normal pressure hydrocephalus (NPH) if the classic combination of urinary incontinence + gait disturbance is seen.[1]

TABLE **1.7** Correlating Physical Exam Findings With Pathologic Conditions

Body System	Physical Exam Finding	Associated Clinical Condition
Head and neck	Pupillary reaction	Medication induced
	Dilatation/lack of dilatation	TBI, ICH
CV	Murmur	HF, severe AS, endocarditis
	Muffled heart sounds/distant	Pericarditis, tamponade
MSS	Mottled skin	Sepsis, elevated lactate, hypoperfusion
	Clubbing of nails	Chronic pathology such as pancreatitis, hepatitis, endocarditis, heart failure, cystic fibrosis
Abdomen	RUQ tenderness; hepatomegaly	Hepatitis/hepatic failure
	Diffuse tenderness with involuntary guarding	SBP

AS, aortic stenosis; CV, cardiovascular; HF, heart failure; ICH, intracranial hemorrhage; MSS, musculoskeletal system; RUQ, right upper quadrant; SBP, spontaneous bacterial peritonitis; TBI, traumatic brain injury.

Diagnostic Plan

LABS

- CBC: Evaluate for infection/sepsis, anemia.

> **CLINICAL PEARL:** An elevated white blood cell (WBC) count and elevated serum lactate level should prompt consideration of sepsis. Consider infectious etiologies, such as urinary tract infection, pneumonia, meningitis, or encephalitis, as these patients may present with acute delirium.

- BMP: Evaluate for hyponatremia, hypoglycemia, acute uremic syndrome with elevated BUN/creatinine. Hypercalcemia can cause confusion and lethargy.
- Serum magnesium and phosphorus: Altered levels may be contributing to patient's presentation.
- Urinalysis: Evaluate for proteinuria indicating declining renal function, nitrates and evidence of infection, glucose, and ketones in DKA.
- Toxicology and urine drug screen: Evaluate for ingestion of substances, including cocaine, opiates, phenobarbital, Tylenol, aspirin.

- Arterial blood gas: Evaluate for evidence of acidosis or alkalosis related to AMS, especially if the patient requires rapid resuscitation, is in a hypoxic or hypercapnia state from respiratory failure, or there is concern of CO poisoning.

> **CLINICAL PEARL:** Consider anticholinergic agents, sedative-hypnotics, selective serotonin reuptake inhibitors (SSRIs), and polypharmacy in the setting of AMS. Some of these agents cannot be measured by serum concentration but rather through historical investigation.

- Serum ammonia: Elevation indicates hepatic encephalopathy
- Serum lactate: Elevated in the setting of sepsis or metabolic acidosis
- Serum alcohol: Elevation indicates alcohol intoxication

> **CLINICAL PEARL:** Serum alcohol should be measured in the setting of AMS. Both acute alcohol ingestion and alcohol (or drug withdrawal) can present as delirium.

Diagnostic Imaging

- Head CT without contrast: Evaluate for intracranial bleed, evidence of skull fracture, epidural/subdural bleed, central nervous system (CNS) mass lesion.
  - ○ NOTE: If patient has a history of hydrocephalus and presents with AMS, you will need to do an abdominal imaging series and a shunt series to check patency of the ventricular drainage device.
- Chest x-ray (CXR): Evaluate for infiltrate, pneumothorax, evidence of pulmonary congestion, widened mediastinum, mass.

> **CLINICAL PEARL:** Patients with congestive heart failure (CHF), an acute myocardial infarction (MI), a pulmonary embolus, hypoxia, or carbon dioxide narcosis may present with acute delirium.

Initial Management

- The cardinal rule in EM when managing patients with altered mentation is to maintain patency of airway, a mean arterial pressure that allows for efficient cardiac output (normal range 70–110 mmHg), and a pulse ox above 95%.
- If the patient demonstrates evidence of hypovolemia or hypotension, administer IV fluids through a large-bore peripheral or central venous access line unless contraindicated (e g., in the setting of heart failure).

- If a patient has AMS related to a CVA and symptoms are within the 3-hour window, a head CT should be done to rule out intracranial bleed and tissue plasminogen activator (tPA) should be initiated as per advanced cardiac life support (ACLS) stroke protocol.

- For patients who present with a fever, administer antipyretics to combat the fever and maintain fluid hydration to ensure they do not become dehydrated.

- If a patient has an intracranial bleed, call neurosurgery to consult for possible evacuation.

- If a patient has evidence of hepatic encephalopathy, with an elevated serum ammonia level, he or she should receive lactulose.

- Evaluate for and treat all other electrolyte abnormalities, including a point-of-care glucose test. The treatment for hypercalcemia is fluid hydration.

DELIRIUM

Because the etiology of delirium can be broad, including drug withdrawal to an organic intracranial condition, treatment is directed at the underlying cause. If there is a need for sedation, haloperidol is an initial choice at a dose of 5 to 10 mg PO, intramuscularly (IM), or IV with a reduced dose for the elderly of 1 to 2 mg.[1] Benzodiazepines can be used alone or as an adjunct to haloperidol, with caution in the elderly. The key is to facilitate psychosocial support until the patient can be stabilized and further investigation as to the etiology of the delirium can be achieved.

DEMENTIA

All types of dementia are treatable, at least to some degree, by environmental or psychosocial interventions.[1] It is a disease of chronicity with progression over time. Because this patient requires around-the-clock care for his or her own safety and that of those around him or her, communication is a key factor in managing this particular etiology of AMS. Monitor the patient's behavior, understanding what some triggers may be. Ensure patients have safety parameters in place. The use of a call bell or a live-in aide may be required for the wandering patient.

As the etiology of vascular dementia is hypertension, managing blood pressure is important. For patients with dementia secondary to normal pressure hydrocephalus, using an interventional diagnostic therapeutic approach in the form of a lumbar puncture or even ventricular shunting are options.

REFERENCE

1. Huff J. Altered mental status and coma. In: Tintinalli JE, Stapczynski J, Ma O, et al., eds. *Tintinalli's Emergency Medicine: A Comprehensive Study Guide.* 8th ed. New York, NY: McGraw-Hill; 2016: 1156–1160.

CHEST PAIN

Chest pain is the second most common reason patients in the United States present to the ED. This common complaint accounts for approximately 6.9 million visits per year, constituting nearly 5% of all ED visits in the United States.[1] Etiologies of chest pain vary widely and range from those that are immediately life-threatening to nonurgent entities.

Differential Diagnosis

The majority of patients with chest pain will fall into one of four categories: cardiovascular, pulmonary, musculoskeletal, or gastrointestinal causes. Although it is important to consider psychiatric and other miscellaneous causes of chest pain, many of these are diagnoses of exclusion and should only be considered when other, more life-threatening causes have been ruled out. The differential diagnosis for chest pain is broad and includes many body systems (Table 1.8). When evaluating the patient with chest pain in the ED, it is important to keep the following life-threatening conditions in mind:

- Acute coronary syndrome (ACS)
- Aortic dissection
- Cardiac tamponade
- Pulmonary embolism (PE)
- Tension pneumothorax
- Mediastinitis/esophageal rupture

TABLE 1.8 Differential Diagnosis of Chest Pain by Body System

Cardiovascular	Pulmonary
ACS	PE
Aortic dissection	Tension pneumothorax/pneumothorax
Cardiac tamponade/pericardial effusion	Pneumonia/respiratory infection
Acute heart failure	Chronic Obstructive Pulmonary Disease
Pericarditis/myocarditis/endocarditis	(COPD) or Asthma exacerbation
Valvular Disease (eg aortic stenosis, mitral	Pulmonary hypertension
valve prolapse)	Malignancy
Cardiomyopathy	Pleural effusion
	Pleuritis

Musculoskeletal	Gastrointestinal
Chest wall contusion	Mediastinitis/esophageal rupture (Boerhaave
Intercostal muscle strain	syndrome)
Costochondritis	Gastroesophageal reflux disease (GERD)
Rib fracture	Esophagitis
	Esophageal spasm
	Hiatal hernia
	Peptic ulcer disease

(continued)

TABLE **1.8** Differential Diagnosis of Chest Pain by Body System (*continued*)

Other	
Psychiatric/anxiety	Substance abuse
Anemia	Herpes zoster
Acute chest syndrome/Sickle Cell Anemia	Inflammatory/collagen vascular disease

ACS, acute coronary syndrome; COPD, chronic obstructive pulmonary disease; GERD, gastroesophageal reflux disease; PE, pulmonary embolism.

History

The initial evaluation of the patient with chest pain begins with obtaining a focused history from the patient. The pneumonic "OPQRST" can be a helpful tool in eliciting important historical details from the patient.

- Onset: The onset of chest pain associated with ACS generally starts gradually and increases over time or with exertion. Sudden onset of chest pain is usually associated with PE, aortic dissection, or pneumothorax. Pain that begins after trauma may be associated with traumatic pneumothorax, rib fracture/chest wall injury, or traumatic pericardial effusion. Onset of pain following eating or vomiting may indicate gastroesophageal reflux disease (GERD) or esophageal disease.

- Provocation/alleviating factors: Pain that worsens with physical exertion is typically associated with ACS, heart failure, or PE. Pain that worsens with deep inspiration (pleuritic) is typical of PE, pneumonia, or pneumothorax. Pain from GERD is usually worsened by laying supine, particularly after eating. Pericarditis is usually associated with pain that is improved when leaning forward and worsened when supine. Musculoskeletal or traumatic causes of chest pain are usually worse with palpation or movement.

> **CLINICAL PEARL:** Although pain that is relieved with nitroglycerin may be associated with ACS, this is not a reliable diagnostic tool in determining cardiac ischemia from other etiologies of chest pain.[2] Likewise, pain alleviated with antacid medications should not be assumed to be from GERD or other gastrointestinal causes.

- Quality: Pain associated with ACS is generally described as squeezing, pressure, or fullness. Chest tightness is common in chronic obstructive pulmonary disease (COPD) and asthma exacerbations. Pain described as sharp and pleuritic is usually associated with a pulmonary etiology such as pneumothorax, PE, or pneumonia. Tearing or ripping quality of pain is associated with aortic dissection. Pain described as burning may be associated with GERD or esophageal disease.

- Radiation/location: Pain located in the mid- to left sternal region that radiates to the left arm/shoulder, jaw, back, or neck is common in ACS. Pain from aortic dissection may be felt in the chest or the back and can radiate to the arms, chest, or abdomen depending on the location of the dissection. Pain beginning in the epigastric abdominal region, radiating up toward the chest is common in GERD and esophageal disease, but can also signify ACS.
- Severity: Pain from an aortic dissection, PE, pneumothorax, and esophageal rupture is usually described as immediately severe. Pain from ACS generally increases in severity gradually.
- Timing: Episodic pain, particularly related to physical activity, cold, or stress, tends to be related to ACS. ACS pain typically worsens gradually over 20 to 30 minutes, pain may last for longer in the setting of a myocardial infarction (MI).[3] Pain from GERD is also episodic, usually related to food intake. Pain from esophageal rupture or aortic dissection is usually constant. PE or pneumothorax causes pain that is usually worse during deep inspiration.

> **CLINICAL PEARL:** Not all patients with ACS will have "classic" chest pain symptoms. Patients who are elderly, female, or those with a history of diabetes may present with atypical symptoms of ACS such as dyspnea or weakness.[2]

Past Medical History Specific to Complaint

Other important historical factors to consider when evaluating risk for specific diseases include

- Age
  - Age greater than 65 years in men and women increases risk for ACS, aortic stenosis, heart failure
  - Age greater than 60 years (men) increases risk for aortic dissection
  - Age greater than 50 years increases risk for herpes zoster
- Gender
  - Male: ACS, aortic dissection, pneumothorax
  - Female: PE (pregnancy, hormonal contraceptives), pleuritis (systemic lupus erythematosus [SLE])
- Underlying disease
  - Hyperlipidemia: ACS, heart failure, aortic dissection
  - Hypertension: ACS, heart failure, aortic dissection
  - Diabetes mellitus: ACS
  - Connective tissue disorder (Marfan's syndrome, Ehler–Danlos): aortic dissection, pneumothorax

- ○ Collagen vascular/systemic inflammatory disease: PE, aortic dissection, pericardial disease, pleuritis
  - ○ Malignancy: PE, pericardial effusion
- Family history
  - ○ First-degree relative age younger than 55 (males), younger than 65 (females) with heart disease: ACS
  - ○ Familial coagulopathy: deep vein thrombosis (DVT), PE
  - ○ Family history of hypertrophic cardiomyopathy or sudden cardiac death
- Comorbid conditions
  - ○ Obesity: ACS, GERD
  - ○ Sedentary lifestyle: ACS, heart failure, PE

It is important to ask about associated symptoms such as

- General
  - ○ Fever: Malignancy, pneumonia, pericarditis or myocarditis, PE
  - ○ Weakness: ACS, heart failure (particularly in the elderly), anemia
  - ○ Diaphoresis: ACS, heart failure, aortic dissection
  - ○ Syncope: Pericardial tamponade, aortic stenosis, arrhythmia, anemia, PE
- Respiratory
  - ○ Cough: Heart failure, COPD/asthma, pulmonary infection, pericarditis, myocarditis
  - ○ Hemoptysis: PE, malignancy, pneumonia
  - ○ Dyspnea: ACS, PE, pneumothorax, pulmonary infection, heart failure, COPD/asthma
- Gastrointestinal
  - ○ Nausea/vomiting: ACS, esophageal rupture, GERD
- Extremities
  - ○ Lower extremity edema: Heart failure, PE/DVT
  - ○ Limb temperature discrepancy or paresthesias: Aortic dissection, PE/DVT

Patients can also be predisposed to certain disease risk based on recent life events such as

- Trauma: Cardiac tamponade, traumatic aortic dissection, rib fracture, chest wall contusion, PE, pneumothorax
- Surgery: PE, mediastinitis, cardiac surgery, pneumonia
- Diagnostic procedures: Mediastinitis, pneumonia
- Prolonged immobility: PE
- Travel: Pneumothorax, PE
- SCUBA diving: Pneumothorax
- Recent upper respiratory infection (URI)/viral infection: Pneumonia, pericarditis, myocarditis, pleurisy

- Pregnancy: PE, aortic dissection, peripartum cardiomyopathy

  It is important to obtain a thorough social history, including

- Smoking tobacco: ACS, aortic stenosis, pneumothorax, aortic dissection, malignancy, COPD
- Alcohol abuse: Esophageal rupture, GERD, esophageal varices
- Substance abuse
  - ○ Cocaine: ACS
  - ○ IV drug use: Endocarditis, myocarditis, septic emboli

> **CLINICAL PEARL:** Make sure to explicitly ask your patient about tobacco, alcohol, and drug use; do not make social history assumptions based on your patient's appearance or age.

Be sure to ask your patient about all medications and supplements that he or she is taking as both prescription, and over-the-counter medications and supplements can increase your patient's risk for certain diseases. For example, oral contraceptives/estrogen supplements increase the risk for PE.

Lastly, recent testing that a patient may have had can help you to determine whether or not a specific diagnosis is more or less likely

- **Stress test**: ACS
- **Cardiac catheterization**: ACS, heart failure, pulmonary hypertension
- **Radiologic imaging**: Recent echocardiography, CT, MRI, or other ultrasonography for purpose of monitoring known disease entities

> **CLINICAL PEARL:** Although less than15% to 30% of nontraumatic chest pain in the ED is related to ACS, the 28-day mortality rate is 10%.[2] It is important to risk stratify your patient when considering ACS as a potential cause of chest pain as these patients may appear well with normal vital signs. When you are evaluating a patient with chest pain, keep in mind the risk factors for ACS (Box 1.1) as these will help guide you in the appropriate disposition of your patient. Heart disease remains the leading cause of death in adults in the United States.[4]

Box 1.1 Risk Factors for Coronary Artery Disease

1. Patient risk factors
   - ▫ Age >55 years (men) >65 years (women)
   - ▫ Male gender

(continued)

Box 1.1 Risk Factors for Coronary Artery Disease (*continued*)

- □ Family history: First-degree relative age <55 (males), <65 (females) with CAD
2. Comorbid conditions
   - □ Hypertension
   - □ Diabetes mellitus
   - □ Hyperlipidemia
   - □ Chronic kidney disease
3. Lifestyle factors
   - □ Smoking tobacco
   - □ Sedentary lifestyle
   - □ Obesity
   - □ Diet (low fiber, high animal fat intake)
   - □ Psychosocial stress

CAD, coronary artery disease.

Physical Examination

Physical exam of a patient with chest pain in the ED should be focused while carefully evaluating general appearance, skin, cardiovascular, pulmonary, extremities, and peripheral vascular systems. Although the most helpful information guiding your diagnostic workup will come from taking a good history, the physical exam may help to further include or exclude certain disease processes from your differential diagnosis.

> **CLINICAL PEARL:** Remember that time is of the essence in examining a critically ill patient. Oftentimes a more comprehensive physical exam may be limited by the need for immediate diagnostic testing or therapeutic interventions. Physical examination of the patient may take place simultaneously as your team assists in obtaining an EKG, blood work, or IV access.

It is possible to obtain important information regarding your patient's condition within seconds to minutes of your initial evaluation. Although the physical exam may be deceivingly normal in some conditions, such as PE or ACS, it is important to keep certain exam findings in mind during your evaluation (Table 1.9).

> **CLINICAL PEARL:** **Beck's triad** found in cardiac tamponade consists of hypotension, distended neck veins, and muffled heart sounds.

TABLE **1.9** Physical Exam Findings in Specific Disease Conditions

Body System	Physical Exam Finding	Associated Clinical Condition
General Appearance	Diaphoretic	ACS, aortic dissection, PE
	Pallor	ACS, aortic dissection, anemia
	Anxious	ACS, PE, aortic dissection
	Severe painful distress	Aortic dissection, esophageal rupture
	Wasting	Malignancy
	Obtunded	Heart failure, COPD
	Cyanosis	Heart failure, COPD
	Fever	Malignancy, pneumonia, pericarditis or myocarditis, PE
Vital Signs	Hypotension	Aortic dissection, pericardial tamponade, ACS/MI with cardiogenic shock
	Hypertension	ACS, aortic dissection, heart failure
	Asymmetric blood pressure	Aortic dissection
	Pulsus paradoxus	Pericardial effusion/cardiac tamponade
	Pulses alternans	Left ventricular failure
	Weak, thready pulse	Heart failure, cardiac tamponade, cardiogenic shock
	Tachycardia	PE, ACS, heart failure, cardiac tamponade, cardiogenic shock
	Bradycardia	ACS/inferior wall MI
	Tachypnea	PE, pneumothorax, pneumonia, pericardial effusion/cardiac tamponade, COPD, asthma
	Hypoxia	PE, pneumothorax, heart failure, COPD, asthma, respiratory failure, toxic ingestion
Cardiovascular	Jugular venous distention	Heart failure, cardiac tamponade, tension pneumothorax, massive PE
	S3, S4	Heart failure
	Systolic murmur	Aortic stenosis (ejection murmur radiating to carotids), mitral regurgitation, hypertrophic cardiomyopathy
	Diastolic murmur	Aortic regurgitation (aortic dissection involving proximal aorta/aortic valve), mitral stenosis
	Pericardial friction rub	Pericardial disease

(continued)

TABLE **1.9** Physical Exam Findings in Specific Disease Conditions
(*continued*)

Body System	Physical Exam Finding	Associated Clinical Condition
Pulmonary	Tracheal deviation	Tension pneumothorax (away from affected side), pleural effusion (toward affected side)
	Pectus excavatum	Marfan's syndrome/connective tissue disorder aortic dissection
	Reduced breath sounds	Pneumothorax (unilateral), COPD/asthma (diffusely), pleural effusion
	Wheeze	Heart failure, COPD, asthma
	Rales (crackles)	Heart failure, pneumonia, pleural effusion
	Pleural rub	Pleuritis
	Mediastinal crunch (Hamman sign)	COPD, mediastinitis/esophageal rupture
	Subcutaneous emphysema	Mediastinitis/esophageal rupture
	Dullness to percussion	Pleural effusion, pneumonia
	Hyperresonance to percussion	Pneumothorax, COPD/asthma
Skin	Ecchymosis/abrasion/signs of trauma	Chest wall contusion, rib fracture
	Vesicular rash	Herpes zoster
Musculoskeletal	Chest wall tenderness	Chest wall injury/rib fracture, costochondritis
Extremities	Unilateral upper or lower extremity edema	DVT → PE
	Bilateral lower extremity edema	Heart failure
	Asymmetric pulses; weakened or absent lower extremity pulses	Aortic dissection
	Clubbing	Chronic lung disease/hypoxia
Neurologic	Stroke or altered mental status (with extension to carotid arteries)	Aortic dissection
	Horner syndrome (involvement of superior cervical sympathetic ganglion)	Aortic dissection
	Hoarseness (compression of left recurrent laryngeal nerve)	Aortic dissection
	Acute paraplegia (spinal cord ischemia)	Aortic dissection

ACS, acute coronary syndrome; COPD, chronic obstructive pulmonary disease; DVT, deep vein thrombosis; MI, myocardial infarction; PE, pulmonary embolism.

Diagnostic Plan

LABS

- CBC: anemia, infection, inflammatory processes
- Troponin: ACS, myocarditis
  - Troponin I will be elevated within 3 hours of an acute MI, an initial set of negative cardiac biomarkers is not sufficient to rule out ACS. Typically, serial assays will be taken at 0-, 3-, and 6-hour intervals during evaluation.
- B-type natriuretic peptide (BNP): Heart failure
  - Levels higher than 100 pg/mL are highly sensitive for acute heart failure, levels lower than 50 pg/mL have a high negative predictive value for acute heart failure.[2]
- D-dimer: PE, aortic dissection
  - D-dimer has a very high sensitivity and negative predictive value in evaluation of patients with a low-pretest probability for PE.

> **CLINICAL PEARL:**   You can use scoring systems such as pulmonary embolism rule-out criteria (PERC) or Well's to determine need for D-dimer testing in ruling out PE.

  - Baseline D-dimer levels can be elevated in elderly or pregnant patients and in those with malignancy, sepsis, and recent trauma or major surgery[2]
  - D-dimer levels of less than 500 ng/mL have been shown to have high sensitivity and negative predictive value in screening patients for aortic dissection and may be useful to identify those patients who do not have aortic dissection
- Erythrocyte sedimentation rate (ESR) or C-reactive protein are used in inflammatory processes such as pericarditis/myocarditis.

DIAGNOSTIC IMAGING STUDIES

- EKG: One of the most important tools in the evaluation of the patient with chest pain; a 12-lead EKG should be obtained for any patient with remote suspicion of or risk factors for ACS; although specific EKG findings may be present in other disease entities presenting with chest pain, it is the most important diagnostic test in evaluating patients with ACS

> **CLINICAL PEARL:**   The American College of Cardiology and American Heart Association guidelines state that an EKG should be obtained and interpreted within 10 minutes of arrival to the ED for any patient with suspected ACS.[2]

○ ST-elevation MI (STEMI): New ST elevation of at least 1 mm in two contiguous leads (in all leads other than V2 and V3) with or without reciprocal ST depressions[5] (Figure 1.1)

○ Non–ST-elevation MI (NSTEMI)/unstable angina: Horizontal or down-sloping ST depression of at least 0.5 mm in two contiguous leads (Figure 1.2); T wave inversion of 1 mm in two contiguous leads (Figure 1.3)[5]

○ Hyperacute T waves in early MI

○ Nonspecific ST–T wave abnormalities in aortic dissection

○ New left bundle branch block (LBBB): Rule out acute MI

○ Arrhythmias: Ventricular tachycardia or ventricular fibrillation due to cardiac ischemia; electrical alternans or low voltage patterns suggestive of pericardial effusion/cardiac tamponade

> **CLINICAL PEARL:** A normal EKG does not exclude ACS; patients with a concerning history or risk factors should be further evaluated with troponin levels or admission to an observation unit for cardiac imaging/stress testing/catheterization. History, EKG, age, risk factors, and troponin (HEART) Score or thrombolysis in myocardial infarction (TIMI) score can be helpful in the decision-making process.

○ Diffuse ST elevation with or without PR depression: Pericarditis

○ S1Q3T3: Large S wave in lead I, deep Q wave in lead III, and inverted T wave in lead III (Figure 1.4) are indicative of right heart strain that can be found in patients with PE

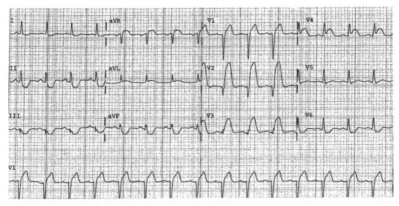

FIGURE 1.1   Anterior wall ST-elevation myocardial infarction with reciprocal changes in inferior leads.

Source: Knechtel MA. *EKGs for the Nurse Practitioner and Physician Assistant.* 2nd ed. New York, NY: Springer Publishing Company; 2017.

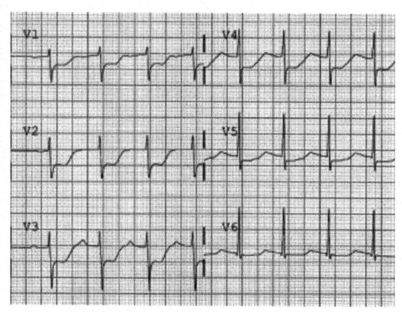

FIGURE 1.2 Diffuse ST depression.

Source: Knechtel MA. *EKGs for the Nurse Practitioner and Physician Assistant.* 2nd ed. New York, NY: Springer Publishing Company; 2017.

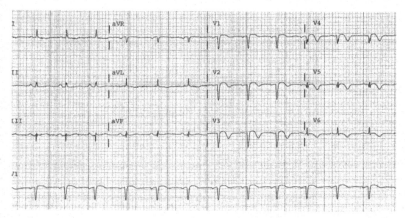

FIGURE 1.3 T-wave inversions in anterior and lateral leads.

Source: Knechtel MA. *EKGs for the Nurse Practitioner and Physician Assistant.* 2nd ed. New York, NY: Springer Publishing Company; 2017.

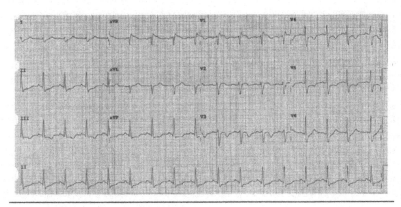

FIGURE 1.4 S1Q3T3 in pulmonary embolism.
Source: Knechtel MA. *EKGs for the Nurse Practitioner and Physician Assistant.* 2nd ed. New York, NY: Springer Publishing Company; 2017.

> **CLINICAL PEARL:** Although the right-heart-strain pattern of S1Q3T3 on EKG is classically associated with PE, the **most common** EKG abnormality in patients with PE is sinus tachycardia.

- ○ Low voltage or electrical alternans in pericardial effusion or cardiac tamponade
- Chest x-ray (CXR): Most useful for evaluating patients with chest pain from pulmonary processes but may also be helpful in the rapid diagnosis of other life-threatening conditions. Evaluate for
  - ○ Tracheal deviation, loss of lung markings, deviation of the visceral pleural line away from the chest wall (Figure 1.5) in pneumothorax

> **CLINICAL PEARL:** Treatment of a suspected tension pneumothorax should not be delayed to obtain CXR; immediate needle decompression or chest tube placement is warranted in the unstable patient.

  - ○ Enlarged cardiac silhouette in pericardial effusion (Figure 1.6) or heart failure

> **CLINICAL PEARL:** At least 200 to 300 mL of pericardial fluid must accumulate before cardiac silhouette abnormalities appear on CXR.

  - ○ Widened mediastinum in aortic dissection (>6–8 cm in diameter)
  - ○ Hampton's hump: A wedge-shaped opacity with its base along the pleural surface in the peripheral lung, and Westermark's sign, segmental

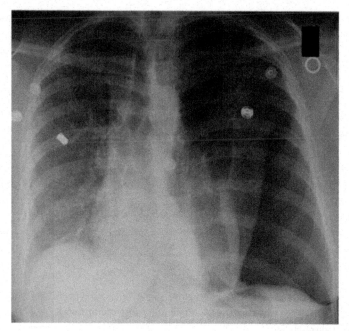

FIGURE 1.5 Pneumothorax.
Source: Courtesy of James Heilman, MD.

distribution of a distinct cutoff of pulmonary vessels with distal hypoperfusion, may be seen in PE
- ○ Mediastinal air in esophageal rupture
- ○ Pulmonary vascular congestion and pleural effusions in heart failure
- ○ Infiltrates: Lobar pneumonia
- ○ Extravasation of oral contrast following contrast esophagram: Esophageal rupture/perforation
- CT
  - ○ CT angiography (chest/abdomen/pelvis): Aortic dissection (Figure 1.7)
  - ○ CT angiography (chest): PE
  - ○ CT without IV contrast: Pneumothorax, esophageal rupture
  - ○ CT coronary angiography: ACS

CLINICAL PEARL: Patients with known IV contrast allergies or severe renal impairment may not be able to receive IV contrast dye. Patients who are on metformin should have their metformin held prior to administration of iodinated contrast dye and should not resume taking it for 48 to 72 hours to avoid precipitating lactic acidosis.

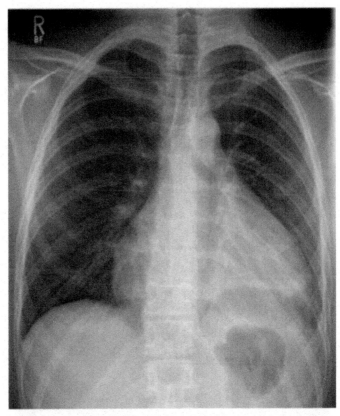

FIGURE **1.6** Pericardial effusion in chest x-ray.
Source: Hellerhoff. Wikimedia Commons. https://commons.wikimedia.org/wiki/File:29-01-Perikarderguss_20_Jahre_Perimyokarditis_pa_Clostridien.png

- Bedside ultrasonography
  - ○ Cardiac ultrasonography/echocardiography: Pericardial effusion/cardiac tamponade (Figure 1.8): Fluid visualized in the pericardial sac in pericardial effusion; right ventricular (RV) collapse visualized in cardiac tamponade
  - ○ PE: RV strain and failure, dilatation or signs of pulmonary artery hypertension
  - ○ Transthoracic echocardiography (TTE): Evaluate for aortic dissection in patients who are not stable enough for CT angiography
  - ○ Evaluate for traumatic pneumothorax as part of the extended focused assessment with sonography in trauma (FAST) exam. Findings include absence of sliding sign and presence of barcode/stratosphere sign.

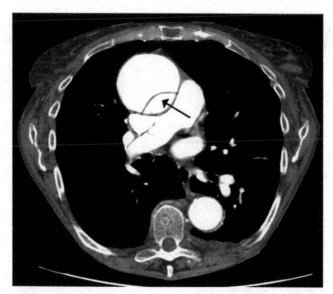

FIGURE 1.7 Aortic dissection on CT angiography (arrow).
Source: Courtesy of James Heilman, MD.

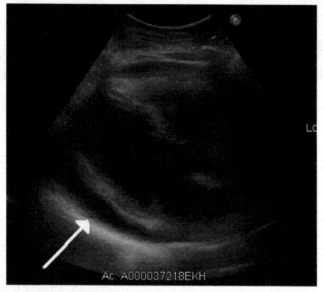

FIGURE 1.8 Pericardial effusion.
Source: Courtesy of James Heilman, MD.

- Nuclear medicine
  - Ventilation/perfusion lung scan (VQ Scan) to evaluate for PE
- Scoring systems
  - TIMI (www.mdcalc.com/timi-risk-score-ua-nstemi; www.mdcalc.com/timi-risk-score-stemi) and HEART (www.mdcalc.com/heart-score-major-cardiac-events) scoring systems may be used to further risk stratify and manage patients with suspected ACS.
  - Wells criteria (www.mdcalc.com/wells-criteria-pulmonary-embolism) and PERC rule (www.mdcalc.com/perc-rule-pulmonary-embolism) scoring systems may be used to risk stratify patients with suspected thromboembolic disease/PE.

Initial Management

The care of most patients, particularly those who are critically ill, begins with securing an airway, delivering oxygen, obtaining IV access, and use of continuous cardiac/hemodynamic monitoring. Immediate intervention for hemodynamic instability, airway compromise, treatment of life-threatening arrhythmias or other general decompensation takes precedence over any other diagnostic or therapeutic intervention. Certain disease processes may require immediate activation of and collaboration with other medical team members, such as cardiology, trauma surgery, cardiac, or cardiothoracic surgery, to coordinate timely transfer of care in the ED.

Initial management of specific disease entities presenting with chest pain is discussed in Table 1.10 and Chapter 2, Common Disease Entities in Emergency Medicine, "Chest Pain" section.

TABLE 1.10 Overview of Diagnosis and Management of Specific Disease Entities

	EKG Findings	Laboratory Studies	Imaging	Initial Treatment
ACS (STEMI)	ST elevations	Troponin I		ASA, P2Y12-I, oxygen (if SPO$_2$ <94%), nitroglycerin, beta-blocker, anticoagulant; PCI/cardiac catheterization within 90 min; fibrinolytic therapy if PCI not available within 120 min
Aortic dissection	Nonspecific ST changes, LV hypertrophy	D-dimer	CT angiography, TTE/TEE	Blood pressure and heart rate control; immediate cardiac surgical consultation for type A

(continued)

TABLE 1.10 Overview of Diagnosis and Management of Specific Disease Entities (*continued*)

	EKG Findings	Laboratory Studies	Imaging	Initial Treatment
Cardiac tamponade	Electrical alternans, low voltage		Echocardiography	Percutaneous or surgical pericardiocentesis
PE	Sinus tachycardia, S1Q3T3	D-dimer	CT angiography, echocardiography	Anticoagulation therapy, thrombolytic therapy
Tension pneumothorax			CXR, bedside ultrasound	Immediate needle or thoracostomy tube decompression
Mediastinitis/ esophageal rupture			CXR/contrast esophagram, CT chest and abdomen	NPO, IV antibiotics (skin and GI flora +/- MRSA), surgical consultation

ACS, acute coronary syndrome; ASA, aspirin; CXR, chest x-ray; DVT, deep vein thrombosis; GI, gastrointestinal; IV, intravenous; LV, left ventricular; MI, myocardial infarction; MRSA, methicillin- resistant *Staphylococcus aureus*; NPO, nothing by mouth; PCI, percutaneous coronary intervention; PE, pulmonary embolism; STEMI, ST-elevation myocardial infarction; TEE, transesophageal echocardiography; TTE, Transthoracic echocardiography.

Key Points . . .

- Chest pain is a common complaint for patients presenting to the ED that has a wide variety of causes; a timely, focused history and physical exam are essential in guiding your diagnosis and management plan.
- Although some causes of chest pain are rare, it is important to keep life-threatening causes in your differential diagnosis while evaluating your patient in the ED.
- ACS is relatively common and potentially life-threatening and should be considered in all patients with no clear alternative etiology of chest pain.
- Early detection and timely evaluation of dangerous diagnoses are essential to initiate life-saving treatments.
- EKG and CXR are important tools in aiding the diagnosis of many causes of chest pain.
- Proper risk stratification is of utmost importance to aid in the appropriate disposition of your patient.

REFERENCES

1. Rui P, Kang K. National hospital ambulatory medical care survey: 2014 emergency department summary tables. https://www.cdc.gov/nchs/data/nhamcs/web_tables/2014_ed_web_tables.pdf. Updated September 7, 2017.
2. Hollander JE, Chase M. Evaluation of the adult with chest pain in the emergency department. In: Hockberger RS, ed. *UpToDate*. https://www.uptodate.com/contents/evaluation-of-the-adult-with-chest-pain-in-the-emergency-department. Updated April 30, 2018.
3. Yelland MJ. Outpatient evaluation of the adult with chest pain. In: Aronson MD, ed. *UpToDate*. https://www.uptodate.com/contents/outpatient-evaluation-of-the-adult-with-chest-pain. Updated June 25, 2019.
4. Heron, M. Deaths: leading causes for 2017. *National Vital Statistics Report.* 2019;68(6):9. Retrieved from https://www.cdc.gov/nchs/data/nvsr/nvsr68/nvsr68_06-508.pdf
5. Thygesen K, Alpert JS, Jaffe AS, et al. Third universal definition of myocardial infarction. *Circulation.* 2012;126(16):2020–2035. doi:10.1161/CIR.0b013e31826e1058

HEADACHE

Headache is the fifth most common reason patients in the United States present to the ED, accounting for approximately 4.3 million visits per year.[1] Although the majority of headaches have a benign cause, you must be able to recognize those patients with potentially life-threatening underlying disease. Perform a detailed, yet concise history and physical exam, focusing on the neurologic system. Determining which patients will require immediate diagnostic imaging or procedures is essential as neuroimaging done on low-risk patients has a low yield and may incur unnecessary cost and radiation exposure.

During your evaluation of the patient with headache, it is important to keep "red flag" historical features (Box 1.2) in mind. They may indicate a potentially dangerous, secondary headache and subsequent need for immediate imaging, diagnostic procedure, or consultation.

Box 1.2 Historical "Red Flags" in Evaluation of the Patient With Headache

- Age >50
- Abrupt onset
- Fever or associated infection
- Absence of similar prior headaches
- Seizure

(continued)

> **Box 1.2** Historical "Red Flags" in Evaluation of the Patient With Headache (*continued*)
>
> □ Altered mental status
> □ Neurologic deficit
> □ Immunosuppression
> □ Visual change
> □ Family history of SAH or brain aneurysm
> □ Exertional headache

SAH, subarachnoid hemorrhage.

Although the vast majority of patients presenting to the ED with headache will have a benign, primary cause, a small percentage may have a fatal, secondary cause (Table 1.11). As with other common presenting complaints, it is your job as an ED provider to determine which patients are at high risk for serious underlying disease.

Differential Diagnosis

Headaches can be classified as primary or secondary, as outlined in Table 1.11.

TABLE 1.11 Differential Diagnosis and Classification of Headache

Primary Headache	Secondary Headache
Migraine	Intracranial pathology: ischemic stroke, SAH/ICH, CVT/venous sinus
Tension	thrombosis
Cluster	Hypertensive emergency
Chronic daily	Carotid/vertebral artery dissection
Trigeminal neuralgia	Traumatic injury/intracranial trauma/TBI: subdural hematoma, ICH, epidural hematoma, concussion/postconcussive syndrome
	Idiopathic intracranial hypertension (pseudotumor cerebri)
	CNS infection: Brain abscess, meningitis, encephalitis
	Sinusitis
	Herpes zoster
	Giant cell/temporal arteritis
	Mass lesion/malignancy (primary or metastatic disease)
	Preeclampsia
	Acute angle-closure glaucoma
	Toxic exposure/carbon monoxide poisoning

CNS, central nervous system; CVT, cerebral venous thrombosis; ICH, intracranial hemorrhage; SAH, subarachnoid hemorrhage; TBI, traumatic brain injury.

History

The initial evaluation of the patient with headache begins with obtaining a focused history from the patient. A good patient history will help guide your diagnostic workup. As with other pain-related complaints, the pneumonic "OPQRST" can be a helpful tool in eliciting important historical details from the patient.

- Onset: The abrupt onset of a severe headache (thunderclap) is concerning for subarachnoid hemorrhage (SAH). Other sudden-onset headaches may come from pituitary apoplexy, hypertensive urgency or emergency, acute angle-closure glaucoma, vertebral or carotid artery dissections, hemorrhage from a mass, or vascular malformation. Pain from migraine headaches or tension-type headaches generally begins as mild to moderate pain that progresses over hours. Pain from meningitis or idiopathic intracranial hypertension may also progress gradually.

> **CLINICAL PEARL:** A "thunderclap" headache that reaches peak intensity within seconds to minutes can indicate blood leaking from an aneurysm and may occur before aneurysm rupture. This description of pain requires aggressive investigation.

- Provocation/alleviating factors: Pain that worsens with physical exertion is concerning for intracranial hemorrhage (ICH) and vertebral or carotid artery dissection. Cough or Valsalva maneuver may worsen pain from malignancy or cerebrovascular disease. Pain that is worse with upright body position may indicate cerebrospinal fluid (CSF) leak (e.g., after lumbar puncture [LP] procedure) and pain that is worse with bending over or laying down may be associated with intracranial mass or sinusitis. Cold temperatures or oral intake and tooth brushing may precipitate pain from trigeminal neuralgia.
- Quality: Pain associated with cluster headaches, trigeminal neuralgia, and herpes zoster is generally described as sharp and stabbing. Migraine headaches typically cause throbbing pain. Pain described as pressure or dullness is common with tension-type headaches.
- Radiation/location: Unilateral pain is common with cluster and migraine headaches (with progression to global headache pain), trigeminal neuralgia, temporal arteritis, carotid or vertebral artery dissection, and herpes zoster. Pain from SAH, tension-type headache, or meningitis may radiate down the posterior neck. Pain that is centered around the affected eye is common in cluster headaches and acute angle-closure glaucoma. Pain from trigeminal neuralgia is typically in the distribution of one or more branches of the fifth cranial nerve.
- Severity: Abrupt onset of severe pain can indicate a potentially catastrophic intracranial process such as SAH, ICH, hemorrhage from a mass, trauma, vascular malformation, carotid or vertebral artery dissection, pituitary apoplexy, acute angle-closure glaucoma, or hypertensive emergency.

> **CLINICAL PEARL:** A change in severity from prior similar headaches for patients with a history of chronic headaches warrants further evaluation.

- Timing: A sentinel headache, heralding potentially serious aneurysmal rupture, can have an abrupt onset but may improve after 1 to 2 hours prior to SAH, and occurs 6 to 20 days prior to SAH.[2] Pain from migraine or tension-type headaches generally progress gradually over hours. Pain from cluster headaches occurs periodically throughout the day with discreet episodes of pain lasting 15 to 180 minutes. Trigeminal neuralgia may also cause episodic pain.

> **CLINICAL PEARL:** New onset of pain or lack of similar prior headaches is concerning for potentially serious underlying cause and should warrant further evaluation.

Past Medical History Specific to Complaint

Other important historical factors to consider when evaluating a patient with headache are

- Age
  - ○ Older than 50 years: Brain mass, temporal arteritis, herpes zoster
  - ○ Older than 60 years: Acute angle-closure glaucoma
- Gender
  - ○ Male: Cluster headache
  - ○ Female: Migraine, preeclampsia, idiopathic intracranial hypertension, acute angle-closure glaucoma
- Underlying disease
  - ○ Hyperlipidemia: Ischemic cerebrovascular accident (CVA)
  - ○ Hypertension: Hypertensive emergency, SAH, ICH, ischemic CVA
  - ○ Atrial fibrillation: Embolic CVA
  - ○ Diabetes mellitus: Ischemic CVA
  - ○ Connective tissue disorder (e.g., Marfan's Syndrome, Ehler–Danlos): Vertebral or carotid artery dissection, SAH/aneurysm
  - ○ HIV or other immunosuppression: Infectious process (e.g., brain abscess, meningitis, toxoplasmosis), brain malignancy, ischemic CVA
  - ○ Autosomal dominant polycystic kidney disease: SAH/aneurysm
  - ○ Malignancy: Metastatic disease to brain, central venous thrombosis (CVT)
- Family history
  - ○ First-degree relative with SAH: SAH
  - ○ Familial coagulopathy: CVT
- Comorbid conditions
  - ○ Obesity: Idiopathic intracranial hypertension
  - ○ Sedentary lifestyle: Ischemic CVA

It is important to ask about associated symptoms such as

- Nausea/vomiting: SAH, migraine, acute angle-closure glaucoma, cerebellar stroke

- Altered mental status or seizure: SAH, meningitis/encephalitis, preeclampsia, ischemic CVA, carbon monoxide poisoning
- Neck stiffness: SAH, meningitis
- Neck pain: SAH, tension headache, meningitis
- Fever: Temporal arteritis, brain abscess, meningitis/encephalitis, malignancy
- Syncope: SAH
- Underlying infection: Pneumonia or sinusitis brain abscess, meningitis
- Visual changes: Ischemic or embolic CVA, temporal arteritis, acute angle-closure glaucoma, mass
- Focal neurologic deficit: Ischemic or embolic CVA, SAH/ICH, vertebral or cranial artery dissection, migraine with aura, idiopathic intracranial hypertension, mass
- Vasomotor symptoms (rhinorrhea, lacrimation, miosis): Cluster headache
- Photophobia: SAH, migraine
- Dizziness/ataxia: Cerebellar stroke

Patients can also be predisposed to certain disease risk based on recent life events such as

- Trauma: SAH/ICH, subdural hematoma, epidural hematoma, posttraumatic headache/concussion, tension-type headache, CVT
- Surgery: CVT
- Diagnostic procedures: CSF leak/post-LP headache
- Prolonged immobility: CVT
- Recent upper respiratory infection (URI)/viral infection: Pneumonia or sinusitis brain abscess, meningitis, encephalitis
- Pregnancy: Preeclampsia, CVT
- Toxic exposure: Carbon monoxide poisoning (family members or coworkers with similar headaches)

> **CLINICAL PEARL:** Preecclampsia can develop any time after the 20-week gestational period. Although most postpartum preecclampsia cases develop within 48 hours of delivery, it may develop up to 6 weeks following childbirth.[3]

It is important to obtain a thorough social history, including

- Smoking tobacco: SAH, ischemic CVA, malignancy
- Alcohol abuse: SAH, malignancy
- Substance abuse
  - ○ Cocaine/methamphetamine: Ischemic CVA, SAH/ICH
  - ○ IV drug use: Brain abscess
- Caffeine withdrawal may precipitate headaches

Be sure to ask your patient about all medications and supplements that she or he is taking as both prescription, and over-the-counter medications and supplements can increase your patient's risk for certain disease processes:

- Oral contraceptives/estrogen supplements: Ischemic or embolic CVA, CVT
- Anticoagulants/antiplatelet therapy: SAH/ICH
- Nonsteroidal anti-inflammatory drugs (NSAIDs)/aspirin: SAH/ICH
- Medication-overuse headaches or rebound headaches can occur when patients stop the use of opioids, medications containing butalbital or caffeine, and triptans

Lastly, recent testing that a patient has had can help you to determine whether or not a specific diagnosis is more or less likely

- LP: CSF leak/post-LP headache
- Radiologic imaging: CT, MRI for purpose of monitoring known disease entities such as brain mass, aneurysm, or dissection

Physical Examination

Physical exam of a patient with headache in the ED should involve careful, efficient evaluation of the neurologic system. Although a good history will help guide your diagnostic workup, a thorough neurologic exam may help to localize a lesion or alert you to the need for rapid diagnostic imaging or procedures. Abnormalities on the neurologic exam warrant further evaluation to rule out serious disease and are the best predictor of intracranial pathology.[4]

> **CLINICAL PEARL:** It is important to remember certain diagnoses, such as CVA, SAH/ICH, or meningitis, are time sensitive and require prompt diagnostic and therapeutic measures. You should develop a succinct, yet comprehensive, head-to-toe neurologic exam that you perform on every patient to avoid missing important aspects of the exam or unnecessary delays in care.

The following physical exam findings may help to further narrow your differential diagnosis (Table 1.12).

TABLE 1.12 Physical Exam Findings in Specific Disease Conditions

Body System	Physical Exam Finding	Associated Clinical Condition
General appearance	Confusion/altered mental status/obtunded	Seizure, SAH/ICH, ischemic CVA, meningitis/encephalitis, preeclampsia, carbon monoxide poisoning
	Wasting	Malignancy, HIV
	Toxic appearance	Brain abscess, meningitis, encephalitis, toxic exposure

(continued)

TABLE 1.12 Physical Exam Findings in Specific Disease Conditions (*continued*)

Body System	Physical Exam Finding	Associated Clinical Condition
Vital signs	Hypertension	Hypertensive emergency, SAH/ICH,
	Fever	Brain abscess, meningitis, encephalitis, malignancy
	Toxic appearance	Brain abscess, meningitis, encephalitis, toxic exposure
HEENT	Abrasions, lacerations, contusions to scalp or face; periorbital bruising, nasal trauma, hemotympanum, Battle's sign, tympanic membrane rupture	Trauma/TBI
	Pupil asymmetry; unilateral fixed, dilated pupil	CVA, SAH/ICH
	Fixed, mid-dilated pupil with hazy cornea	Acute angle-closure glaucoma
	Fixed gaze	CVA, SAH/ICH, seizure
	Dysconjugate gaze	CN III, IV, VI palsy
	Papilledema	Idiopathic intracranial hypertension, hypertensive emergency
	Visual field cuts	Mass lesion, CVA, migraine
	Lacrimation, rhinorrhea, miosis, ptosis, eyelid edema, conjunctival injection	Cluster headache
	Horner's syndrome	Carotid artery dissection
	Meningeal signs (Kernig's sign, Brudzinski's sign)	SAH, meningitis
	Conductive hearing loss	Mass lesion, trauma
	Sensorineural hearing loss	CN VIII palsy, mass lesion, trauma
	Sinus tenderness (frontal or maxillary)	Sinusitis
Neurologic: Mental status	Altered mental status	Seizure, SAH/ICH, CVA, meningitis/encephalitis, preecclampsia, carbon monoxide poisoning
Neurologic: Cranial nerves	CN I: Olfactory abnormality	Trauma
	CN II: Abnormal visual acuity, visual field deficit, funduscopic abnormality	CVA, SAH/ICH, mass lesion, migraine, idiopathic intracranial hypertension, hypertensive emergency
	CN III: Abnormal pupil dilation, ptosis, lateral deviation	CVA, SAH/ICH, mass lesion, migraine, trauma

(*continued*)

TABLE **1.12** Physical Exam Findings in Specific Disease Conditions (*continued*)

Body System	Physical Exam Finding	Associated Clinical Condition
	CN IV: Diplopia, impaired inferior gaze, impaired ocular abduction	CVA, SAH, trauma
	CN V: Abnormal clenching or lateral jaw movement (motor), dysarthria; facial sensation along V1, V2, V3 branches; abnormal corneal reflex (sensory)	CVA, SAH/ICH, mass lesion, trauma, trigeminal neuralgia
	CN VI: Diplopia, impaired ocular abduction	CVA, SAH/ICH, mass lesion, trauma, temporal arteritis
	CN VII: Abnormal motor function of eyebrows, eyelids, lips/cheeks, loss of nasolabial fold; abnormal corneal reflex (motor), dysarthria	CVA, SAH/ICH, mass lesion, trauma, Bell's palsy
	CN VIII: Abnormal hearing or conduction	CVA, SAH/ICH, mass lesion, trauma
	CN IX: Vocal hoarseness, impaired swallowing or taste, impaired gag reflex	CVA, SAH/ICH, mass lesion, trauma, vertebral artery dissection
	CN X: Vocal hoarseness, dysarthria, impaired gag reflex, abnormal soft palate movement	CVA, SAH/ICH, mass lesion, trauma, vertebral artery dissection
	CN XI: Inability or weakness of shoulder shrug or turning head	Trauma
	CN XII: dysarthria, abnormal tongue movement or deviation	CVA, trauma
Neurologic: Motor, sensory, reflexes	Strength of upper and lower extremities: Asymmetric weakness or paralysis (hemiparesis or hemiparalysis)	CVA, SAH/ICH, mass lesion, trauma
	Ataxia or wide-based gait, abnormal coordination, point-to-point, rapid alternating movements or inability to walk heel-to-toe	Cerebellar lesion
	Unilateral diminished or loss of sensation	CVA

(*continued*)

TABLE 1.12 Physical Exam Findings in Specific Disease Conditions (*continued*)

Body System	Physical Exam Finding	Associated Clinical Condition
	Hyperreflexia, muscle spasticity, clonus, positive Babinski	CVA: Brainstem
	Hyporeflexia, hypotonic muscles	CVA: Cerebellum
Cardiovascular	Carotid bruit	CVA
Skin	Dermatomal, vesicular rash: CN V, branches 1-3; C2 and C3 dermatomes	Herpes zoster
	Cherry-red skin/lips	Carbon monoxide poisoning

CVA, cerebrovascular accident; CN, cranial nerve; HEENT, head, eyes, ears, nose, and throat; ICH, intracranial hemorrhage; SAH, subarachnoid hemorrhage; TBI, traumatic brain injury.

CLINICAL PEARL: Unilateral facial paralysis/droop that **involves** the forehead of the affected side is common in Bell's palsy and signifies a peripheral injury to CN VII; unilateral facial paralysis droop that **spares** the forehead is common in central injury to CN VII as in CVA. (Stroke spares the forehead.)

CLINICAL PEARL: Always ambulate your patient prior to discharge; patients with no history of ambulatory dysfunction with the inability to walk normally require further evaluation (e.g., MRI or neurology consultation).

SCORING SCALES

- NIH Stroke Scale (www.mdcalc.com/nih-stroke-scale-score-nihss) may help determine stroke severity and predict outcomes. Although it is helpful to familiarize yourself with this assessment tool, it is generally most useful in conjunction with neurology consultation.
- Glasgow Coma Scale (GCS; www.mdcalc.com/glasgow-coma-scale-score-gcs) can be used to objectively define a patient's level of consciousness and responsiveness following trauma.

Diagnostic Plan

LP and CT/computed tomography angiography (CTA) are the predominant testing modalities in the emergent evaluation of headache. MRI and magnetic resonance angiography (MRA) may also have a role in the evaluation of headache; however, immediate availability and length of study time may limit their use in the ED setting. Laboratory studies, particularly blood glucose levels in the setting of stroke-like symptoms, may also aid in the diagnostic evaluation process.

LABS

- Blood glucose: Both hyper- and hypoglycemia can cause stroke-like symptoms
- CBC:
  - ↑WBC: CNS infection
  - ↓Platelets: Increased risk of bleeding → SAH/ICH
- Coagulation studies: May be altered for patients on anticoagulation therapy, increasing risk of bleeding → SAH/ICH
  - Prothrombin time (PT)/international normalized ratio (INR): ↑ with warfarin therapy
  - Activated partial thromboplastin time (aPTT): ↑ with unfractionated heparin therapy
  - Thrombin time (TT): ↑ with unfractionated heparin, low-molecular-weight heparin, direct thrombin inhibitors
- Carboxyhemoglobin: Elevated in cases of carbon monoxide toxicity; may obtain via arterial blood gas or venous sample. Carboxyhemoglobin ranges
  - Nonsmokers: 0% to 3%
  - Smokers: 10% to 15%
  - Carbon monoxide poisoning: >15%
- ESR: Will be markedly elevated (≥50 mm/hr) in temporal arteritis
- D-dimer: May be elevated in CVT (normal level **does not exclude** CVT)
- Severe preecclampsia lab abnormalities
  - ↓Platelets (<100,000/µL)
  - ↑Creatinine (>1.1 mg/dL)
  - ↑ Aspartate aminotransferase (AST)/alanine aminotransferase (ALT; 2x normal rate)
  - Proteinuria: 3+ on a urine dipstick or >5 g/24 hr
- Typical CSF findings in meningitis are discussed in Table 1.13.

TABLE 1.13 Cerebrospinal Fluid Findings in Meningitis

Test	Bacterial	Viral	Fungal
Opening pressure	Elevated	Normal	Elevated (*Crypotococcal*); variable
Gram stain	Positive	Negative	Negative
WBC count	1,000–5,000 cells/L	<250 cells/L	20–200 cells/L
WBC differential	>80% neutrophils	Predominantly lymphocytes	Predominantly lymphocytes, monocytes, or eosinophils
Protein	>200 mg/dL	Elevated up to 150 mg/dL	Elevated up to 250 mg/dL
Glucose	<40 mg/dL	Normal	Low

WBC, white blood cell.

DIAGNOSTIC IMAGING STUDIES

Diagnostic imaging studies for patients with headache are discussed in Table 1.14.

TABLE 1.14 Imaging Modalities of Choice for Specific Disease Processes

Imaging Modality	Imagining Modality With Specific Diagnosis
CT without IV contrast	CVA[a] (Figure 1.9) SAH ICH (Figure 1.10) Hypertensive emergency with severe headache or neurologic abnormality Traumatic injury/intracranial trauma[b] Subdural hematoma (Figure 1.11) Epidural hematoma (Figure 1.12)
CT with IV contrast	Brain abscess (can further delineate with MRI with contrast)
CTA	Carotid or vertebral artery dissection (can further delineate with MRA)
MRI	Suspected mass lesion Malignancy Pituitary apoplexy CVA[c]
MRV	CVT

[a]Timely evaluation and imaging of suspected ischemic or embolic CVA is essential as emergent neurology consultation and possible tissue plasminogen activator (tPA) administration are time sensitive.
[b]Canadian CT Head Injury/Trauma Rule (CCHR), New Orleans/Charity Head Trauma/Injury Rule (NOC), and Nexus II scoring systems can be used to determine the need for CT imaging in the setting of head trauma.
[c]Can also be used in cases of CVA or trauma to further delineate areas of injury, but length of time of study and immediate availability generally limit use in ED settings.
CTA, computed tomography angiography; CVA, cerebrovascular accident; CVT, central venous thrombosis; ICH, intracranial hemorrhage; IV, intravenous; MRA, magnetic resonance angiography; MRV, magnetic resonance venography; SAH, subarachnoid hemorrhage.

CLINICAL PEARL: All patients with history or physical exam suspicious for SAH/ICH should undergo LP if CT of head is negative.[5,6] CTA may be considered in lieu of LP.

CLINICAL PEARL: It is important to consider CVT in your differential diagnosis, particularly in younger, female patients who are pregnant, in the puerperium period, or are taking oral contraceptives. Head CT is often normal in patients with CVT.

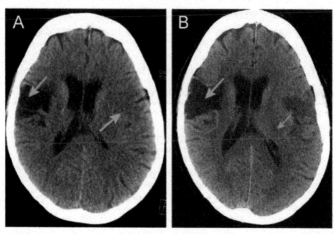

FIGURE **1.9** CT demonstrating: (A) hypodensity from ischemic CVA in the right frontal (downward-pointing arrow) and left temporal (upward-pointingarrow) lobes (B) ischemic CVA in the right frontoparietal (downward-pointing arrow arrow) and left frontoparietal (upward-pointing arrow) CVA, cerebrovascular accident cortices.

Source: 0475ramosk. Wikimedia Commons. https://commons.wikimedia.org/wiki/File:1-s2.0-S0967586810002766-gr2.jpg. Published March 27, 2017.

- LP is the diagnostic test of choice in patients with meningitis, encephalitis, and in whom suspicion is high for SAH/ICH with negative CT results.

> **CLINICAL PEARL:** Empiric antibiotic therapy should be started in any patient with suspected bacterial meningitis and **should not be delayed** in order to obtain LP or imaging studies.[7]

  - Patients at risk for herniation secondary to mass lesions or increased intracranial pressure (ICP) should be screened with CT based on the following risk factors:[8–10]
    - Immunocompromised state (e.g., HIV, immunosuppressive therapy, organ or stem cell transplant)
    - History of prior CNS mass, lesion, stroke, or focal CNS infection
    - New-onset seizure within 1 week of presentation
    - Papilledema
    - Altered mental status
    - Focal neurologic deficit
  - Useful for diagnostic and therapeutic purposes in patients with idiopathic intracranial hypertension

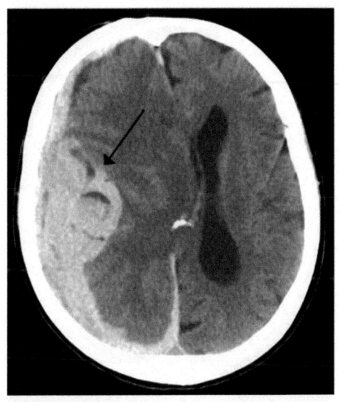

Figure 1.10   Intracranial hemorrhage with significant midline shift.
Source: Heilman JH. Wikimedia Commons. https://commons.wikimedia.org/wiki/File:
Intracranial_bleed_with_significant_midline_shift.png. Published August 29, 2011.

> **CLINICAL PEARL:** MRI/magnetic resonance venography (MRV) should be done **prior to LP** in patients with suspected idiopathic intracranial hypertension to rule out other causes of increased ICP.

- EKG: An EKG should be obtained in all patients suspected of stroke to rule out atrial fibrillation as a potential cause of embolism
- Other helpful tools
  - Tonometer: Normal intraocular pressure is 10 to 20 mmHg and may be elevated in acute angle-closure glaucoma.
  - Slit lamp: A shallow anterior chamber and cloudy cornea can be visualized in acute angle-closure glaucoma.

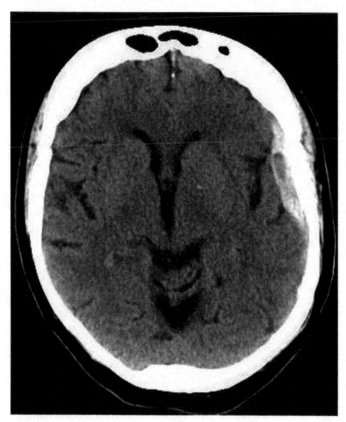

Figure 1.11   Subdural hematoma on CT.
Source: Monfils L. Wikimedia Commons. https://commons.wikimedia.org/wiki/File:Ct-scan_of_the_brain_with_an_subdural_hematoma.jpg. Published July 22, 2008.

Initial Management

The care of most patients, particularly those who are critically ill, begins with delivering oxygen, obtaining IV access, and use of continuous cardiac/hemodynamic monitoring. Immediate intervention for hemodynamic instability, airway compromise, treatment of life-threatening arrhythmias, or other general decompensation takes precedence over any other diagnostic or therapeutic intervention. Certain disease processes may require immediate activation of and collaboration with other medical team members such as neurology, neurosurgery, or OB/GYN.

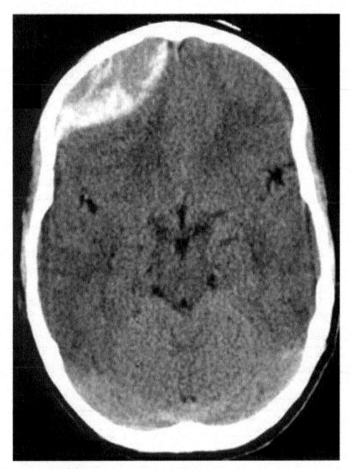

FIGURE 1.12   **Epidural hematoma on CT.**
Source: Jpogi. Wikimedia Commons. https://commons.wikimedia.org/wiki/File:
Traumatic_acute_epidual_hematoma.jpg. Published July 20, 2012.

- CVA
  - Acute ischemic stroke should be managed in conjunction with immediate neurologic consultation in the ED.
  - Once neuroimaging is obtained and hemorrhagic stroke has been ruled out, patients presenting within **3** to **4.5 hours** of symptom onset should receive IV alteplase (tPA) if inclusion/exclusion criteria (Tables 1.15 and 1.16; www.mdcalc.com/tpa-contraindications-ischemic-stroke) are met.

○ Further management is discussed in Chapter 2, Common Disease Entities in Emergency Medicine, "Headache" section.

CLINICAL PEARL: Ischemic CVA is a time-sensitive diagnosis requiring rapid, coordinated evaluation and diagnostic efforts of EMS, ED staff, neurology consultation, and radiology. The goal is to arrive at a treatment decision within 60 minutes of the patient's arrival to the ED.[11]

○ Acute hemorrhagic stroke (SAH/ICH) is also a time-sensitive diagnosis requiring prompt diagnosis and management. Initial management includes
  ▪ Prompt neurosurgical consultation/intervention (e.g., clipping or coiling of aneurysm, evacuation of clots, ventriculostomy placement)
  ▪ Control of hyperglycemia, fever, blood pressure, and reversal of anticoagulation therapy/bleeding diathesis when necessary
  ▪ Further management is discussed in Chapter 2, Common Disease Entitiesin Emergency Medicine, "Headache" section

TABLE 1.15 Inclusion and Exclusion Criteria for Administration of Tissue Plasminogen Activator Within 3 Hours of Symptom Onset

Inclusion Criteria
Diagnosis of ischemic stroke causing measurable neurologic deficit
Onset of symptoms <3 hours prior to administration of treatment
Age ≥18 years

Exclusion Criteria
Significant head trauma within 3 months
Prior stroke within 3 months
Symptoms suggestive of SAH
Arterial puncture at noncompressible site in previous 7 days (e.g., subclavian artery)
History of previous ICH, known intracranial neoplasm, arteriovenous malformation, or aneurysm
Hypertension: Systolic >185 mmHg, diastolic > 110 mmHg[a]
Active internal bleeding
Bleeding diathesis
• Platelet count <100,000/μL
• Heparin therapy within 48 hourswith elevated aPTT
• Anticoagulant therapy with INR >1.7 or PT >15 seconds
• Direct thrombin inhibitor or factor Xa inhibitor therapy with abnormal aPTT, INR, platelet count, or ECT
Blood glucose <50 mg/dL
CT with large or multilobular infarct (hypodensity involving >1/3 of the cerebral hemisphere)

(continued)

TABLE 1.15 Inclusion and Exclusion Criteria for Administration of Tissue Plasminogen Activator Within 3 Hours of Symptom Onset (*continued*)

Relative Exclusion Criteria
Minor or rapidly improving stroke symptoms
Pregnancy
Seizure at onset of symptoms with residual postictal neurologic impairment
Major surgery or trauma within 14 days
Gastrointestinal or urinary tract hemorrhage within 21 days
MI within 3 months

[a] Patients who meet criteria except for blood pressure >185/110 mmHg may receive labetalol or nicardipine (may also consider other agents, e.g., hydralazine, enaliprilat) with continuous blood pressure monitoring.

aPTT, activated partial thromboplastin time; ECT, ecarin clotting time; ICH, intracranial hemorrhage; INR, international normalized ratio; MI, myocardial infarction; PT, prothrombin time; SAH, subarachnoid hemorrhage.
Source: Jauch EC, Saver JL, Adams HP. Guidelines for the early management of patients with acute ischemic stroke: a guideline for healthcare professionals from the American Heart Association/American Stroke Association. *Stroke*. 2013;44(3):870–947. doi:10.1161/STR.0b013e318284056a

TABLE 1.16 Inclusion and Exclusion Criteria for Administration of Tissue Plasminogen Activator Within 3 to 4.5 Hours of Symptom Onset

Inclusion Criteria
Diagnosis of ischemic stroke causing measurable neurologic deficit
Onset of symptoms <4.5 hours prior to administration of treatment

Exclusion Criteria
Age >80 years
Severe stroke (NIHSS score >25)
Oral anticoagulation therapy regardless of INR
History of diabetes **and** prior ischemic stroke

INR, international normalized ratio; NIHSS, National Institutes of Health Stroke Score

Source: del Zoppo GH, Saver FJ, Jauch EC, Adams HP, Jr. Expansion of the time window for treatment of acute ischemic stroke with intravenous tissue plasminogen activator: a science advisory from the American Heart Association/American Stroke Association. *Stroke*. 2009;40(8):2945–2948. doi:10.1161/STROKEAHA.109.192535

- CNS infection
  - ○ Bacterial meningitis: Empiric antibiotic therapy should be started immediately after CSF is obtained or prior to obtaining CSF if suspicion is high and LP is delayed.
  - ○ Further management of meningitis is discussed in Chapter 2, Common Disease Entitiesin Emergency Medicine, "Headache" section.
  - ○ Viral encephalitis
    - ▪ Clinical features and diagnostic workup of viral meningitis, but patients present with altered mental status, seizure, or focal neurologic deficit
      - Empiric treatment against herpes simplex virus (HSV) with IV acyclovir (10 mg/kg q8h); otherwise treat causative agent

○ Brain abscess
  ▪ Empiric antibiotic therapy with neurosurgical intervention +/- IV dexamethasone in cases with mass effect on imaging
● Traumatic brain injury management is discussed in Chapter 2, Common Disease Entities in Emergency Medicine, "Headache" section
● Sinusitis
  ○ Uncomplicated acute viral sinusitis should improve or resolve within 10 days and **does not** require antibiotic therapy.
  ○ Uncomplicated acute bacterial sinusitis may also be treated with observation for 7 to 10 days; patients who are immunocompromised or have worsening symptoms after 10 days may be treated with empiric antibiotics.
    ▪ Amoxicillin–clavulanate (500 mg/125 mg q8h or 875 mg/125 mg q12h) is the treatment of choice.
    ▪ Doxycycline (100 q12h or 200 mg daily), or a third-generation cephalosporin (cefixime 400 mg daily or cefpodoxime 200 mg q12h) plus clindamycin (150–300 g q6h) are alterative regimens.
    ▪ Levaquin (500 mg daily) and moxifloxcin (400 mg daily) should be reserved for patients with no other treatment options.
    ▪ All patients may benefit from symptomatic treatments such as analgesics, decongestants, mucolytics, intranasal steroid sprays, and nasal saline irrigation.
  ○ Complicated acute bacterial sinusitis (e.g., periorbital edema/erythema, vision changes or cranial nerve palsies, altered mental status or meningeal signs) should be evaluated with neuroimaging and immediate otolaryngology consultation
● Herpes zoster
  ○ Uncomplicated herpes zoster in immunocompetent patients may be treated within 72 hours with
    ▪ Valacyclovir (1,000 mg q8h), famciclovir (500 mg q8h), acyclovir (800 mg five times per day)
    ▪ Patients may be treated if presenting >72 hours if new lesions are continuing to appear
    ▪ Treat mild to moderate pain with NSAIDs or acetaminophen; more severe pain may require opioid analgesics

> **CLINICAL PEARL:** Always check patients with herpes zoster affecting the dermatome of the fifth cranial nerve for signs and symptoms of herpes zoster ophthalmicus (HZO). These include conjunctival injection or other signs and symptoms of conjunctivitis, vesicular lesions at the tip of the nose (Hutchinson's sign), and dendritic lesions on fluorescein staining. HZO requires topical steroid drops and consultation with ophthalmology.

Initial management of other less common disease entities causing secondary headache varies widely and may involve consultation with numerous subspecialties (Table 1.17).

TABLE 1.17 Initial Management of Causes of Secondary Headache

Disease	Initial Management	Consultation[a]
Venous sinus thrombosis	Anticoagulation with heparin or LMWH Endovascular thrombolysis or thrombectomy for worsening neurologic status despite anticoagulation	Neurology, interventional radiology
Pituitary apoplexy	Maintain blood pressure with IV fluids and high-dose IV hydrocortisone	Neurosurgery
Acute angle-closure glaucoma	Topical beta-blocker (0.5% timolol), topical alpha-2 agonist (1% apraclonidine), topical pilocarpine (1%–2% pilocarpine)[12] IV acetazolamide (500 mg IV or PO), IV mannitol (1–2 g/kg IV)	Ophthalmology
Hypertensive emergency	Blood pressure control if ≥185/110 mmHg for tPA candidates or if ≥220/120 mmHg in all other patients Lower blood pressure by 10%–20% during first hour in hypertensive encephalopathy Labetalol (10–20 mg IV over 2 min) and nicardipine (5 mg IV over 1 hr) are first-line agents Other agents to consider are clevidipine, nitroprusside, nitroglycerin, fenoldopam, hydralazine, enalaprilat	Consider cardiology consult
Preeclampsia	Term pregnancy (≥37 weeks' gestation): labor induction/delivery Preterm pregnancy: conservative management with monitoring, bed rest, and medical treatment of complications Treat severe hypertension (≥150–160/100–110 mmHg) with labetalol (20 mg IV over 2 min) or hydralazine (5 mg IV over 1–2 min) Postpartum: treat hypertension Seizure prophylaxis with magnesium sulfate (4–6 g over 15–20 min loading dose)	Obstetrics
Carotid/vertebral artery dissection	Thrombolysis (with tPA if within 3–4.5 hr) or endovascular means followed by antithrombotic treatment with either antiplatelet or anticoagulant therapy	Neurology, neurosurgery, vascular surgery
Malignancy	Dependent on disease type (e.g., primary vs. metastatic disease) Steroids and analgesics	Neurosurgery

(continued)

Table 1.17 Initial Management of Causes of Secondary Headache (*continued*)

Disease	Initial Management	Consultation[a]
Temporal arteritis	High-dose steroids: methylprednisolone (1,000 mg daily IV) if vision loss present at diagnosis; prednisone (40–60 mg daily for 2–4 wk followed by taper) if no visual change **Treat as soon as diagnosis is suspected,** do not wait for temporal artery biopsy results to initiate treatment	Rheumatology, ophthalmology
Carbon monoxide poisoning	High-flow oxygen via facemask Hyperbaric oxygen fo carboxyhemoglobin >25% (>20% in pregnant patients), altered mental status or loss of consciousness, metabolic acidosis (pH <7.1), end-organ ischemia (e.g., chest pain, EKG changes)[13]	Poison control/toxicology
Idiopathic intracranial hypertension	Acetazolamide (250–500 mg twice daily) +/- furosemide (20–40 mg daily) Therapeutic LPs no longer recommended for most patients	Neurology

[a] Most consultations will take place immediately upon diagnosis or suspected diagnosis; however, some consultations may be made on a nonurgent basis.

IV, intravenous; LMWH, low-molecular-weight heparin; LP, lumbar puncture; PO, by mouth; tPA, tissue plasminogen activator.

The vast majority of headache patients will fall into the category of benign, primary headache etiologies. Close follow-up with primary care providers and neurology can help prevent ED visits for chronic or recurrent primary headaches; however, severe attacks and breakthrough pain episodes may occur. The most common benign causes of headache and their initial treatment include

- Migraine headache
  - Most patients presenting to the ED with migraine headache will have moderate to severe pain that is unrelieved with the typical medications used for treatment. New-onset migraine headaches require careful evaluation and neurologic follow-up to rule out other disease processes.
  - Management of migraine headache is discussed in further detail in Chapter 2, Common Disease Entities in Emergency Medicine, "Headache" section.
- Cluster headache
  - Initial treatment for severe attacks includes sumatriptan (6 mg subcutaneous injection) and high-flow oxygen (100% via nonrebreather mask at 12–15 L/min) for at least 15 minutes.
  - May consider intranasal lidocaine (1 mL of 4%–10% solution to ipsilateral pain side).

- Tension-type headache
  - ○ The majority of tension-type headaches may be treated with over-the-counter analgesics such as acetaminophen, ibuprofen, aspirin, naproxen, or caffeine-containing combination medications.
- Trigeminal neuralgia is commonly treated with the following medications
  - ○ Carbamazepine (100 mg PO twice daily), oxcarbazepine (300 mg PO twice daily), baclofen (5 mg PO q8h), lamotrigine (400 mg daily)
  - ○ Patients with new-onset trigeminal neuralgia should be started on carbamazepine and referred to neurology for follow-up
  - ○ May consider phenytoin or fosphenytoin (250–1,000 mg IV given at ≤50 mg/min) or lidocaine (100–300-mg IV infusion given over 30 minutes) with continuous cardiac monitoring[14,15]

Key Points . . .

- The most common headache entities will generally have normal neurologic exams, laboratory studies, and imaging tests. You must rely heavily on history and physical exam to determine which patients require further evaluation.
- Keep "red flag" historical features in mind as these may elucidate a potentially dangerous, secondary headache with a need for immediate imaging, diagnostic procedure, or subspecialty consultation.
- Although many causes of secondary headache are rare, it is important to keep life-threatening disease processes in your differential diagnosis while evaluating your patient in the ED.
- Sudden onset of severe headache is a concerning historical feature of headache.
- Early detection and timely evaluation of dangerous diagnoses are essential to initiate life-saving treatments.
- Delay in diagnostic imaging, procedures (head CT or LP), and the initiation of life-saving therapeutics (tPA, IV antibiotics) must be avoided.
- ED evaluation for initial presentations and acute exacerbations of chronic or recurrent headache entities is common. Ensuring proper follow-up and long-term medical management is an essential part of managing these disease processes.
- Detailed discharge instructions and return-to-ED criteria for concerning signs or symptoms should be given to all headache patients who are being discharged from the ED.

References

1. Rui P, Kang K. National hospital ambulatory medical care survey: 2014 emergency department summary tables. https://www.cdc.gov/nchs/data/nhamcs/web_tables/2014_ed_web_tables.pdf. Updated September 7, 2017.
2. Singer RJ, Ogilvy CS, Rordorf G. Aneurysmal subarachnoid hemorrhage: Clinical manifestations and diagnosis. In: Biller J, Edlow JA, eds. *UpToDate*. https://www.uptodate.com/contents/aneurysmal-subarachnoid-hemorrhage-clinical-manifestations-and-diagnosis. Updated July 26, 2019.
3. Mayo Clinic Staff. Postpartum preeclampsia. https://www.mayoclinic.org/diseases-conditions/postpartum-preeclampsia/symptoms-causes/syc-20376646. Updated May 3, 2018.
4. Cutrer FM, Wippold FJ, 2nd, Edlow JA. Evaluation of the adult with non-traumatic headache in the emergency department. In Hockberger RS, Swanson JW, eds. *UpToDate*. https://www.uptodate.com/contents/evaluation-of-the-adult-with-nontraumatic-headache-in-the-emergency-department. Updated June 19, 2019.
5. Vermeulen M, van Gijn J. The diagnosis of subarachnoid haemorrhage. *J Neurol Neurosurg Psychiatry*. 1990;53(5):365–372. doi:10.1136/jnnp.53.5.365
6. Connolly ES Jr, Rabinstein AA, Carhuapoma JR., et al. *Stroke*. Guidelines for the Management of Aneurysmal Subarachnoid Hemorrhage: A Guideline for Healthcare Professionals From the American Heart Association/American Stroke Association 2012;43(6):1711–1737. doi:10.1161/STR.0b013e3182587839
7. Bhimraj A. Acute community-acquired bacterial meningitis in adults: an evidence-based review. *Cleve Clin J Med*. 2012;79(6):393–400. https://www.mdedge.com/ccjm/article/95751/infectious-diseases/acute-community-acquired-bacterial-meningitis-adults-evidence
8. Hasbun R, Abrahams J, Jekel J, Quagliarello VJ. Computed tomography of the head before lumbar puncture in adults with suspected meningitis. *N Engl J Med*. 2001;345(24):1727–1733. doi:10.1056/NEJMoa010399
9. Gopal AK, Whitehouse JD, Simel DL, Corey R. Cranial computed tomography before lumbar puncture: a prospective clinical evaluation. *Arch Intern Med*. 1999;159(22):2681–2686. doi:10.1001/archinte.159.22.2681
10. Tunkel AR, Hartman BJ, Kaplan SL, et al. Practice guidelines for the management of bacterial meningitis. *Clin Infect Dis*. 2004;39(9):1267–1284. doi:10.1086/425368
11. Adams HP, Jr, del Zoppo G, Alberts MJ, et al. Guidelines for the early management of adults with ischemic stroke. *Stroke*. 2007;38(4):1655–1711. doi:10.1161/STROKEAHA.107.181486
12. Walker RA, Adhikari S. Eye emergencies. In: Tintinalli JE, Stapczynski J, Ma O, et al., eds. *Tintinalli's Emergency Medicine: A Comprehensive Study Guide*. 8th ed. New York, NY: McGraw-Hill; 2016:1543ñ1578.
13. Clardy PF, Manaker S, Perry H. Carbon monoxide poisoning. In: Traub SJ, Burns MM, eds. *UpToDate*. https://www.uptodate.com/contents/carbon-monoxide-poisoning. Updated June 6, 2018.
14. McCleane GJ. Intravenous infusion of phenytoin relieves neuropathic pain: a randomized, double-blinded, placebo-controlled, crossover study. *Anesth Analg*. 1999;89(4):985–988. doi:10.1097/00000539-199910000-00030

15. Scrivani SJ, Chaudry A, Maciewicz RJ, Keith DA. Chronic neurogenic facial pain: lack of response to intravenous phentolamine. *J Orafac Pain.* 1999;13(2):89–96. Retrieved from http://www.quintpub.com/journals/ofph/abstract.php?article_id=7268#.XVmMGGGR7nct

Low-Back Pain

Low-back pain (LBP) alone accounts for approximately 3% of all ED visits in the United States.[1] Back pain is the most common musculoskeletal chief complaint and the second most common symptom-related complaint for the primary care provider.[1] Similar to other common EM presentations, the etiology of back pain is typically benign. The key to establishing an accurate diagnosis is doing a thorough yet focused history and physical exam. Many causes of back pain are benign; however, you must be aware of signs and symptoms suggestive of a more serious etiology. Oftentimes, benign etiologies, such as musculoskeletal injury or renal colic, can mimic those that are much more serious, such as a dissecting aortic aneurysm or cauda equina syndrome. Oftentimes, the presence of one key individual finding doesn't correspond to a specific pathology, which is why a complete history and physical exam are crucial.[1]

Differential Diagnosis

The majority of acute back pain is mechanical in origin and includes etiologies such as strains, degenerative changes, discogenic pain, and trauma. In EM, it is prudent to initially entertain a broad differential diagnosis, including

- Acute aortic syndromes-aneurysm dissection/rupture
- Cauda equina syndrome
- Lumbar radiculopathy
- Lower back sprain or strain
- Osteomyelitis
- Epidural abscess
- Malignancy
- Spondyloarthropathies

The differential diagnosis of LBP can be further narrowed based on OPQRST.

O: Onset

- Sudden onset is common with renal colic or muscle spasm. Ask what the patient was doing when the pain started. Back pain secondary to musculoskeletal origin may have occurred with heavy lifting, or immediately following a sneezing or coughing episode. Pain from degenerative disc disease or lumbar strain may be unilateral and radiate down the back through the buttocks and into the posterior thigh. Patients may also report that bed rest alleviates the pain of degenerative joint disease (DJD)/lumbar strain.

- Gradual onset over several days: Consider cauda equina syndrome or muscle spasm.
- Gradual onset over several weeks should prompt consideration of
  - Spinal infection (tuberculosis [TB])
  - Herniated disc/facet
  - AAA
  - Neoplasm
  - Spinal/epidural abscess/hematoma

P: PALLIATIVE/PROVOCATING FACTORS
- Heavy lifting precipitates pain: Herniated disc/herniated facet
- Sneezing/coughing with sudden onset: Muscle spasm
- Pain after lifting/twisting: Increased with degenerative disc disease/lumbar strain

Q: QUALITY
- Burning pain/nerve pain: Herniated disc/herniated facet or sciatica
- Sharp, stabbing pain: Renal colic
- Tearing pain: AAA

R: RADIATION
- Pain that radiates from the back to the lower extremities is suggestive of radiculopathy from a herniated disc. Cauda equina syndrome should also be excluded as this is a medical emergency.

S: SEVERITY
- Ask the patient to rate the pain on a scale of 1 to 10. Severe pain may be suggestive of a more significant underlying pathology.

T: TIMING
- Inquire whether the pain is constant or whether it comes and goes. Timing of pain can be delineated along with onset, as described earlier, particularly in terms of what provokes the pain.

Associated symptoms to inquire about include:

- Paresthesias or incontinence to bowel or bladder: This may indicate spinal cord compression secondary to cancer, trauma, or cauda equina syndrome.
- Fever or chills can be present with epidural abscess.

Past Medical History Specific to the Complaint
- Ask about a patient's occupation. Some patients with laborious occupations, such as landscaping, construction, or factory work, may develop back pain due to the demands of their job.
- IV drug use is a risk factor for spinal canal infections, and back pain may be the sole presenting complaint.
- TB can manifest in the spine, and is referred to as *Pott's disease*. Inquire about a personal and family history of TB.

- History of osteoporosis may indicate compression fracture of a vertebral body.
- Inquire about medications and a history of familial blood disorders. The use of anticoagulants or a history of a bleeding disorder can be a risk factor for a spinal or epidural hematoma. Steroid use can also predispose patients to vertebral body fractures.[1]
- Onset of pain after recent chiropractic interventions, manipulations, and acupuncture may indicate a complication of the intervention.
- Any history of Crohn's colitis, inflammatory diseases, or autoimmune conditions should be documented as these patients may be at risk for joint arthritis, spondylolisthesis, or ankylosing spondylitis.

Physical Examination

A focused physical examination, led by a thorough history, can help determine the etiology of back pain. Physical examination findings with their associated clinical conditions are outlined in Table 1.18.

TABLE 1.18 Correlating Physical Exam Findings With Pathologic Conditions

Body System	Physical Exam Finding	Associated Clinical Condition
General/vitals	Fever (+/- tachycardia/hypotension)	Spinal abscess/epidural abscess, pyelonephritis
	BP in the lower extremities is lower compared to the upper extremities (findings of discrepancy)	Aortic dissection, coarctation of aorta
	<40 years old + back pain	Infection, primary tumor, spondylolisthesis; ankylosing spondylitis
	>40 years old + back pain	Dissecting aortic aneurysm, metastatic spine mass
	Geriatric population + back pain	Vertebral body compression fracture
Peripheral vascular	Absent or diminished DP and PT pulses, cold lower extremity	Vascular compromise or arterial occlusion
Musculoskeletal	(+)SLR	Herniated disc (ipsilateral side)/facet disease
	(+)CSLR[a]	Herniated disc (contralateral side)/facet disease
	Multijoint arthritis	Autoimmune condition such as ankylosing spondylitis or Crohn's colitis/ulcerative colitis

(continued)

TABLE 1.18 Correlating Physical Exam Findings With Pathologic Conditions (*continued*)

Body System	Physical Exam Finding	Associated Clinical Condition
Back/spine	Palpation of the back/spine leading to tenderness	Paralumbar muscle spasm, herniated disc, radiculopathy, psoas abscess, degenerative disc disease
	(+)tenderness to the sacroiliac joints	Ankylosing spondylitis
	(+)tenderness to palpation to the midgluteal region	Sciatica
	(+)CVA tenderness	Pyelonephritis
	Limited range of motion of the spine	Herniated discs/facets may have difficulty with flexion of the spine (ask patient to touch his or her toes)
Neurological	Saddle anesthesia (perineal sensory deficit) and/or decreased rectal tone	Spinal cord compression/cauda equina syndrome
	Loss of sensation unilaterally down one leg following the S1 nerve root pattern	Herniated disc/facet conditions
	DTRs	Spinal infections or tumors due to compression of the spinal canal; also consider the same in patients with acute trauma to the back or a history of cancer; disc rupture with significant canal stenosis

^aThis is a physical exam maneuver during which the provider passively lifts the patient's leg on the ipsilateral side of pain to 45° and then dorsiflexes the foot, eliciting pain on the ipsilateral side of the back. That is considered a (+)SLR. Doing so with the contralateral leg, inducing pain on the affected side, is known as a *CSLR*.

BP, blood pressure; CSLR, crossed straight leg raise; DTR, deep tendon reflexes; DP, dorsalis pedis; PT, posterior tibialis; SLR, straight leg raise.

Diagnostic Plan

Some of the more common nonemergent etiologies of LBP include Disc disease, facet syndrome, thoracic or lumbar strains, and thoracic or lumbar sprains from acute injury

These are primarily diagnosed based on presentation and do not often require imaging or further diagnostics. An MRI is generally warranted in the presence of any "red flags" discussed earlier. Other diagnostic testing to consider include:

LABS
- CBC with differential
  - WBCs may be elevated in spinal infection, TB, intravenous drug use (IVDU) with spinal infection, meningitis secondary to non-TB pathogen

- ○ Hemoglobin and hematocrit (HGB/HCT) may be decreased in dissecting AAA requiring packed red blood cell (PRBC) infusion intraoperatively, spinal hematoma
- ESR/CRP may be elevated in inflammatory conditions leading to arthritis/inflammation of the joints such as Crohn's colitis, ulcerative colitis, ankylosing spondylitis; use in conjunction with physical examination to consider the presence of discitis or abscess, which can influence imaging choice
- BMP: Elevated BUN/creatinine with renal compromise may occur in the presence of an obstructing stone or advanced pyelonephritis
- Urinalysis
  - ○ Pyuria in infected renal colic, pyelonephritis
  - ○ Hematuria in renal colic or dissecting AAA
  - ○ Urine drug screen for IVDU to note use of illicit agents

DIAGNOSTIC IMAGING

- EKG: ST elevation/changes are indicative of acute MI
- CT scan abdomen/pelvis without contrast: Best imaging for renal colic
- CT scan abdomen/pelvis with contrast (CT angiogram) to confirm AAA
- CT/MRI with contrast: To confirm spinal/epidural hematoma/abscess or compression syndrome
- X-ray of the thoracic/lumbar to view vertebral body compression fracture, evidence of "step off" indicating vertebral malalignment, and x-ray are also part of the comprehensive approach for patients who suffer work-related injury, and may be a mandate for some workman's compensation situations.
- Ultrasound: The use of ultrasound is becoming more commonplace in the ED setting due to the rapidity of test results and the ability to perform the test at the bedside. This is particularly helpful for unstable patients, such as those with suspected AAA.

Initial Management

- If a patient presents with acute LBP, take caution in moving the patient. If he or she arrives on a backboard in cervical spine immobilization, only move the patient by means of a logroll with the assistance of other members of the ED team. In the trauma setting, cervical spine immobilization should be maintained until clinically/radiologically cleared by a provider. After the logroll, in-line positioning should be maintained while doing the physical exam.
- For lumbar strain and degenerative disc disease, treatment is aimed at managing symptoms. This includes administering NSAIDs or acetaminophen. Patients should maintain activities of daily living as tolerated, and physical therapy should be initiated.
- Epidural compression syndrome is a true medical emergency in which patients may present with the red flags mentioned earlier. If this

diagnosis is likely, the first-line treatment is immediate steroid therapy with dexamethasone 10 to 100 mg IV while awaiting imaging confirmation and in conjunction with consultation with a neurosurgeon.

- Other treatment options are initiated based on the ultimate diagnosis. Management of specific etiologies of LBP is discussed in detail in Chapter 2, Common Disease Entities in Emergency Medicine.

Key Points . . .

- As with other chief complaints, always take a thorough history. Mechanical LBP is made worse with movement. Back pain due to organic etiologies, such as renal colic or AAA, generally does not change or improve with position.
- Have a strong suspicion for "the worst-case scenario" in elderly patients with LBP, particularly for AAA in the setting of cardiovascular morbidity and mortality risk.
- Perform a thorough lower extremity examination. Always have patients remove clothes, change into a gown, and remove socks and shoes.
- In the setting of compromised immune status, IVDU, or untreated TB, maintain a high index of suspicion for spinal abscess/epidural abscess or Pott's disease.
- If possible, observe your patient as he or she ambulates. Assess his or her gait to help determine the severity of back pain.
- Always ask how your patients arrived to the ED. If they drove themselves, giving them opioids or muscle relaxants is not appropriate unless they can get a ride home.

REFERENCE

1. Waterman BR, Belmont PJ, Schoenfeld AJ, Jr. Low back pain in the United States: incidence and risk factors for presentation in the emergency setting. *Spine J.* 2012;12:63. doi:10.1016/j.spinee.2011.09.002

TRAUMATIC INJURY

Trauma and injury-related complaints are the 10th most common reason patients in the United States present to the ED, accounting for approximately 2.6 million visits per year.[1] Some of the most common injuries seen in the ED include

- Fractures, dislocations, sprains, strains, head and facial injuries, burns, and soft-tissue injuries, including abrasions, lacerations, contusions, and bite wounds.

- You may also encounter trauma from gunshot or stab wounds, electrical injuries, or environmental injuries such as frostbite.

The majority of these injuries will occur in the setting of sports or leisure activities, motor vehicle collisions (MVCs), falls, and workplace or domestic accidents; however, violent crime, sexual assault, and domestic abuse injuries are also commonly evaluated in the ED setting. Careful examination looking for less obvious injuries is essential in the assessment of all patients, even in the setting of minor trauma. Developing a systematic approach to the evaluation of patients with specific injury-related complaints will help you avoid common pitfalls and missed diagnoses. The differential diagnosis should be constructed based on the mechanism and location of injury.

History

The initial evaluation of the injured patient begins with obtaining a focused history from the patient, including when and how the injury occurred, what treatments/wound care have already been administered, whether or not intoxication with drugs or alcohol was involved, and whether there is potential for associated injury. Certain cases may require inquiry about loss of consciousness, tetanus vaccination status, hand dominance, ability to ambulate, whether or not wounds were self-inflicted, and potential for body fluid exposure, wound contamination from a bite or other contamination source, or foreign body. Information about the injury from family members, coworkers, or other witnesses may also be helpful.

Important historical factors to consider when evaluating risk for specific injuries include:

- **Age**
  - Age greater than 65 years increases risk for fractures due to decreased bone density and fall risk, and TBI
  - Young adults: TBI (age 15–34),[2] MVC (age 18–29)[3]

- **Gender**
  - Male: Higher risk of TBI[2]
  - Female: Domestic abuse, sexual abuse[4]

- **Past medical history**
  - Diabetes mellitus and/or peripheral vascular disease: Delayed wound healing, wound infection
  - Osteoporosis: Fractures
  - Movement disorders (e.g., Parkinson's disease): Increased fall risk
  - Cognitive impairment (e.g., Alzheimer dementia): Increased fall risk

It is important to ask about associated symptoms, as outlined in Table 1.19.

TABLE **1.19** Pertinent Review of Systems With Corresponding Diagnosis

System	Signs/Symptoms	Diagnosis
General	Fever	Wound infection
HEENT	Headache, visual changes	Head injury
Cardiovascular	Palpitations	Electrical injury
	Chest pain	Chest trauma
	Cold extremity	Vascular compromise
Pulmonary	Dyspnea	Chest trauma, traumatic pneumothorax
GI	Nausea/vomiting	Head injury, pain response
	Abdominal pain	Blunt trauma, internal injury/bleeding
GU	Hematuria	Kidney injury
Musculoskeletal	Inability to ambulate/bear weight	Sprain, strain, fracture
	Weakness, decreased range of motion	Muscle or tendon injury
	Swelling, bruising	Sprain, strain, fracture, contusion
Neurologic	Numbness, paresthesias, weakness	Nerve injury
	Loss of consciousness	Head trauma: Consider that syncope could be the cause of trauma

GI, gastrointestinal; GU, genitourinary; HEENT, head, ear, eye, nose, and throat.

CLINICAL PEARL: It is always important to ask patients about contact lens use in the evaluation of eye injury.

- Social history
  - Occupation: Patients can also be predisposed to certain injuries based on occupational hazards, such as heavy lifting, repetitive movements, welding, electrical work, environmental exposures, chemical burns, and eye injuries

CLINICAL PEARL: Although it will not change the level of care your patient receives, it is important to clarify whether an injury is work related as this will ensure that the patient's initial care and follow-up visits are covered by workman's compensation insurance.

  - Smoking tobacco: Delayed wound healing, wound infection
  - Alcohol abuse: Increased fall/accident risk, masking of pain/other injury
  - Substance abuse: Increased fall/accident risk, masking of pain/other injury

- Medications and supplements, particularly those that can increase the risk for bleeding/further injury
  - Anticoagulants: Increased risk of bleeding/bruising; head trauma, intra-abdominal bleeding, pelvic/long bone bleeding with fracture
  - Chronic steroid use: Delayed wound healing
- Injury-specific historical information to inquire about and document
  - MVC Injury: Driver/passenger, front/back seat, vehicle damage, airbag deployment,restrained or unrestrained, site of car impact, low speed or high speed impact, ability to self-extricate/ambulate on scene, significant injury or death in other vehicle, drug or alcohol intoxication
  - Use of protective equipment: Use of helmets or other protective clothing/gear in athletes or patients involved in motorcycle or bicycle accidents
  - Wound/laceration/abrasion injury: Contamination (dirt, debris, animal or human bite); what caused the injury (wood, glass, metal); potential for foreign body in the wound; tetanus vaccination status; vaccination status of source patient or source animal in bite wounds/body fluid exposure; how long ago wound occurred; abnormal sensation, circulation, or range of motion to affected area

> **CLINICAL PEARL:** Tetanus toxoid vaccine (Td or Tdap) should be given if date of last vaccination was 10 or more years for clean, minor wounds and if more than5 years for all other contaminated or complicated wounds. Tetanus immune globulin should be given for contaminated or complicated wounds in patients who have unknown tetanus vaccination status or who have received fewer than three doses of tetanus vaccinations/boosters.[5]

  - Musculoskeletal injury: Ability to bear weight; range of motion; hand dominance; prior injury, surgery, or hardware/prosthesis to affected area; paresthesias, weakness, abnormal circulation, or sensation to affected area; neurologic symptoms that correspond to a specific spinal level or dermatome
  - Head/facial injury: Loss of consciousness; anticoagulant use; vomiting; altered mental status; visual change; hearing loss or other focal neurologic deficit; seizure activity; eye, ear, nose, or dental injury; mandibular range of motion; neck pain or injury
  - Burn: What substance caused burn, material safety data sheet (MSDS) information (for chemical burn), potential for inhalation injury, body surface area involvement
  - Frostbite: Exposure to cold environmental temperatures or substance (metal); exposure to halogenated hydrocarbons (Freon)
  - Electrical injury: Amount and type of current, duration and location of contact, voltage

- ○ Trauma: Height of fall, type of injury (blunt vs. penetrating), vehicle or machinery involvement, anticoagulation use, altered mental status
- ○ Domestic abuse/violent crime/sexual assault: Time/date/location of assault, does patient feel safe at home/have a safe place to be discharged to, are the police involved/does the patient want to file a report

CLINICAL PEARL: Remember to keep in mind that domestic abuse may involve children, intimate partners, family members, and the elderly. Abusers may be significant others, family members, acquaintances, or other caregivers. Abuse may be emotional, physical, financial, sexual, or take the form of neglect.

- ○ Sexual assault: Has patient bathed or changed clothing, drug or alcohol involvement, type of sexual contact that occurred, potential for body fluid exposure, condom use; victims of sexual assault should be evaluated with a trained provider

PHYSICAL EXAM

Physical examination of a patient with an injury-related complaint in the ED should be focused on the area of injury while carefully evaluating for associated injuries. Any patient with fall, MVC, or other trauma-related injury should be thoroughly examined, from head to toe. Specific exam findings are discussed in Tables 1.20 and 1.21.

TABLE 1.20 Physical Exam Findings in Specific Disease Conditions by Body System

	Physical Exam Finding	Associated Clinical Condition
General appearance	Diaphoresis/pallor	Trauma with internal bleeding or significant blood loss
	Anxious/severe painful distress	Trauma with internal bleeding or significant blood loss
	Obtunded/altered mental status	Head trauma, trauma with internal bleeding or significant blood loss
	Cyanosis, pallor	Vascular injury
Vital signs	Weak, thready pulse	Trauma with internal bleeding or significant blood loss
	Tachycardia	Trauma with internal bleeding or significant blood loss, shock, cardiac tamponade, contusion
	Asymmetric pulses, weakened or absent lower extremity pulses	Traumatic aortic dissection, other peripheral vascular injury
	Pulsus paradoxus	Cardiac tamponade

(continued)

TABLE **1.20** Physical Exam Findings in Specific Disease Conditions by Body System (*continued*)

	Physical Exam Finding	Associated Clinical Condition
	Hypertension	Severe head injury (traumatic SAH/ICH); traumatic aortic dissection
	Hypotension	Trauma with internal bleeding or significant blood loss, traumatic aortic dissection
	Asymmetric blood pressure	Traumatic aortic dissection
	Hypoxia	Traumatic pneumothorax, hemothorax
	Tachypnea	Traumatic pneumothorax, hemothorax, or pericardial effusion; cardiac tamponade
HEENT	Abrasions, lacerations, contusions to scalp or face; periorbital bruising, nasal trauma, hemotympanum, Battle's sign	TBI, skull or facial bone fractures
	Pupil asymmetry; unilateral fixed, dilated pupil; fixed gaze	Traumatic SAH/ICH, concussion
	Dysconjugate gaze	Traumatic cranial nerve III, IV, VI palsy
	Papilledema	Traumatic intracranial hypertension
	Visual changes or decreased visual acuity	TBI, ocular injury, concussion syndromes
	Conjunctival injection, tearing, photophobia	Corneal abrasion, chemical/UV conjunctivitis or keratitis
	Uptake on fluorescein staining	Corneal abrasion/laceration (linear or slightly irregular uptake), UV keratitis (punctate uptake)
	Persistent lacrimation	Lacrimal apparatus injury, chemical conjunctivitis
	Periorbital swelling, ecchymosis, subconjunctival hemorrhage, or chemosis	Periorbital contusion or fracture, ocular injury
	Impaired EOM, upward gaze palsy	Orbital floor fracture with entrapment of extraocular muscles
	Unilateral afferent pupil defect; teardrop pupil, extrusion of vitreous, prolapse of uvea, tenting of the cornea or sclera, Seidel sign[a]	Globe rupture
	Infraorbital hypesthesia or anesthesia	Facial bone fracture (zygoma) or laceration with infraorbital nerve injury

(*continued*)

TABLE **1.20** Physical Exam Findings in Specific Disease Conditions by Body System (*continued*)

	Physical Exam Finding	Associated Clinical Condition
	Conductive hearing loss	TBI or ear canal/barotrauma
	Sensorineural hearing loss	CN VIII palsy, mass lesion, trauma
	TM rupture	TBI or ear canal/barotrauma
	Epistaxis, septal hematoma[b]	TBI, nasal injury/fracture
	Singed nasal hairs, soot in nasal passages or oropharynx	Inhalation injury
	Facial bone tenderness, ecchymosis or swelling	Facial bone fracture
	Intraoral bleeding, loose dentition, mandibular tenderness or decreased ROM	Dental fracture[c], intraoral laceration, mandibular fracture
Cardiovascular	Pericardial friction rub	Traumatic pericardial effusion, cardiac tamponade
	Jugular venous distention	Tension pneumothorax, cardiac tamponade
	Pulsating bleeding of bright-red blood, active hemorrhage, or diminished pulse	Arterial injury
Pulmonary	Reduced breath sounds	Pneumothorax, hemothorax
	Tracheal deviation	Tension pneumothorax (away from affected side), pleural effusion/hemothorax (toward affected side)
	Mediastinal crunch (Hamman sign)	Mediastinitis/traumatic esophageal rupture
	Subcutaneous emphysema	Mediastinitis/traumatic esophageal rupture
	Dullness to percussion	Hemothorax
	Hyperresonance to percussion	Traumatic pneumothorax
	Ecchymosis/abrasion/signs of trauma	Chest wall contusion, rib fracture, other chest trauma
	Chest wall tenderness	Chest wall contusion, rib fracture, other chest trauma
	Flail chest (paradoxical chest wall movement with respiration of part of the chest wall)	Multiple contiguous rib fractures increases likelihood
Skin	Ecchymosis	Contusion, fracture, sprain, internal bleeding/injury
	Contusions or abrasions in area of seatbelt restraint ("seatbelt sign")	Potential for underlying vascular injury (e.g., vertebral artery) or internal chest or abdominal injury

(*continued*)

TABLE **1.20** Physical Exam Findings in Specific Disease Conditions by Body System (*continued*)

	Physical Exam Finding	**Associated Clinical Condition**
	Superficial epidermal injury	Abrasion, laceration, burn
	Dermal, subcutaneous fat, fascial, or muscle injury	Superficial, moderate, deep laceration
	Muscle or tendon exposure[d]	Deep laceration
	Visible bony fragments, tenting of skin	Open fracture, dislocation or grossly displaced fracture
	Puncture wounds, abrasions lacerations associated with ecchymosis	Bite wound
	Erythema, blisters, eschar	Burn[e] (see Chapter 2, Common Disease Entities in Emergency Medicine, "Burns" section for further details on burn classification), frostbite
	Burn with entrance and exit wound	Electrical injury
	Penetrating wound with entry and exit wounds; deep penetrating wound[f]	GSW; stab wound or other penetrating injury
	Focal pallor or cyanosis	Vascular injury, frostbite
GI	Contusions/abrasions/tenderness/palpable masses to abdomen or flank[g,h]	Internal organ injury (e.g., rupture, hemorrhage, laceration, contusion of organs)
	Cullen's sign (periumbilical ecchymosis), Grey Turner's sign (flank ecchymosis)	Intraperitoneal bleeding often develops later in course
	Rigidity, distention, tympany, guarding, rebound tenderness	Intraperitoneal air from ruptured viscous or intraperitoneal hemorrhage
	Rectal bleeding	GI/GU injury, sexual assault[i]
	Decreased rectal tone	Spinal cord injury of sacral roots
GU	Suprapubic tenderness	Bladder injury
	Gross or microscopic hematuria, blood at the urethral meatus	Kidney, ureteral, bladder, or urethral injury
	Priapism	Spinal cord injury of sacral roots
	Urinary retention or incontinence	Spinal cord injury of sacral roots
	Scrotal, testicular, perineal, or penile ecchymosis/laceration/abrasion/deformity	Pelvic fracture or other genitourinary trauma, sexual assault
	Labial, vaginal, or perineal ecchymosis, laceration/abrasion/deformity	Pelvic fracture or other genitourinary trauma, sexual assault

(*continued*)

TABLE 1.20 Physical Exam Findings in Specific Disease Conditions by Body System (*continued*)

	Physical Exam Finding	**Associated Clinical Condition**
Extremities	Pallor, mottling, or discoloration; temperature or pulse asymmetry; abnormal pulse; delayed capillary refill (> 2 sec)	Vascular injury, fracture or dislocation with vascular compromise, frostbite
	Swelling, inability to bear weight	Contusion, sprain/strain, fracture
Neurologic	Stroke-like symptoms or altered mental status	TBI, traumatic aortic dissection
	Horner syndrome (involvement of superior cervical sympathetic ganglion)	Traumatic aortic dissection
	Hoarseness (compression of left recurrent laryngeal nerve)	Traumatic aortic dissection, cervical injury
	Weakness, asymmetric strength or paralysis (hemiparesis or hemiparalysis)	Peripheral nerve injury, spinal cord trauma, traumatic aortic dissection
	Sensory abnormality, paresthesias, abnormal two-point discrimination	Peripheral nerve injury

[a] Clinical Pearl: Seidel sign is the streaming of fluid noted away from the puncture site on fluorescein staining.

[b] Clinical Pearl: All head/facial trauma patients should be evaluated for nasal septal hematoma. If found, nasal septal hematoma requires immediate drainage by ED provider or ENT specialist to prevent permanent nasal septal injury/damage/deformity.

[c] Clinical Pearl: Dental fractures are classified using the Ellis fracture classification system, which divides injuries into eight categories: enamel infraction, enamel fracture, enamel–dentition fracture, enamel–dentin-pulp fracture, crown–root fracture without pulp exposure, crown–root fracture with pulp exposure, root fracture, and alveolar bone fracture.

[d] Clinical Pearl: Tendon tissue appears as shiny white, flat tissue that will move in associated extremity movement in a partial tear or will remain immobile in a complete tear/laceration.

[e] Clinical Pearl: Circumferential full-thickness burns around an extremity can predispose a patient to developing compartment syndrome in that extremity.

[f] Clinical Pearl: An attempt to locate entrance and exit wounds in cases of GSW can help determine the path of the bullet and whether or not the bullet is retained. In cases of stab wounds, size of penetrating object can potentially help determine size and depth of wound.

[g] Clinical Pearl: LUQ tenderness or ecchymosis in a pregnant patient or patient with recent history of mononucleosis or symptoms suggestive of mononucleosis should be screened for splenic injury or rupture.

[h] Clinical Pearl: It is always important to determine whether a female patient of childbearing age is pregnant when assessing for trauma, particularly abdominal trauma.

[i] Clinical Pearl: It is important to treat all sexual assault patients in a caring, nonjudgmental, and professional manner. Notify the sexual assault examiner immediately in all cases of suspected sexual assault if the patient consents to examination for forensic purposes. Most states will perform a forensic examination for all patients presenting within 72 hours of assault, some states will perform examination up to 96 hours after assault.[6] Do not have the patient change into a hospital gown as clothing may contain evidence for the forensic examination.

CN, cranial nerve; ENT, ear, nose, and throat; EOM, extraocular muscles; GI, gastrointestinal; GSW, gunshot wound; GU, genitourinary; HEENT, head, ear, eye, nose, throat; ICH, intracranial hemorrhage; LUQ, left upper quadrant; ROM, range of motion; SAH, subarachnoid hemorrhage; TBI, traumatic brain injury; TM, tympanic membrane; UV, ultraviolet.

TABLE **1.21** Physical Exam Findings in Specific Disease Conditions:
Musculoskeletal Complaints

Musculoskeletal System	Physical Exam Finding	Associated Clinical Condition
General	Tenderness overlying bone, joint, or muscle	Contusion, sprain/strain, fracture
	Decreased ROM, pain with ROM	Sprain/strain, fracture, dislocation, tendon rupture or injury
	Pain out of proportion to exam	Compartment syndrome[a]
	Asymmetric muscle contour, swelling, gross deformity	Sprain/strain, fracture, dislocation, tendon rupture or injury
Spine	Midline cervical, thoracic, or lumbar spine tenderness	Spinal contusion, fracture
	Palpable paraspinal muscle spasm or paraspinal tenderness	Torticollis, muscle strain/spasm
	Positive straight leg raise test	Sciatica
Shoulder	Clavicular tenderness/deformity	Clavicular fracture
	AC tenderness/deformity	AC separation/"separated shoulder"
	Tenderness overlying scapula, decreased ROM of shoulder	Scapular fracture (generally high-force injury or from direct trauma, requires further investigation of associated injury)
	Decreased sensation to lateral shoulder; weakened shoulder flexion, extension, internal/external rotation of shoulder	Axillary nerve injury (shoulder dislocation/humerus fracture)
	Weak external rotation, positive Neer's, Hawkin's, or drop-arm tests	Rotator cuff injury/impingement/tear
	Held in slightly abducted/externally rotated position, loss of rounded appearance	Anterior shoulder dislocation
	Held in slightly adducted/internally rotated position, shoulder appears prominent posteriorly and flattened anteriorly	Posterior shoulder dislocation
	Humerus ecchymosis, swelling, tenderness, and decreased ROM of shoulder	Humerus fracture
Elbow	Distal humerus/elbow tenderness, swelling, limited ROM	Supracondylar fracture (uncommon in adults), intercondylar fracture

(continued)

TABLE **1.21** Physical Exam Findings in Specific Disease Conditions: Musculoskeletal Complaints (*continued*)

Musculoskeletal System	Physical Exam Finding	Associated Clinical Condition
	Gross deformity with prominent olecranon posteriorly; elbow tenderness, swelling, limited ROM	Posterior elbow dislocation
	Elbow held partially flexed, close to body in pronation; child generally refuses to use affected arm	Radial head subluxation (Nursemaid's elbow)
	Tenderness overlying lateral elbow or antecubital fossa; decreased ROM, particularly supination/pronation	Radial head fracture
	Tenderness, erythema, swelling to lateral elbow; pain with wrist extension	Lateral epicondylitis (tennis elbow)
	Tenderness, erythema, swelling to medial elbow; pain with wrist flexion	Medial epicondylitis (golfer elbow)
	Tenderness, swelling overlying olecranon process with pain on ROM of elbow	Olecranon fracture, olecranon bursitis (may have associated overlying erythema and warmth)
Forearm	Tenderness, swelling, ecchymosis to midforearm; decreased ROM	Midshaft radius fracture and/or midshaft ulnar fracture (nightstick fracture)
Wrist	Tenderness, swelling, ecchymosis to distal forearm/wrist; decreased ROM	Distal radius fracture, distal ulnar fracture, wrist contusion or sprain
	Tenderness, swelling/ecchymosis over dorsal aspect of radial side of wrist	Scapholunate dissociation injury, perilunate and lunate dislocation
	Wrist drop, weakness of wrist extension	Radial nerve injury ("Saturday night palsy")
	Weakness of wrist flexion or flexion of fourth and fifth digits	Ulnar nerve injury
	Weakness of wrist flexion or flexion of thumb, second and third digits and opposition/abduction of thumb	Median nerve injury
Hand	Tenderness, swelling, ecchymosis, decreased ROM	Fracture, sprain/strain[b]
	Positive Finkelstein test	De Quervain's tenosynovitis
	Snuffbox tenderness, pain on axial compression loading of the thumb	Scaphoid fracture
	Positive Tinel's or Phalen's sign, atrophy or weakness of thenar eminence	Carpal tunnel syndrome

(*continued*)

TABLE 1.21 Physical Exam Findings in Specific Disease Conditions: Musculoskeletal Complaints (*continued*)

Musculoskeletal System	Physical Exam Finding	Associated Clinical Condition
	Swelling, ecchymosis, tenderness to dorsal aspect of fourth or fifth metacarpals	Metacarpal neck fracture (boxer's fracture[c])
	Laxity of UCL with valgus stress to thumb	Gamekeeper's thumb/skier's thumb/UCL injury
	Tenderness to base of thumb/first carpometacarpal joint	Intra-articular fracture/dislocation (Bennett's fracture), sprain
	Inability to extend DIP	Mallet finger/extensor tendon injury
	Boutonniere deformity	Central slip injury
	Nail or nail margin abrasion/laceration, nail bed exposure	Nail fold or nail bed laceration, partial or complete nail avulsion
	Ecchymosis to distal phalanx or under nail	Subungual hematoma, tuft fracture
Pelvis	Tenderness, swelling, ecchymosis along anterior, lateral, or posterior pelvic region; may have signs of intra-abdominal/pelvic organ trauma as earlier	Pelvis fracture
Hip	Inability to walk; groin pain; hip/pelvic pain; shortened, externally rotated lower extremity	Hip fracture
	Severe pain, tenderness, swelling, gross deformity, loss of ROM, shortened and rotated; may have signs of other associated trauma as indicated fornative hip dislocations	Hip dislocation (posterior dislocation is most common in both native and prosthetic hips)
	Weakened hip flexion or knee extension	Femoral nerve injury
Thigh	Severe pain, tenderness, swelling, and gross deformity; may have signs of other associated trauma	Femoral fracture
	Pain with weight-bearing, difficulty with weight-bearing and ROM; overlying tenderness, ecchymosis	Hamstring strain, quadriceps strain
Knee	Pain with weight-bearing or inability to bear weight, instability of knee joint, significant swelling, positive anterior drawer test, positive Lachman test	ACL tear

(*continued*)

TABLE **1.21** Physical Exam Findings in Specific Disease Conditions: Musculoskeletal Complaints (*continued*)

Musculoskeletal System	Physical Exam Finding	Associated Clinical Condition
	Pain with weight-bearing or inability to bear weight, instability of knee joint, significant swelling, positive posterior drawer test	PCL tear
	Laxity on valgus stress	Medial collateral ligament injury
	Laxity on varus stress	Lateral collateral ligament injury
	Tenderness along medial or lateral joint line, positive McMurray test (medial meniscus injury)	Medial or lateral meniscus injury
	Severe pain, tenderness, swelling, and gross deformity; may have signs of other associated trauma	Knee dislocation (tibiofemoral dislocation)
	Moderate to severe pain; tenderness overlying anterior knee, gross deformity/displacement of the patella from the trochlear groove (more commonly laterally); loss of ROM of knee	Patellar dislocation
	Moderate to severe pain; tenderness, swelling overlying anterior knee; decreased ROM	Patellar fracture
	Instability during knee extension, positive patellar apprehension test	Patellar subluxation
	Pain with flexion or extension, tenderness to superior (quadriceps) or inferior (patellar) pole of patella	Quadriceps or patellar tendinitis
	Pain with flexion or extension, swelling, tenderness to anterior knee; palpable defect in complete tear of quadriceps tendon; inability to extend knee to 180° or hold knee in full extension against gravity	Quadriceps or patellar tendon tear
	Erythema, swelling, tenderness to anterior knee	Bursitis
	Swelling and tenderness to anterior knee/proximal tibia, pain with weight-bearing or inability to bear weight	Tibial plateau fracture
Lower leg	Swelling and tenderness to anterior knee/proximal tibia	Tibial tuberosity injury, stress fracture, medial tibial stress syndrome (shin splints)

(*continued*)

TABLE **1.21** Physical Exam Findings in Specific Disease Conditions: Musculoskeletal Complaints (*continued*)

Musculoskeletal System	Physical Exam Finding	Associated Clinical Condition
	Swelling, tenderness to proximal fibula; swelling, tenderness, and decreased ROM of ankle in Maisonneuve fracture	Fibular head fracture
	Swelling, tenderness, ecchymosis to lower leg; inability to bear weight (tibia fracture) or pain with weight-bearing	Tibia and/or fibular fracture
Ankle	Swelling, tenderness, ecchymosis; gross deformity; inability to bear weight or perform ROM	Ankle dislocation
	Swelling, tenderness, ecchymosis; difficulty or inability to bear weight	Sprain/strain, ligament injury, fracture
	Foot drop	Common peroneal nerve injury
Foot	Swelling, tenderness, ecchymosis overlying posterior ankle/Achilles; positive Thompson test and palpable defect (complete tear); difficulty or inability to perform plantar flexion or raise onto tip toes	Achilles injury
	Swelling, tenderness, ecchymosis overlying heel; difficulty or inability to bear weight	Calcaneus fracture
	Swelling, tenderness, ecchymosis to midfoot	Lisfranc injury
	Swelling, tenderness, ecchymosis; difficulty or inability to bear weight	Metatarsal fracture, toe fracture
	Swelling, tenderness, ecchymosis to base of fifth metatarsal	Fifth metatarsal fracture, avulsion fracture (Dancer's fracture), fracture between base and metaphasis (Jones fracture)
	Ecchymosis to distal phalanx or under nail	Subungual hematoma, tuft fracture

[a] Clinical Pearl: Compartment syndrome typically develops in the extremities following a long bone fracture but may also develop in the setting of crush injuries, burns, bleeding diathesis, prolonged limb compression, and minor trauma. In addition to pain out of proportion to exam, pain with passive stretching of muscles, and tense tissue or firmness of compartment on exam, the six "Ps" of compartment syndrome may also be noted

[b] Clinical Pearl: Be sure to isolate each metacarpophalangeal and interphalangeal joint to check for flexor and extensor tendon injuries in your evaluation of hand and finger trauma.

[c] Clinical Pearl: It is important to examine skin for abrasions or signs of a "fight bite" for all patients with boxer's fractures to identify those who are at risk for infection. Any patient with suspected injury caused by a tooth should have aggressive wound irrigation and be given antibiotic prophylaxis.

pain, pallor, paresthesias, pulselessness, paralysis, poikilothermia (injured limb is cooler than unaffected tissue

AC, acromioclavicular; ACL, anterior cruciate ligament; DIP, distal interphalangeal joint; PCL, posterior cruciate ligament; ROM, range of motion; UCL ulnar collateral ligament.

> **CLINICAL PEARL:** All trauma patients should be changed into a hospital gown to allow for proper exposure of skin for thorough examination, keeping in mind patient modesty and potential cultural/religious needs.

Patients may arrive to the ED with a cervical immobilization collar in place on a rigid backboard. Such patients should be log rolled while maintaining spinal alignment and immobilization to check for potential spinal injury, and patients should be removed from the backboard as quickly as possible. Nexus criteria (www.mdcalc.com/nexus-criteria-c-spine-imaging) and Canadian C-spine rules (www.mdcalc.com/canadian-c-spine-rule) can be used to determine which patients may safely have cervical immobilization collars removed based on history and physical exam without the use of imaging to rule out injury.

Wounds should be irrigated and bleeding controlled to facilitate thorough wound exploration to assess for depth of injury, potential tendon or nerve involvement, and whether or not contamination or foreign bodies are present. Careful examination of the skin, musculoskeletal, vascular, and neurologic systems is important for most patients, particularly those with extremity injuries. It is important to keep in mind limb-threatening injuries and disease processes such as neurovascular injury or compartment syndrome. Thorough investigation of the body system involved in the trauma as well as surrounding areas is essential to avoid missing associated injuries or becoming preoccupied with distracting injuries. The patient history and mechanism of injury should guide your physical examination.

> **CLINICAL PEARL:** Perform and document a detailed examination of cranial nerves, eyes, eyelids, lacrimal system, nose, ears, and mouth, including dental and salivary gland structures, for all patients with head and facial trauma. These are potentially high-risk injuries that may require emergent consultation with ophthalmology, oral/maxillofacial surgery, or plastic surgery. If missed, they may have long-term functional, neurologic, and cosmetic consequences and lead to poor patient outcomes.

Any patient with a potentially severe traumatic injury or mechanism of injury may be evaluated on arrival to the ED in conjunction with members from a trauma surgery team in centers where field activation of these teams is done by EMS. It is important to activate a trauma surgery team in centers where immediate consultation is available as soon as severe traumatic injury is suspected based on physical exam or FAST examination. Delay in performing a detailed physical exam or delay in obtaining advanced imaging, such as CT or MRI, may result in deterioration of your patient's condition. Patents with high suspicion for certain injuries may be transferred directly for immediate operative care, bypassing advanced imaging when it may cause unnecessary delay of life-saving treatment.

Diagnostic Plan

LABS

- CBC: Evaluate for anemia from blood loss; a decrease in hemoglobin from acute blood loss takes approximately 6 hours; evaluate for elevated WBC in wound infection
- Blood type and screen: Needed when there is severe blood loss in trauma requiring blood transfusion
- Coagulation studies needed for patients on anticoagulation therapy
- D-dimer: Consider in suspected aortic dissection: D-dimer levels of <500 ng/mL have been shown to have high sensitivity and negative predictive value for screening patients for aortic dissection and may be useful to identify those patients who do not have aortic dissection
- Arterial blood gas (ABG): Evaluate for metabolic abnormalities in chest trauma, inhalation injury/burn injury, hemorrhagic shock
- Carboxyhemoglobin: Elevated in cases of carbon monoxide toxicity (see Chapter 3, Diagnostic Testing in Emergency Medicine)
- Creatine phosphokinase (CPK): Elevated in rhabdomyolysis from burn, crush, or electrical injuries
- Urine myoglobin: Elevated from rhabdomyolysis in burn, crush, or electrical injuries
- Troponin: Elevated in cardiac injury sustained in high-voltage electrical injury
- Lactate: Elevated in hemorrhagic shock, burn injury
- Blood alcohol or urine drug screen testing: Order in suspected cases of intoxication
- Pregnancy testing: For cases of sexual assault, risk stratification of mother/fetus, anticipation of potential imaging studies for radiation exposure (CT)
- Sexually transmitted infection (STI) testing: In cases of sexual assault
- Comprehensive metabolic panel may show abnormalities in glucose, liver function tests, or BUN, but are generally nonspecific; electrolyte abnormalities may develop due to large fluid shifts in burn and electrical injury patients; baseline renal function should be established for patients being monitored for potential acute kidney injury (rhabdomyolysis)

DIAGNOSTIC IMAGING

- EKG to evaluate for
  - Arrhythmia in electrical injury
    - Most arrhythmias are benign
    - Ventricular and atrial arrhythmias, bradyarrhythmias, and QT-interval prolongation are more common in high-voltage injuries

- Direct current and lightning-strike injuries may cause cardiac arrest due to asystole; alternating current injury may cause ventricular fibrillation[7]
  - ○ Arrhythmia or ST elevation or depression in patients with significant chest trauma
  - ○ Arrhythmia or heart block for cases in which syncope is cause of trauma
- CT imaging without IV contrast
  - ○ Occult fracture if suspicion is high and x-ray is normal. This is particularly helpful in cases of vertebral fractures, distal radius, femoral neck, radial head, scaphoid, and supracondylar fractures in pediatric patients
  - ○ Head injury/TBI: Findings on noncontrast CT may include blood in the meninges as in SAH or into the brain parenchyma in ICH (see Figure 1.10); CT findings of subdural hematoma will appear as blood accumulation in the subdural spaces, generally with a crescent or concave shape (see Figure 1.11); epidural hematoma will appear as blood accumulation in a convex pattern between the skull and outermost layer of the dura (see Figure 1.12)
  - ○ Facial bone fractures: Nondisplaced nasal bone fractures, sinus injury, orbital injury, zygoma injury, maxilla or mandibular injury
  - ○ Cervical spine injury: Vertebral fracture or dislocation; patients with significant mechanism of injury or high suspicion for cervical injury (fracture or dislocation as in Figure e3.1) should have CT imaging done as plain radiography is often inadequate in completely evaluating the cervical spine[8]
    - Canadian CT Head Injury/Trauma Rule (CCHR), New Orleans/Charity Head Trauma/Injury Rule (NOC), and Nexus II scoring systems can be used to determine the need for CT imaging in the setting of head trauma. NEXUS Criteria and Canadian C-Spine Rule can be used to determine which patients with cervical spine injuries need imaging studies.
- CT with IV contrast for chest, abdominal, or pelvic injury in setting of trauma; CT may demonstrate more subtle findings and associated injuries better than x-ray; chest CT may show rib fractures (see Figure e3.2), pneumothorax, or hemothorax; other findings may include pulmonary contusion (see Figure e3.2), sternal fracture, scapular fracture, mediastinal/esophageal injury

CLINICAL PEARL: Many chest injuries are easily visualized on chest CT without IV contrast; however, in the trauma setting it is common to image the chest/abdomen/pelvis simultaneously. Therefore, IV contrast that illuminates abdominal and pelvic injuries is commonly administered at the same time.

- ○ CT of abdomen/pelvis may show liver, splenic, renal, or pancreas lacerations or contusions; perforated viscus; hemoperitoneum; pneumoperitoneum; bladder or urethral injury; pelvic fractures
- CT angiography (CTA) for
  - ○ Vascular injury: CTA of the head/neck may demonstrate vertebral/carotid artery dissection; CTA of the chest/abdomen/pelvis may demonstrate aortic dissection (see Figure 1.7)
- MRI for
  - ○ Occult fractures: MRI should be used in patients with high suspicion of hip fracture with normal x-rays
  - ○ Spinal injury: Acute spinal cord injury, epidural hematoma, intervertebral disk, or ligamentous injury of the spine
  - ○ Extremity ligamentous or tendon injury (e.g., anterior cruciate ligament [ACL] tear): Unlikely to be obtained in ED setting
- X-ray, evaluate for musculoskeletal injury (fractures/dislocations) as seen in Table 1.22

TABLE 1.22 X-ray Indications and Findings

Anatomic Area and Trauma	Specific Findings to Evaluate
Spine	Fracture of cervical, thoracic, or lumbar vertebrae (see Figure e3.3): Dislocation/subluxation of vertebrae
Chest	Pneumothorax (see Figure 1.5), pericardial effusion (see Figure 1.6), widened mediastinum from aortic dissection, pneumomediastinum, or rib fractures (see Figure e3.4)
Clavicle	Clavicular fracture (see Figure e3.5), sternoclavicular or acromioclavicular dislocation (normal coracoclavicular distance is 11–13 mm)
Scapular fracture	Generally these are high-force injuries, further investigation with CT to rule out chest trauma is recommended
Humerus fracture	Proximal, midshaft, supracondylar in pediatric patients, intercondylar in adults; proximal humerus fracture (see Figure e3.6)
Shoulder dislocation: Anterior, posterior	Evaluate for presence of associated fracture in both pre- and postreduction x-rays Anterior shoulder dislocations (see Figure e3.7) constitute the vast majority of shoulder dislocations; humeral head will appear anterior, medial, and inferior to glenoid fossa Presence of the "light bulb sign" on x-ray in posterior shoulder dislocation
Elbow	Supracondylar fracture (most common in pediatric patients) may demonstrate anterior humeral line displacement relative to the capitellum (should intersect the middle 1/3 of the capitellum) Intracondylar fracture in adults may demonstrate separation of the condyles

(continued)

Table **1.22** X-ray Indications and Findings (*continued*)

Anatomic Area and Trauma	Specific Findings to Evaluate
	Posterior elbow dislocation may be seen; radial head fracture (see Figure e3.8) may be obvious or may only demonstrate posterior fat pad and/or anterior sail sign (see Figure e3.8) in occult fractures Observe for olecranon fracture
Forearm: Radius and/or ulnar midshaft fracture	Midshaft ulnar fracture/"nightstick fracture" Galeazzi fracture demonstrates a midshaft radial fracture with distal radioulnar joint instability/dislocation Monteggia fracture demonstrates fracture of the proximal 1/3 of the ulna with associated radial head dislocation (see Figure e3.9)
Wrist	Distal radius fracture with dorsal displacement of distal fragment (Colles's fracture; see Figure e3.10) or ventral displacement of the distal fragment (Smith's fracture) Observe for intra-articular involvement (Barton's fracture) or associated styloid process fracture; radial styloid process fracture with or without lunate or scapholunate dissociation (Hutchinson's fracture/"chauffer's fracture")
Hand	Scapholunate dissociation injury: >3 mm distance between scaphoid and lunate on AP view of hand x-ray; a scaphoid fracture is seen in Figure e3.11 Metacarpal neck fracture/"boxer's fracture" (see Figure e3.12) Bennett's fracture demonstrates intra-articular fracture with dislocation of the first carpometacarpal joint Deformity at the DIP/inability to extend DIP in mallet finger (see Figure e3.13) Hyperflexion of the PIP joint and hyperextension of the DIP joint in Boutonniere's deformity Phalangeal fractures: Observe for displacement, intra-articular involvement, distal phalanx involvement (tuft fracture)
Pelvis	May involve the iliac wing, rami, acetabulum, disruption of the pelvic ring, or widening of the pubic symphysis
Sacrum/coccyx	Fractures may involve neural foramina, obtain MRI for neurologic impairment/bowel or bladder dysfunction
Hip fracture	May involve femoral neck (most common, see Figure e3.14), femoral head, intertrochanteric, or subtrochanteric regions;anterior or posterior constitute the most common hip dislocations
Femur	Femoral shaft fracture, distal femur/femoral condyle fractures (less common)
Knee	Tibiofemoral dislocation (rare); evaluate for displacement of the femur (posterior, anterior, medial, lateral, or rotational) to the tibia

(continued)

TABLE **1.22** X-ray Indications and Findings (*continued*)

Anatomic Area and Trauma	Specific Findings to Evaluate
Patella fracture	Dislocation or subluxation may be visualized on x-ray (see Figure e3.15); may visualize tendon defect or avulsion fracture of the patella in quadriceps or patellar tendon rupture; a high-riding patella ("patella alta") may be seen in patellar tendon tear (see Figure e3.16)
Tibia	Tibial plateau fracture (see Figure e3.17), tibial tuberosity avulsion fracture or stress fracture, more common in adolescent athletes, and tibial shaft fracture or tibia/fibula fracture
Fibula	Fibular head fracture may be visualized either in isolation or in association with ankle injury (Maisonneuve fracture)
Ankle	Fracture or dislocation of the tibia, fibula (see Figure e3.18) or both (see Figure e3.19) may be visualized on x-ray; note whether there is any disruption to the ankle mortise; Achilles tendon injury may demonstrate tendon defect, soft tissue swelling, and/or loss of the pre-Achilles fat pad
Foot	Calcaneus: Most common fracture of the body (usually associated with fall from a height) extending intra-articularly, stress fractures, less common are avulsion fractures Lisfranc injury Dislocation of one of the tarsometatarsal joints with (see Figure e3.20) or without fracture
Metatarsal fracture	May occur in any of the metatarsals, generally in the midshaft region of metatarsals 1–4. Observe for significant displacement or intra-articular involvement; multiple metatarsal shaft fractures (typically from crush injuries) are considered unstable; the most common metatarsal injury is the proximal fifth metatarsal and may involve Avulsion of the proximal tuberosity/styloid ("Dancer's fracture"; see Figure e3.21) Proximal diaphyseal extending toward the intertarsal joint ("Jones fracture,"; see Figure e3.22), or stress fractures
Phalanx fracture	Observe for displacement, intra-articular involvement, distal phalanx involvement (tuft fracture)
Foreign body	X-ray may detect radiopaque foreign bodies (e.g., glass, metal); may help determine presence of debris in a wound, location/size/orientation of foreign body, possibility of retrieval of foreign body, postprocedural removal of foreign body
Complex fractures or penetrating injury	Evaluate for open fractures, subcutaneous air, intra-articular air in penetrating injuries (note CT can provide further detail for complex wounds and may be required after initial x-ray)

AP, anteroposterior; DIP, distal interphalangeal joint; PIP, proximal interphalangeal.

> **CLINICAL PEARL:** All patients with snuffbox tenderness on exam with negative x-ray should have repeat hand x-ray in 7 to 10 days to rule out occult scaphoid fracture with immobilization using a thumb spica splint until fracture can be ruled out. MRI or bone scan may also be considered for repeat imaging.

- Ultrasound:
  - Traumatic injury with the FAST and extended FAST exam; bedside cardiac ultrasonography/echocardiography, chest injuries, pericardial effusion (see Figure 1.8), traumatic aortic dissection; can also be used for hemothorax, rib fractures, cardiac injuries
  - Foreign bodies: May be helpful adjunct in foreign-body detection
  - Musculoskeletal ultrasound for muscle tears or tendon ruptures: Biceps tendon rupture; hamstring, quadriceps, gastrocnemius muscle, or tendon injury
- Arteriography/ankle–brachial Index (ABI): Evaluate for vascular involvement in extremity injury; ABI, CTA, arterial duplex ultrasonography may be used

> **CLINICAL PEARL:** Evidence of obvious arterial injury, including weak or absent pulses, neurologic deficit, rapidly expanding hematoma, or arterial bleeding, should be immediately assessed by trauma or vascular surgery for possible immediate surgical intervention.

- Manometry (e.g., Stryker) testing: Can be performed by orthopedics to evaluate tissue pressures in cases of suspected compartment syndrome

Initial Management

Hemodynamic instability, airway compromise, general decompensation of the patient's condition, and life- or limb-threatening injuries require immediate intervention and take precedence over any other diagnostic or therapeutic measures. All patients with potentially severe traumatic injury or mechanism of injury should be evaluated on arrival to the ED in conjunction with members from a trauma surgery team when such resources are available. Patients with suspected severe injury based on physical exam findings or FAST examination results may require immediate surgical intervention. Delays in care for further examination or advanced imaging may result in the deterioration of your patient's condition and should be avoided. Detailed discussions of particular injuries can be found in corresponding sections of Chapter 2, Common Disease Entities in Emergency Medicine and e-chapter 10. Specific wound care instructions can be found in Chapter 6, Common Procedures in Emergency Medicine.

- Wound care
  - Initial management includes controlling bleeding, thorough wound irrigation, and debridement
- Soft tissue and musculoskeletal injuries
  - General principles of management include
    - Pain control
      - Patients should be offered oral or IV pain medication; severity of injury and potential need for urgent or emergent surgical intervention (therefore keeping patient on nothng per os [NPO status]) should be considered
      - Pain may be safely and adequately controlled with peripheral nerve and hematoma block techniques
      - Common pain medication regimens include oral acetaminophen, NSAID, or opiates; IV NSAIDs or opiates
      - Ice and elevation/stabilization of injured area
    - Management of neurologic, vascular, or joint capsule injury with prompt surgical consultation
    - Splinting and immobilization with proper after care instructions
- Facial and head, eyes, ears, nose, and throat (HEENT) injuries
  - Certain facial and HEENT injuries require specific management and prompt treatment in the ED to avoid poor outcomes, permanent disability, or long-term complications; consultation with ophthalmology, plastic surgery, oral maxillary facial surgery (OMFS), or otolaryngology may be needed to ensure prompt evaluation in the ED or to arrange close follow-up for these injuries
- Environmental injuries
  - Burn care: Moderate and severe thermal burns
    - Patients with suspected significant inhalation injury or respiratory distress should undergo rapid sequence intubation (RSI) prior to onset of airway edema; high-flow oxygen should be given for cases of carbon monoxide poisoning
    - Initiate fluid resuscitation immediately in cases of severe burns, which can result in large fluid shifts and hypoperfusion
      - The Parkland formula can be used to calculate initial fluid resuscitation needs (www.mdcalc.com/parkland-formula-burns)
      - Body surface area can be calculated using the rule of nines
    - Chemical burns
      - Thoroughly decontaminate your patient if this has not been done prior to arrival with removal of contaminated clothing and thorough irrigation of infected areas with water or normal saline; keep in mind your safety and the safety of the ED area and staff during decontamination process
  - Electrocution/lightning strike
    - Treat all life-threatening cardiopulmonary and neurologic injuries

- Obtain immediate trauma, neurosurgical, or orthopedic consultation for severe traumatic, limb-threatening or neurovascular injuries
- Patients with low-voltage injuries (<1,000 V) do not need further cardiac monitoring if initial EKG is normal[9]
- Begin aggressive fluid resuscitation for patients with severe soft-tissue or burn injuries
- Neurologic injury
  - Spinal cord injury
    - Manage any life-threatening conditions and maintain spinal immobilization
    - Patients with high cervical spine injury may require intubation to maintain airway and breathing
    - Monitor for and treat neurogenic shock
    - Patients stable enough for imaging should undergo CT
    - Obtain immediate neurosurgical consultation
      - Discussion with neurosurgery regarding the use of methylprednisolone is warranted as its use in acute spinal cord injury is controversial[10,11]
  - Peripheral nerve injury
    - Complete neurologic evaluation should be performed before and after all procedures and splinting
    - Depending on the location and type of the injury, peripheral nerve injury may require consultation in the ED or close follow-up with ophthalmology, otolaryngology, plastic surgery, orthopedics, neurosurgery, or neurology
  - Vascular injury
    - Aortic injury
      - Traumatic aortic injury or dissection can be immediately life-threatening and requires prompt diagnosis and surgical management for hemodynamically unstable patients.
      - Monitoring of airway, breathing, and circulation should be initiated; aggressive management of hypotension with IV fluids or blood transfusion and RSI may be indicated in unstable patients.
      - Immediate consultation with trauma, cardiac, and vascular surgery depending on location of aortic injury.
      - Stable patients may undergo CT or CTA imaging.
      - Mechanism of injury typically involves penetrating or blunt-force trauma (high-speed MVC or fall from significant height) to thoracic cavity or abdomen and should be ruled out in any patient with chest, back, or abdominal pain with significant mechanism of injury.
    - Vertebral and carotid artery injury
      - Mechanism of injury typically involves penetrating or significant blunt-force trauma (seatbelt) to neck.

- Cervical spine immobilization and airway monitoring should be initiated; significant injury or respiratory distress should be treated with RSI.
- Immediate consultation by trauma surgery for transfer of care to operating room for unstable patients is needed.
- Stable patients may undergo CT or CTA imaging.
- Peripheral artery injury
  - Complete vascular evaluation should be performed before and after all procedures and splinting.
  - Application of direct pressure or tourniquet may be needed to control bleeding.
  - Close monitoring of hemodynamic status should be initiated.
  - Blood transfusion may be necessary for patients with severe blood loss.
  - Extremity injuries involving dislocations of major joints and displaced or open fractures (particularly of the humeral or femoral shaft) can cause serious vascular injury or compromise.
  - Immediate consultation with orthopedics or vascular surgery should be obtained when vascular injury is suspected.
  - Fractures should be stabilized and joint dislocations should be reduced as quickly as possible with transfer of care for operative management.
  - Stable patients may undergo CTA, ABI, or arterial duplex sonography.
  - Compartment syndrome
    - Most often develops following long bone fracture, crush injury, burns (particularly circumferential), vascular injury, or injury causing significant swelling.
    - Pain out of proportion to exam, pain with passive stretching, and significant tissue swelling/induration are generally present (see 6 Ps in footnote to Table 1.21).
    - Control pain; remove any constrictive splints or casts; place affected extremity at level of heart.
    - Immediate orthopedic consultation needed for suspected cases of emergent fasciotomy.
    - Confirmation is made with manometry testing.
    - All patients with injuries or splinting at risk for developing compartment syndrome should be given clear discharge and return-to-ED instructions for any signs or symptoms of compartment syndrome.
- Management based on specific mechanism of injury
  - Concussion and TBI
    - Clear instructions for follow-up with primary care provider or neurology and return to activity/driving/sports/work should be given.
- Violent crime
  - Penetrating and blunt-force-injury wounds

- Patients with penetrating wounds from gunshot or stab wounds should be stabilized and life-threatening injuries should be evaluated immediately.
- It is important to take a good history from patients with blunt-force injuries if possible as many of these injuries may have subtle physical exam findings.
  - Significant head, chest, back, abdominal, or extremity tenderness should be evaluated with further imaging as appropriate.
- The majority of these injuries will require immediate consultation and collaboration with trauma surgery, neurosurgery, thoracic surgery, and orthopedics.

> **CLINICAL PEARL:** Patients with significant traumatic injury will require collaborative care from physicians, nurses, PAs, and other ancillary staff in the ED. Never be afraid to ask for help if you feel your patient's condition is deteriorating or requires a higher level of care.

- Unstable patients may require immediate operative management; stable patients will likely require CT imaging to further evaluate injuries.
- Initial stabilization and management of penetrating wounds may involve initiating or maintaining cervical spine immobilization; RSI; obtaining large-bore IV access for fluid resuscitation; preparation for blood transfusion; needle thoracostomy or chest tube placement, application of direct pressure, hemostatic dressings, or tourniquets.
  - ○ Sexual assault
    - Sexual assault cases should be examined by a trained forensic examiner if patient consent is given.
    - Authorities should be notified if patient wishes to file a report and has not already done so.
    - Patients should be given information about local resources.
    - Urine pregnancy test should be done prior to initiation of treatment.
    - Prophylaxis for STIs, including HIV, hepatitis B and C, and emergency contraception should be offered to the patient if it is started within 72 hours of exposure, immediate dose may be given in the ED if available.
    - Postexposure treatment regimens are as follows:[12]
      - HIV postexposure prophylaxis: Emtricitabine/tenofovir disloproxil (Truvada) 200 mg/300 mg qd + raltegravir (Isentress) 400 mg qd OR dolutegravir (Tivicay) 50 mg qd
      - Chlamydia prophylaxis: Azithromycin 1 g × 1 dose; doxycycline 100 mg PO BID × 7
      - Gonorrhea prophylaxis: Ceftriaxone 250 mg IM × 1 dose
      - Trichomonas: Metronidazole 2 gm PO × 1 dose

- Pregnancy prevention: Three treatment options exist, may choose one of the following:[13]
    - Levanorgestrel (Plan B) 1.5 mg PO × 1 dose or 0.75 mg PO q12h × 1 d
    - Combined estrogen-progestin: Ethinyl estradiol 100 mcg + 0.5 mg levonorgestrel PO q12h × 1 d
    - Ulipristal acetate (Ella/Fibristal) 30 mg PO × 1 dose
    - Patients should be prescribed antiemetics for all emergency contraception regimens to ensure tolerability
- Hepatitis B:[6] Patients without known or documented hepatitis B immunity should be given hepatitis B vaccine and hepatitis B immune globulin if source patient is known to be infected with chronic hepatitis B or if hepatitis B status is unknown and vaccines are administered within 12 to 24 hours
- Baseline hepatitis B (baseline hepatitis B surface antibody, hepatitis B core antibody, and hepatitis B surface antigen) and hepatitis C (hepatitis C antibody) titer testing needed to guide future treatment and monitoring either in the ED or in close follow-up with a primary care provider

> **CLINICAL PEARL:** Serologic testing without rapid results should only be ordered from the ED if systems are in place to contact patients and provide results and clear follow-up instructions are available to avoid loss of follow-up with important testing information. If consistent follow-up cannot be assured, testing should be deferred to the health department or primary care provider to ensure appropriate follow-up and management of results.

- Patients should be referred to primary care providers, gynecologists, or other local health departments for comprehensive STI testing if unavailable in the ED.
- Patients should be advised to have repeat confirmatory testing 6 months from initial exposure.

Key Points . . .

- Careful history taking, including details of mechanism of injury, and thorough head-to-toe physical exam with complete exposure of your patient are essential.
- Life-threatening injuries involving airway, breathing, or circulatory compromise must be treated immediately, often in close consultation with trauma surgery for potential immediate operative management.

- Severe burn injuries may require transfer of care to designated burn centers upon stabilization to maximize care.
- Thorough neurovascular examination before and after reduction and splinting procedures is important to avoid limb-threatening complications. Patients at high risk for developing compartment syndrome should be admitted for frequent neurovascular examinations or given clear return-to-ED instructions for signs or symptoms of neurovascular complications.
- Proper initial wound care in the ED followed by detailed discharge and follow-up instructions for the patient are necessary to maximize healing and improve patient outcomes. Patients at high risk for developing wound infections (e.g., contaminated wound, history of immunocompromise) should be given prophylactic antibiotics as appropriate and clear follow-up instructions on wound checks and return-to-ED instructions for signs and symptoms of infection.
- Severe traumatic injury and certain high-risk injuries (e.g., facial, eye, hand) may require immediate consultation with specialists for management in the ED and to arrange close follow-up to avoid poor outcomes and long-term disability.
- It is important to consider patient safety (e.g., mobility, ambulation) and possible work or activity restrictions upon discharge.
- Patients who are victims of assault should be treated in an understanding, empathetic, nonjudgmental manner. It is important to ensure patient safety in the ED and upon disposition. Involvement of social workers, case managers, law enforcement, and other local organizations may be necessary.

REFERENCES

1. Rui P, Kang K. National hospital ambulatory medical care survey: 2014 emergency department summary tables. https://www.cdc.gov/nchs/data/nhamcs/web_tables/2014_ed_web_tables.pdf. Updated September 7, 2017.
2. Evans RW, Whitlow CT. Acute mild traumatic brain injury (concussion) in adults. In Aminoff MJ, Moreira ME, eds. *UpToDate*. https://www.uptodate.com/contents/acute-mild-traumatic-brain-injury-concussion-in-adults. Updated March 8, 2019.
3. Raja A, Zane RD. Initial management of trauma in adults. In Moreira ME, ed. *UpToDate*. https://www.uptodate.com/contents/initial-management-of-trauma-in-adults. Updated May 30, 2018.
4. Breiding M, Smith S, Basile K, et al. Prevalence and characteristics of sexual violence, stalking, and intimate partner violence victimization—National Intimate Partner and Sexual Violence Survey, United States, 2011. *MMWR Surveill Summ*. 2011;63(SS08):1–18. https://www.cdc.gov/mmwr/preview/mmwrhtml/ss6308a1.htm

5. Singer AJ, Hollander JE. Postrepair wound care. In: Tintinalli JE, Stapczynski J, Ma O, et al., eds. *Tintinalli's Emergency Medicine: A Comprehensive Study Guide.* 8th ed. New York, NY: McGraw-Hill 2016 :320–324.

6. Moreno-Walton L. Female and male sexual assault. In: Tintinalli JE, Stapczynski J, Ma O, et al, eds. *Tintinalli's Emergency Medicine: A Comprehensive Study Guide.* 8th ed. New York, NY: McGraw-Hill; 2016:1983–1987.

7. Lown B, Neuman J, Amarasingham R, Berkovits B. Comparison of alternating current with direct current electroshock across the closed chest. *Am J Cardiol.* 1962; 10:223–233. doi:10.1016/0002-9149(62)90299-0

8. Gale SC, Gracias VH, Reilly PM, Schwab CW. The inefficiency of plain radiography to evaluate the cervical spine after blunt trauma. *J Trauma.* 2005;59(5):1121–1125. doi:10.1097/01.ta.0000188632.79060.ba

9. Bailey C. Electrical and lightning injuries. In: Tintinalli JE, Stapczynski J, Ma O, et al., eds. *Tintinalli's Emergency Medicine: A Comprehensive Study Guide.* 8th ed. New York, NY: McGraw-Hill; 2016:1411–1418.

10. Hurlbert RJ, Hadley MN, Walters BC, et al. Pharmacological therapy for acute spinal cord injury. *Neurosurgery.* March 2013;72(suppl 3):93–105. doi:10.1227/NEU.0b013e31827765c6

11. American Academy of Emergency Medicine. Steroids in acute spine care injury. https://www.aaem.org/resources/statements/position/steroids-in-acute-spinal-care-injury. Published February 23, 2003.

12. Aberg JA, Daskalakis DC. Management of nonoccupational exposures to HIV and hepatitis B and C in adults. In: Bartlett JG, Sax PE, eds. *UpToDate.* https://www.uptodate.com/contents/management-of-nonoccupational-exposures-to-hiv-and-hepatitis-b-and-c-in-adults. Updated May 24, 2019.

2

Common Disease Entities in Emergency Medicine

Introduction

Although the emergency medicine (EM) rotation allows students to see a wide range of conditions from routine medical care to high-acuity conditions, there are disease states that are more commonly encountered than others. The most common disease entities you can expect to see on your EM rotation are presented in this chapter and grouped by a common presenting complaint.

1. Abdominal pain: Appendicitis, cholelithiasis, diverticulitis, ectopic pregnancy, gastritis/peptic ulcer disease, gastroenteritis, renal colic, urinary tract infection
2. Altered mental status: Diabetic ketoacidosis, hepatic encephalopathy, hypoglycemia, seizure
3. Chest pain: Acute coronary syndrome, aortic dissection, musculoskeletal chest pain, pericarditis, pneumothorax, pulmonary embolus
4. Dyspnea: Asthma, chronic obstructive pulmonary disease (COPD) exacerbation, heart failure, pneumonia, pulmonary edema
5. Headache: Acute angle-closure glaucoma, cerebrovascular accident, meningitis, migraine, temporal arteritis, tension type, traumatic brain injury
6. Low-back pain: Abdominal aortic aneurysm, compression fracture, epidural abscess, neoplasm, sciatica, thoracic/lumbar strain
7. Traumatic injury: Bite wounds, burns, foreign bodies, fracture, lacerations, joint dislocations, sprains and strains

ABDOMINAL PAIN

APPENDICITIS

Etiology
Fecalith (hard stool) is the most common cause of nonperforated appendicitis, leading to 65% of cases, followed by appendicoliths (calcified deposits).[1]

Epidemiology
Appendicitis is the most common cause of acute abdominal pain requiring operative intervention in patients younger than 50 years old.[1] Risk factors associated with appendicitis include male gender, White ethnicity, and age younger than 30 years old.

Clinical Presentation
The classic presentation of appendicitis is periumbilical pain with radiation into the right lower quadrant (RLQ) over McBurney's point. This evolution and migration of pain is a distinct feature of the disease. Patients who have inflammation at just the tip of the appendix may present with back pain or pelvic pain. Some cases may have additional positive symptoms of nausea, anorexia, or vomiting. Low-grade fever may be present. Physical exam findings may reveal tenderness over McBurney's point. Evaluate for signs of peritoneal irritation such as Blumberg's sign (rebound tenderness), Rovsing sign, obturator sign, and psoas sign. Referred rebound tenderness is noted if the patient has pain in the RLQ with removal of pressure in the left lower quadrant (LLQ). These patients often report that the ride into the ED was difficult because of the bumps in the road.

> **CLINICAL PEARL:** Tip appendicitis can be missed on imaging and should be considered if a patient presents with persistent pain despite administration of analgesic pain medication.

Diagnosis
The differential diagnosis of appendicitis is vast, especially in women, in whom reproductive pathologies can mimic appendicitis. The diagnosis should be suspected based on history and physical examination findings, and confirmed by laboratory investigation and imaging.

LABS
- Complete blood count (CBC): White blood cell (WBC) count alone cannot diagnose or exclude appendicitis, but if elevated, is suggestive of it.

- C-reactive protein (CRP) is a nonspecific marker for inflammation synthesized by the liver. Because of its lack of specificity, an elevated CRP can be seen in many other conditions causing inflammation or infection and is usually used to trend response to intervention or antibiotics. An elevated CRP (>8–10 mg/L) may be useful in predicting severity of disease and likelihood of complications.[1]
- Basic metabolic panel (BMP) should be ordered to evaluate for any electrolyte imbalances as a result of vomiting or diarrhea associated with the disease. Baseline liver function testing may be helpful if administering hepatically metabolized medications.
- Urinalysis allows for assessment of possible urinary tract infection, if clinically suggested.
- In women of reproductive age, a urine pregnancy test must be done to confirm pregnancy. Because ectopic pregnancy and appendicitis can mimic one another and the former is a life-threatening condition, it must be ruled out.

DIAGNOSTIC IMAGING
- Routine x-rays provide no benefit in the diagnosis of appendicitis.
- Ultrasound may confirm the diagnosis of appendicitis, while eliminating exposure to ionizing radiation and limiting the time to diagnosis.
- The diagnostic study of choice is a CT scan of the abdomen and pelvis with intravenous (IV) contrast to evaluate for appendicitis. CT is accurate and consistent in diagnosing appendicitis and decreasing the negative appendectomy rate.[1]

CT findings diagnostic of appendicitis may include any of the following: periappendiceal fat stranding, signs of a fecalith, acute tip luminal edema, and enlargement of the appendix.

Management

Once the diagnosis is confirmed, administer parenteral broad-spectrum and anaerobic antibiotics immediately. For nonperforated cases, recommendations include the following:

- Ciprofloxacin 400 mg IV + metronidazole 500 mg IV
- Levofloxacin 400 mg IV + metronidazole 500 mg IV
- Rocephin 1 g IV + metronidazole 500 mg IV

  For perforated appendicitis

- Piperacillin/tazobactam 3.375 mg IV
- Cefipime 2 gm IV
- Imipenem/cilastatin 500 mg IV

Definitive treatment depends on the extent of disease. Nonperforated appendicitis with no complications can be treated with antibiotic administration and percutaneous drainage through interventional radiology. The traditional model has been to administer IV antibiotics with surgical resection of the appendix. Perforated appendicitis requires operative intervention.

REFERENCES

1. Cole MA, Huang RD. Acute appendicitis. In: Walls RM, Hockberger RS, Gausche-Hill M, et al., eds. *Rosen's Emergency Medicine: Concepts and Clinical Practice*. 9th ed. Philadelphia, PA: Elsevier; 2018:1121–1127.
2. O'Brien MC. Acute abdominal pain. In: Tintinalli JE, Stapczynski J, Ma O, et al., eds. *Tintinalli's Emergency Medicine: A Comprehensive Study Guide*. 8th ed. New York, NY: McGraw-Hill; 2016: 481–488.

CHOLELITHIASIS/CHOLECYSTITIS

Etiology

Cholelithiasis refers to the presence of gallstones within the gallbladder. *Cholecystitis* refers to inflammation of the gallbladder, typically caused by obstructing gallstones.[1] This is more specifically referred to as *calculous chole-cystitis*. Gallstone formation is multifactorial and involves supersaturation of bile components, crystal nucleation, and gallbladder dysmotility.[1]

Epidemiology

In the United States, the prevalence of gallstones is 8% among men and 17% among women.[2] The prevalence increases with age and body mass. Patients who have undergone bariatric surgery with a resulting rapid weight change are also at risk for gallstone development. Frequently, patients who have gallstones do not exhibit symptoms until the gallstones cause an obstruction within the gallbladder or the bile duct.

Clinical Presentation

Symptoms of biliary colic are the most common presentation of gallstone disease.[1] Early cholecystitis may cause vague midline epigastric pain that progresses to sharp right upper quadrant (RUQ) pain as localized peritoneal irritation develops.[1] The timing of pain is typically gradual, steady, and often postprandial, occurring over several hours. Provoking factors include heavy, fatty meals. As the disease develops, patients may develop increased symptoms with less fatty meals. One of the physical findings synonymous with acute cholecystitis is a positive Murphy's sign, which is cessation of inspiration during deep palpation of the RUQ.[3]

Fever is usually absent in patients with biliary colic, but may be present in patients with acute cholecystitis. Jaundice in the setting of gallbladder disease typically indicates common bile duct obstruction from choledocolithiasis or extrinsic compression of the bile duct by an impacted cystic duct, gallbladder stone, or adjacent inflammation (Mirizzi's syndrome).[1]

> **CLINICAL PEARL:** Cholangitis is a more severe ascending infection involving the biliary tract. The classic presentation of cholangitis is Charcot's triad: fever, RUQ pain and jaundice, and patients who appear acutely ill.

Diagnosis

LABS

- Patients with classic biliary colic do not have abnormalities in laboratory testing.
- In the setting of acute cholecystitis, there may be evidence of leukocytosis, with WBC count higher than 10, 000 mm.^{3}
- Liver function tests, including bilirubin, aspartate aminotransferase (AST), and alanine aminotransferase (ALT), may be normal or elevated in acute cholecystitis but are more likely to be elevated in bile duct obstruction/acute choledocolithiasis. In order to rule out gallstone pancreatitis, a serum lipase should be ordered as well.

DIAGNOSTIC IMAGING

- The imaging modality of choice for acute cholecystitis is abdominal ultrasound, which has the advantages of a short study time, lack of ionizing radiation, and excellent sensitivity for gallstones.[1]
  - Findings on ultrasound suggestive of acute cholecystitis include gallbladder wall thickening, pericholecystic fluid, and evidence of gallstones or gallbladder sludge. The ultrasound reading from the technician may report a "positive sonographic Murphy's sign," which indicates cessation of inspiration when the ultrasound probe was used to image the gallbladder.
- A CT scan is insensitive for gallstones and is therefore usually reserved for exclusion of other diagnoses.
- Patients who display history and physical exam findings consistent with acute cholecystitis, but whose initial imaging studies demonstrate nonvisualization of the gallbladder, a hepatoiminodiacetic acid (HIDA) scan can facilitate the diagnosis. HIDA can also be helpful in diagnosing acalculous cholecystitis due to other causes.
- Magnetic resonance cholangiopancreatography (MRCP) is the study of choice to visualize the biliary tree.

Management

- Patients with asymptomatic gallstones do not require treatment and an elective cholecystectomy can be scheduled for a later time.
- Patients with biliary colic should undergo diet modification to avoid triggers, have pain management on an outpatient basis, and undergo elective cholecystectomy. ED management of biliary colic includes fluid hydration, administration of antiemetics such as ondansetron 4 mg IV every

4 hours, metaclopromide 10 mg IV, and nonsteroidal anti-inflammatory drugs (NSAIDS). Opioids may cause some degree of spasm of the sphincter of Oddi, but the resultant resolution of pain outweighs the minimal occurrence of sphincter spasm.

- Patients with acute cholecystitis should receive a surgical consult, as the treatment of choice is a laparoscopic cholecystectomy.[1] Antibiotics should be administered and include carbapenems, third- generation cephalosporins or a combination of metronidazole IV + flouroquinolone IV. Endoscopic retrograde cholangiopancreatography (ERCP) may be performed to decompress the gall bladder prior to removal.

- Cholangitis is a life-threatening emergency and requires urgent biliary decompression, aggressive parenteral fluid administration, pain management, and consultation with a gastrointestinal (GI) surgeon or gastroenterologist.

REFERENCES

1. Besinger B, Stehman C. Pancreatitis and cholecystitis. In: Tintinalli JE, Stapczynski J, Ma O, Yealy DM, Meckler GD, Cline DM, eds. *Tintinalli's Emergency Medicine: A Comprehensive Study Guide*. 8th ed. New York, NY: McGraw-Hill; 2016: 517–524

2. Goldman L, Schafer Al, eds. *Goldman–Cecil Medicine*. 25th ed., Vol 2. Philadelphia, PA: Elsevier Health Sciences; 2016.

3. O'Connell K, Brasel K. Bile metabolism and lithogenesis. *Surg Clin North Am.* 2014;94:361–375. doi:10.1016/j.suc.2014.01.004

DIVERTICULITIS

Etiology

Diverticulosis occurs when there is a protrusion of the colonic wall. When the area becomes inflamed and infected, this is referred to as *diverticulitis*. A true diverticulum involves all the layers of the colonic wall and a false diverticulum involves only the mucosal and submucosal layers.

Epidemiology

Diverticular disease is common in Western diets, and in patients who consume little dietary fiber. As the population ages, the incidence of diverticular disease increases. In most patients, diverticular disease is an incidental finding.[1]

Clinical Presentation

The clinical presentation of diverticulitis is divided into the uncomplicated variant and the complicated variant. This is relevant because it determines the treatment protocol. When abscess, phlegmon, microperforation, or bacterial translocation occur, the diverticulitis is considered to be complicated.[2]

The typical pain related to diverticulitis occurs in the LLQ, due to sigmoid involvement, but can be suprapubic in younger patients. In cases in which diverticular disease affects the ascending colon, the pain is often right sided.

For patients who present with RLQ pain, appendicitis must be ruled out. Associated symptoms include changes in bowel habits in the days leading up to presentation, such as diarrhea or constipation. Patients may also complain of fever, tenesmus, or urinary symptoms if the diverticulitis is proximal to the bladder.

> **CLINICAL PEARL:** If a patient presents with presumed diverticulitis and has vomiting as well, this suggests complication.[3]

Vital signs may reveal fever and tachycardia. Physical exam usually reveals tenderness in the LLQ; however, right-sided diverticulitis can occur. For patients with complications such as a bleed, there may be hemoccult-positive stool on rectal exam. Females of reproductive age with LLQ pain should undergo a pelvic exam to rule out tubo-ovarian abscess and ovarian cysts. A urine pregnancy test should be ordered to evaluate for ectopic pregnancy.

Diagnosis

LABS

- Urine pregnancy test if female of childbearing age
- CBC: Up to 45% of patients may have a normal WBC count, but an elevated WBC is suggestive of the diagnosis[3]
- For patients presenting with diarrhea and/or vomiting, a basic metabolic panel (BMP) should be done to rule out electrolyte imbalances, particularly hypokalemia
- Urinalysis may reveal a sterile pyuria, or the presence of WBCs in the absence of bacteria

DIAGNOSTIC IMAGING

- The diagnostic procedure of choice is a CT scan of the abdomen and pelvis with by mouth (PO) and IV contrast. Ensure the blood urea nitrogen (BUN)/creatinine is normal in these patients if IV contrast will be administered. If IV contrast is being used in a patient on metformin, he or she should be instructed to avoid taking it for 48 to 72 hours and aggressive fluid hydration should be maintained after IV contrast administration to prevent lactic acidosis.
- CT findings consistent with diverticulitis include bowel wall thickening, pericolic fat stranding, and possible microperforations or abscess formation if these complications are present.

Management

Treatment for diverticulitis depends on whether it is complicated or uncomplicated.

- In the setting of uncomplicated diverticulitis, patients should remain on a clear liquid diet and advance to a low-residue diet after 3 to 4 days.

Antibiotics should be administered with Gram-negative and anaerobic coverage. Metronidazole plus either a flouroquinolone or trimethoprim-sulfamethoxazole (TMP-SMX) combination therapy is recommended. Alternatively, moxifloxacin or amoxicillin–clavulanic acid can be used in a monotherapy approach. It may be reasonable to treat uncomplicated diverticulitis conservatively without antibiotics. These patients should be closely followed to monitor for resolution, with possible colonoscopy in 6 to 8 weeks.

- Patients with complicated diverticulitis should remain on nothing per os (NPO) status to promote bowel rest and receive aggressive parenteral fluid resuscitation and parenteral antibiotics. Monotherapy with piperacillin/tazobactam or imipenem can be initiated. The use of multiple agents, such as metronidazole plus flouroquinolone or third-generation cephalosporin, can be started as an alternative. These patients should not have colonoscopy for 6 to 8 weeks so as to avoid perforation during this acute time period. If there is evidence of complication, such as microperforation or abscess development, surgery or interventional radiology should be consulted to facilitate management.

References

1. Collins SP, Storrow AB. Acute heart failure. In: Tintinalli JE, Stapczynski J, Ma O, et al., eds. *Tintinalli's Emergency Medicine: A Comprehensive Study Guide.* 8th ed. New York, NY: McGraw-Hill; 2016: 366–372. http://accessmedicine.mhmedical.com/content.aspx?bookid=1658&sectionid=109428688

2. Morris AM, Regenbogen SC, Hardiman KM, et al. Sigmoid diverticulitis: a systematic review. *JAMA.* 2014;311:287. doi:10.1001/jama.2013.282025

3. McAninch S, Smithson CC, 3rd. Gastrointestinal emergencies. In: Stone C, Humphries RL, eds. *Current Diagnosis & Treatment: Emergency Medicine.* 8th ed. New York, NY: McGraw-Hill; 2017: 597–635. http://accessmedicine.mhmedical.com/content.aspx?bookid=2172&sectionid=165065027

Ectopic Pregnancy

Etiology

An ectopic pregnancy occurs when an embryo implants outside of the uterine cavity. The fallopian tubes are a common site of implantation. Inflammatory insults, such as previous sexually transmitted infections, and prior surgical manipulation can be contributing factors.

Epidemiology

Risk factors include a history of ectopic pregnancy, history of pelvic inflammatory disease (PID), surgical history significant for tubal ligation or tubal sterilization, and confirmed conception despite having an intrauterine device. Patients with advanced maternal age between 35 and 44 are at higher risk, as are those who have had previous induced abortions. According to the Centers for Disease Control and Prevention (CDC), ectopic pregnancy is a leading cause of maternal death in the first trimester of pregnancy.[1]

Clinical Presentation

The most common symptom of ectopic pregnancy is abdominal pain or discomfort.[2] The pain is often located in the lower pelvic region and is unilateral, sharp, and severe. Patients may also present with vaginal bleeding in the absence of abdominal pain. Syncope can also be present in ectopic pregnancy and should be considered in a patient of childbearing age.

It is important to closely monitor the blood pressure (BP) and heart rate of patients of childbearing age presenting with acute abdominal pain. Patients with ectopic pregnancy may decompensate quickly and become hypotensive or tachycardic in the setting of rupture. A thorough abdominal and pelvic exam should be performed. On pelvic exam, you may appreciate unilateral adnexal tenderness or a mass along with blood at the cervical os. The cervical os may also have a characteristic blue appearance to it, which is a normal finding in patients who are pregnant. It is difficult to diagnose ectopic pregnancy based on physical exam alone. The combination of a suggestive history, a positive urine pregnancy test, and physical exam findings should facilitate the differential diagnosis.

Diagnosis

Pregnancy tests are performed using urine beta-human chorionic gonadotropin (beta-HCG). It can be detected as early as 1 week prior to an expected menstrual cycle. A beta-HCG is considered positive when the concentration is greater than or equal to 20 mIU/mL in the urine and greater than or equal to 10 mIU/mL in serum. A positive test implies that beta-HCG is present. Table 2.1 provides an overview of beta-HCG levels after conception.[3] Ectopic pregnancy is commonly diagnosed between 6 and 10 weeks' gestation.

TABLE 2.1 Beta-Human Chorionic Gonadotropin Levels After Conception

Postconception Week	Beta-HCG Levels (mIU/mL)
<1 week	5–50
2–3 weeks	100–5,000
4–5 weeks	1,000–50,000
6–8 weeks	15,000–200,000
8–12 weeks	10,000–100,000

Beta-HCG, human chorionic gonadotropin.
Source: Heaton HA. Ectopic pregnancy and emergencies in the first 20 weeks of pregnancy. In: Tintinalli JE, Stapczynski J, Ma O, et al., eds. *Tintinalli's Emergency Medicine: A Comprehensive Study Guide.* 8th ed. New York, NY: McGraw-Hill; 2016:628–635. http://accessmedicine.mhmedical.com/content.aspx?bookid=1658§ionid= 109434141

If a urine pregnancy test is negative at bedside but ectopic pregnancy is still suspected, then perform a quantitative serum pregnancy test. Confirmation should still be performed by ultrasound. Vaginal examination in stable women presenting with first-trimester bleeding may add little to the clinical diagnosis; some providers are moving away from routine use of vaginal examinations in the initial patient assessment as long as transvaginal ultrasound can be obtained.[4]

> **CLINICAL PEARL:** If pregnancy is detected, ectopic pregnancy must remain in the differential diagnosis until it can be either confirmed or excluded with conviction.[3]

Diagnosis is made when there is an embryo visualized outside of the uterus. Some terms for ultrasound findings that may be documented include any of the following to confirm diagnosis: *confirmed pelvic mass or free pelvic fluid in the setting of an empty uterus, combination of an echogenic adnexal mass with free fluid in the setting of an empty uterus*, an *extrauterine gestational sac*.[3]

> **CLINICAL PEARL:** It is possible to have an ectopic pregnancy in addition to intrauterine pregnancy, which is referred to as heterotropic pregnancy. This is rare in natural conception cycles.

Management

The treatment for an ectopic pregnancy in the ED setting includes:

- Stabilization of the patient. Place two large-bore V lines; keep the patient on NPO status) in case she requires surgery; obtain blood work, including type and screen; and consult the OB/GYN team as soon as possible.
- Decide whether or not the patient can be medically managed or requires surgical treatment. This is a decision made by the OB/GYN team.
- The most common medical approach for patients with unruptured stable ectopic pregnancy is administration of methotrexate. Methotrexate can be administered as an intramuscular (IM) injection or as a direct injection into the ectopic gestational sac. Contraindications to methotrexate administration include
  - Peptic ulcer disease; active pulmonary disease; renal or hepatic dysfunction; breastfeeding; hemodynamic instability; cytopenias, including low WBC, hemoglobin (HGB), hematocrit (HCT) or platelets; evidence of an intrauterine pregnancy (IUP); or immunocompromised status.
  - Patients should receive instructions that stomatitis and/or abdominal pain can persist for up to 1 week following administration.
- The most common surgical approach is to perform a laparoscopic salpingostomy.
- If the patient is hemodynamically unstable, the treatment of choice is laparotomy.
- Regardless of treatment approach, beta-HCG levels should be followed every 48 hours until they are nondetectable.
- Both the American College of Emergency Physicians (ACEP) and American College of Obstetricians and Gynecologists (ACOG) recommend treatment with 50 mcg of RhoGAM for Rh-negative women

with ectopic pregnancy when diagnosed prior to 12 weeks' gestation due to the small volume of red cells in the fetoplacental circulation.[3]

REFERENCES

1. Centers for Disease Control and Prevention. Ectopic pregnancy—United States, 1990–1992. *JAMA*. 1995;273:533. doi:10.1001/jama.1995.03520310027023

2. Clayton HB, Schieve LA, Peterson HB, et al. Ectopic pregnancy risk with assisted reproductive technology procedures. *Obstet Gynecol*. 2006;107:595. doi:10.1097/01.AOG.0000196503.78126.62

3. Heaton HA. Ectopic pregnancy and emergencies in the first 20 weeks of pregnancy. In: Tintinalli JE, Stapczynski J, Ma O, et al., eds. *Tintinalli's Emergency Medicine: A Comprehensive Study Guide*. 8th ed. New York, NY: McGraw-Hill; 2016:628–635. http://accessmedicine.mhmedical.com/content.aspx?bookid=1658&sectionid=109 434141

4. Johnstone C. Vaginal examination does not improve diagnostic accuracy in early pregnancy bleeding. *Emerg Med Aust*. 2013;25:219. doi:10.1111/1742-6723.12068

GASTRITIS/PEPTIC ULCER DISEASE

Etiology

Gastritis is defined as chronic gastric mucosal inflammation that has various etiologies. If acute in presentation, it can occur as a result of overeating or as alcoholic gastritis. Peptic ulcer disease (PUD) is a chronic illness manifested by recurrent ulcerations in the stomach and proximal duodenum.[1] The majority of PUDs is related directly to *Helicobacter pylori* infection or use of NSAIDs.[2]

Epidemiology

Uncomplicated PUD has an incidence of more than five cases per 1,000 persons per year, and about 10% of people living in the Western world will experience a peptic ulcer at some point during their lives.[3,4] Risk factors for PUD not related to NSAID use or *H. pylori* infection include stress, use of antiplatelet agents, cytomegalovirus, Crohn's colitis, Zollinger-Ellison syndrome (ZES), cirrhosis with portal hypertension (HTN), older age, and African American ethnicity.[2]

Clinical Presentation

Patients often present with burning epigastric pain. Specific historical components to inquire about include sharp or dull pain, the sense of a "hunger pang" feeling, and relief or worsening of pain with antacids or food. Patients with gastritis may present with epigastric pain and nausea/vomiting but the most common presentation is GI bleed.[2]

PUD includes both gastric and duodenal ulcers. A gastric ulcer typically manifests with pain 1 to 2 hours postprandially and patients may be afraid to eat. Pain due to a duodenal ulcer generally subsides with eating, but returns 2 to 3 hours postprandially. A duodenal ulcer may also wake the patient up at night. Symptoms of both gastric and duodenal ulcers typically recur over weeks to months.

Physical exam may reveal epigastric tenderness, but can also be normal. If there is evidence of perforation, this will cause a rigid abdomen, often with tachycardia and fever. If hemoccult-positive blood is present on rectal exam, there should be high suspicion of a bleeding ulcer, in which case patients may also report melena.

Diagnosis
Labs and Diagnostic Imaging

- Due to the frequency of GI bleeding, decreased HGB and HCT and hemoccult-positive stool is often seen with gastritis and ulcers.
- The gold standard for diagnosing PUD is by upper GI endoscopy.[1]
- Because infection due to *H. pylori* has been implicated in the development of PUD, testing for the pathogen can be done through endoscopic testing or through a rapid urease test, urea breath test, and stool antigen test. The latter two are less invasive.
- An EKG should be done in the ED to rule out a cardiac etiology for the patient's pain.

Management

The goal of managing PUD is to heal the ulcer, manage symptoms, and prevent further complications. If the PUD is related to NSAID use, patients should be instructed to discontinue the offending agent. Therapy is usually multimodal with the use of H2 blockers, proton-pump inhibitors (PPIs), or antacids. Sucralfate is also a useful agent. In the ED setting, giving patients a trial of a PPI or H2 blocker and then referring them to a GI specialist or primary care provider for further investigation is the appropriate management. If treatment of *H. pylori* is indicated, patients should receive the triple therapy approach: PPI + clarithromycin + amoxicillin or metronidazole for 10 to 14 days. The treatment of gastritis is similar and centers around reducing stomach acid, healing inflammation, and avoiding triggers.

Clinical Pearl: If there is high clarithromycin resistance, patients may require a quadruple therapy with documentation of appropriate follow-up.[1]

When discharging patients home with a diagnosis of PUD or gastritis, advise them to avoid potential trigger foods and avoid NSAID use if that was implicated in the diagnosis. As patients' symptoms improve, they may wish to discontinue medication. If antibiotics were given for the potential eradication of *H. pylori*, it is important to tell them not to discontinue the antibiotics but rather complete the course regardless of symptom eradication. Patients should also receive instructions to return for signs of perforation such as tachycardia, fever, worsening pain despite intervention, vomiting to the point where they are unable to tolerate PO intake, and blood in the stool.

REFERENCES

1. Gratton MC, Bogle A. Peptic ulcer disease and gastritis. In: Tintinalli JE, Stapczynski J, Ma O, et al., eds. *Tintinalli's Emergency Medicine: A Comprehensive Study Guide.* 8th ed. New York, NY: McGraw-Hill; 2016:514–516. http://accessmedicine.mhmedical.com/content.aspx?bookid=1658&sectionid=109 430430 Accessed July 25, 2019.

2. Mendelson M. Esophageal emergencies. In: Tintinalli JE, Stapczynski J, Ma O, et al., eds. *Tintinalli's Emergency Medicine: A Comprehensive Study Guide.* 8th ed. New York, NY: McGraw-Hill; 2016:508–513.

3. Banerjee S, Cash BD, Dominitz JA, et al. The role of endoscopy in the management of patients with peptic ulcer disease. *Gastrointest Endosc.* 2010:71–663. doi:10.1016/j.gie.2009.11.026

4. Barkun A, Leontiadis G. Systematic review of the symptom burden, quality of life impairment and costs associated with peptic ulcer disease. *Am J Med.* 2010;123:358. doi:10.1016/j.amjmed.2009.09.031

GASTROENTERITIS

Etiology

Inflammation of the stomach and intestines that manifests as vomiting and diarrhea, typically due to viral or bacterial etiology, is known as *gastroenteritis*. The most common cause is viral with the most common virus being norovirus. Others include rotavirus and enteric adenovirus. Bacterial etiologies typically have a more severe clinical presentation with the most common being *Salmonella*, which is found in ground turkey, chicken, eggs, and romaine lettuce.

Epidemiology

The CDC estimates that foodborne diseases cause one in six Americans to get sick, leading to 128,000 hospitalizations and 3,000 deaths in the United States each year.[1,2]

Clinical Presentation

Patients usually present with symptoms of vomiting (nonbloody), frequent watery diarrhea, and fever. There may also be report of other household members with the same symptoms. Ask about recent travel, camping and hiking, eating out at public venues or restaurants, and contact with food handlers. If there are children in the house, ask whether they go to day care. Determine whether there is any potential for immunocompromised status such as long-term steroid use, HIV infection, cancer with chemotherapy administration, or other immunosuppressive disorders. Inquire whether the patient has been able to tolerate any oral intake in order to get an idea of the patient's disease severity.

Be sure to evaluate and document signs and symptoms of dehydration. Physical examination should note any of the following, if present:

General: Evaluate for acute distress

Vital signs: Tachycardia, fever, hypotension

Skin: Poor turgor, jaundice

Head, eyes, ears, nose, and throat (HEENT): Conjunctival pallor, dry mucous membranes

Abdomen: Mild tenderness to the abdomen throughout the quadrants, hypoactive bowel sounds

Diagnosis

Gastroenteritis is typically a diagnosis of exclusion, and most patients do not require diagnostic testing. The history and clinical presentation are usually sufficient to make the diagnosis. In some cases, a CBC and BMP can be sent to evaluate for potential blood loss and electrolyte disturbances. An elevated WBC count does not require further imaging or studies as this may be expected with an acute infectious process. Routine stool culture is not indicated. If patients are undergoing chemotherapy, or are immunocompromised, stool culture and sensitivity may be considered.

Management

- Most patients with gastroenteritis can be managed with supportive treatment. This includes aggressive parenteral fluid resuscitation, administration of antiemetics if there is vomiting, and acetaminophen for fever.
- Use of antimotility agents is not recommended as most cases are caused by viruses, and this can prolong the illness.
- The use of empiric antibiotic therapy is not typically recommended. If patients are immunocompromised or require hospitalization due to volume depletion, they may receive ciprofloxacin 500 mg twice daily or levofloxacin 500 mg once daily for 3 to 5 days.[3] An alternative agent is azithromycin 500 mg once daily for 3 days.[3]
- Patients are stable to go home once they can tolerate PO fluid intake with a PO fluid challenge in the ED, vital signs are stable, and patients report improved symptoms.
- Upon discharge, recommend the banana/bread, rice, applesauce, toast (BRAT) diet and fluid hydration with the use of a glucose-containing fluid such as Pedialyte.
- If others in the house are infected, cleaning household items, such as toys and door knobs, with a mild bleach solution or cleaning wipes is recommended.
- Patients should be instructed to return to the ED if they have continued fever, are unable to tolerate PO intake, have increased abdominal pain, or altered mental status.

REFERENCES

1. Schar RL. Economic burden from health losses due to foodborne illness in the United States. *J Food Prot.* 2012;75:123–131. doi:10.4315/0362-028X.JFP-11-058

2. Centers for Disease Control and Prevention. Incidence and trends of infection with pathogens transmitted commonly through food–Foodborne Diseases Active Surveillance Network, 10 U.S. Sites, 1996-2012. *MMWR Morb Mortal Wkly Rep.* 2013;62:283.https://www.cdc.gov/mmwr/preview/mmwrhtml/mm6215a2.htm

3. Mendelson M. Esophageal emergencies. In: Tintinalli JE, Stapczynski J, Ma O, et al., eds. *Tintinalli's Emergency Medicine: A Comprehensive Study Guide.* 8th ed. New York, NY: McGraw-Hill; 2016:508–513.

GASTROESOPHAGEAL REFLUX DISEASE

Etiology

Gastroesophageal reflux disease (GERD) occurs secondary to reflux of gastric contents into the esophagus. The primary etiology is a transient relaxation of the lower esophageal sphincter (LES) with normal tone in between periods of relaxation.[1]

Epidemiology

Patients who are prone to GERD include those with decreased esophageal motility, such as those with diabetes mellitus and scleroderma, in addition to those with prolonged gastric emptying, such as those with diabetic gastroparesis. Dietary factors can lead to decreased pressure of the LES . These include a high-fat diet, alcohol, caffeine, and pregnancy. Medications can also contribute, including nitrates, calcium channel blockers, estrogens, and anticholinergics.

Clinical Presentation

The classic symptom of GERD is heartburn. However, patients can also present with chest discomfort, midepigastric abdominal pain radiating bilaterally, nausea, excess eructation, dysphagia, and odynophagia. For patients who present with a persistent dry cough, GERD should be considered. GERD symptoms can mimic cardiac chest pain with symptoms of diaphoresis, pallor, nausea, vomiting, and radiation of pain down the arms. Therefore, a cautious approach is warranted.[2]

Diagnosis

The diagnosis of GERD is primarily clinical. An outpatient endoscopy can be done for patients who continue to have symptoms despite intervention, or to rule out other gastroesophageal etiologies of symptoms. GERD is a diagnosis of exclusion in the ED. Therefore, an EKG and test of cardiac enzymes should be considered depending on the presentation to rule out a cardiac cause of the symptoms.

Management

The treatment of GERD is multifactorial, including diet and lifestyle modifications. In addition to staying upright after a meal, avoid sleeping for at least 3 hours after eating, and sleeping with the head of the bed elevated 30 degrees. Patients should be advised to keep a diary of symptoms and potential triggers, such as caffeine, nicotine, alcohol, fatty foods, and chocolate. Antacids or an H2 blocker may be recommended initially, but PPIs arethe mainstay of therapy.[2]

REFERENCES

1. Manthey DE, Nicks BA. Urological stone disease. In: Tintinalli JE, Stapczynski J, Ma O, et al., eds. *Tintinalli's Emergency Medicine: A Comprehensive Study Guide.* 8th ed. New York, NY: McGraw–Hill; 2016:609–612.
2. Scales CD, Smith A, Hanley JM, et al. Prevalence of kidney stones in the United States. *Eur Urol.* 2012;62:160. doi:10.1016/j.eururo.2012.03.052

RENAL COLIC

Etiology

Nephrolithiasis is the existence of stones in the urinary system. The pain with which the patient presents is defined as *renal colic* (similar to biliary colic in patients with gallstones).

Renal colic occurs when a renal calcification develops and attempts to pass through the ureter. Pain occurs when the stone interacts with a narrow part of the ureter or a junction (i.e., ureterovesicular junction). The majority of renal stones are calcium oxalate, making up 80% of stone composition.[1]

Medications that have been implicated in the development of nephrolithiasis include the protease inhibitor indinavir, used to treat HIV, and the carbonic anhydrase inhibitor, triamterene. Laxative abuse can also lead to renal stone development.

Epidemiology

Renal stones are more common in men compared to women with a prevalence of 10.6% to 7.1%.[2] Renal stone development is strongly associated with obesity and diabetes. Risk factors for nephrolithiasis include low urine volume, excess dietary meat and sodium, metabolic syndrome, a family history of nephrolithiasis, gout, and prolonged immobilization.[1]

Clinical Presentation

Renal colic is described as sudden-onset, sharp or "knifelike" pain that is intermittent. It typically originates in the flank with radiation to the groin. Patients struggle to find a position of comfort and may have guarding. Half of patients will have associated nausea and vomiting.[1] Eighty-five percent of patients may also have associated hematuria.[1]

> **CLINICAL PEARL:** Abdominal aortic aneurysm presentation can mimic renal colic.[1]

Diagnosis

The diagnosis of renal colic is primarily clinical and is supported by the presence of hematuria.

LABS

- Order a urine pregnancy test in all women of childbearing age.
- Urinalysis should be ordered to confirm hematuria and to evaluate for the presence of infection.
- Check a BMP to evaluate for renal function.

DIAGNOSTIC IMAGING

- The imaging study of choice is the noncontrast helical CT scan. Imaging not only confirms the diagnosis but also allows for evaluation of ureteral obstruction, evidence of pyelonephritis such as perinephric stranding, assessment of the size of the stone to determine interventional treatment, and for assessment of renal parenchyma.

> **CLINICAL PEARL:** Stones produced by indinavir are radiolucent on plain x-ray and CT scan, making the diagnosis difficult.

- Approximately 90% of urinary calculi are radiopaque because calcium phosphate and calcium oxalate stones have a density similar to that of bone.[1] As a result, a plain film is not recommended to identify a stone but can be used to track a stone once it has been identified on CT scan.
- Ultrasound can be used, but if a stone is less than 5 mm in diameter, it may be missed.

Management

The goal of treatment for patients suffering from renal colic is primarily to manage symptoms.

- Patients should receive IV fluid hydration due to limited oral intake and also to support rehydration in the setting of vomiting.
- NSAIDs are the primary choice in pain relief and can be administered parenterally in the form of ketorolac 30 mg IV. NSAIDS should not be used if patients have hypersensitivity, coagulopathy, or use aspirin or other anticoagulants.
- For patients who may not have relief with NSAIDs alone, hydromorphone 0.5 to 2.0 mg or morphine 1 to 4 mg can be used, but with caution due to opiate effects.

- For nausea and vomiting, metoclopramide can be given 10 mg IV.[1] Ondansetron 4 mg IV can also be given and may be less sedating.
- Alpha-blockers have been documented to facilitate stone expulsion, specifically for stones in the distal third of the ureter.[1] Agents include tamsulosin 0.4 mg by mouth once daily, terazosin 5 to 10 mg once daily, or doxazosin 4 mg once daily.
- If there is evidence of associated urinary tract infection, patients can be treated with gentamycin or tobramycin IV. Piperacillin–tazobactam IV is used if the patient is being admitted. If patients are stable for discharge, they can receive a flouroquinolone. In cases of high-grade obstruction and infection, the patient will require urgent stenting.
- Discharge instructions should include taking medications as needed for pain and encouragingoral fluid hydration. Send patients home with a urine strainer to catch the stone for analysis, and follow-up with a urologist. Reasons to return to the ED include symptoms of vomiting in which the patient is unable to tolerate oral intake, development of fever or frank hematuria, or pain not relieved with oral medications.

References

1. Manthey DE, Nicks BA. Urological stone disease. In: Tintinalli JE, Stapczynski J, Ma O, et al., eds. *Tintinalli's Emergency Medicine: A Comprehensive Study Guide*. 8th ed. New York, NY: McGraw-Hill; 2016:609–612.
2. Scales CD, Smith A, Hanley JM, et al. Prevalence of kidney stones in the United States. *Eur Urol.* 2012;62:160. doi:10.1016/j.eururo.2012.03.052

Urinary Tract Infection

Etiology

Infections of the urinary tract are defined and identified by their anatomical location. Infection of the urethra is described as urethritis in males and a urinary tract infection (UTI) in females. When the infection ascends to the bladder, it is referred to as *cystitis*. Further ascent into the renal system involving the upper urinary tract (ureters and kidneys) is known as *pyelonephritis*. Due to its increased frequency in presentation, this section only covers uncomplicated UTIs. The most common pathogen implicated in the development of a UTI in adults is *Escherichia coli*. Over the course of the past 30 years, community-acquired β-lactamase-producing *E. coli* has emerged as a small but growing source of antibiotic resistance in UTI.[1,2]

Clinical Pearl: Complicated UTI/cystitis is infection involving a functional or anatomically abnormal urinary tract or infection in the presence of comorbidities that place the patient at risk for more serious adverse outcomes or if a patient has not responded to recent treatment on an outpatient basis.[3]

Epidemiology

In 2010, UTI was the sixth most common diagnosis in women aged 15 to 64 years and the fourth most common diagnosis in women aged 65 years and older presenting to the ED.[4] UTI is more common in women compared to men. After the age of 66, the incidence increases in men due to prostatic hypertrophy and the use of instrumentation in elderly men.[4]

Clinical Presentation

Symptoms of a UTI include dysuria, urinary frequency, urgency, and hematuria. Because the female urethra is shorter in comparison to the male anatomy, recurrence is a concern. Ask whether patients have been treated for UTI in the past, how long ago it was, and what antibiotic was given. If the patient was treated within the past month, a different agent may be preferable.

In obtaining a sexual history, ask whether the patient urinates immediately following intercourse with vaginal penetration as that is a risk factor for UTI. Document any history of sexually transmitted infections (STIs) as *Chlamydia* can cause UTI. In young males, urethritis presents as dysuria with urethral discharge.

Cystitis symptoms include frequency, urgency, hematuria, and suprapubic tenderness. Fever is not typically present with cystitis. Older patients with urosepsis often present with fever, tachycardia, increased respiratory rate. Labs often show leukocytosis on CBC along with a positive urinalysis. Patients may present from long-term-care facilities, have recently had instrumentation, or have a history of being bedbound for an extended period of time.

> **CLINICAL PEARL:** Consider UTI in an elderly patient with acute mental status changes.

Diagnosis

A clinical diagnosis of uncomplicated UTI can be made based on history in the absence of vaginal discharge, no other risk factors for alternative diagnoses, and no recurrence.[5] Diagnosis of a UTI can be confirmed with either a urine dipstick or urinalysis. The urine specimen obtained for the sample should be midstream and clean catch. A catheterized specimen should be obtained from patients who are unable to provide an uncontaminated specimen. UTI often results in a positive test for protein, leukocyte esterase, and nitrites. A urine culture is not generally required for patients with a positive urinalysis or urine dipstick test. A culture is recommended for patients who have complicated UTI, are pregnant, adult males, patients with recurring symptoms despite treatment, and patients who are septic.[3]

Management

Treatment is typically initiated based on

- The patient's history of previous infections, comorbidities, the cost of antibiotics, and the development of antibiotic resistance in the geographic location.
- For adult females with uncomplicated UTI/cystitis, the first-line treatment is nitrofurantoin 100 mg twice daily × 5 days or trimethoprim–sulfamethoxazole (TMP–SMX) DS (160/800 mg) twice daily × 3 days. Patients may also be given fosfomycin 3 g in a single dose if available or pivmecillinam 400 mg twice daily × 5 days.[3]
- If patients have uncomplicated urethritis, the recommendation is ceftriaxone 250 mg IM + azithromycing 1 g.
- If the patient is penicillin-allergic, give doxycycline 100 mg twice daily × 7 days.
- Patients with complicated cystitis can receive a flouroquinolone (ciprofloxacin 500 mg twice daily × 7 days or levofloxacin 750 mg once daily × 5 days). If the subsequent urine culture shows sensitivity to either TMP–SMX or amoxicillin–clavulanate, they can be switched to those medications.

REFERENCES

1. Doi Y, Park YS, Rivera JI, et al. Community-associated extended-spectrum β-lactamase–producing *Escherichia coli* infection in the United States. *Clin Infect Dis.* 2013;56:641. doi:10.1093/cid/cis942
2. Meier S, Weber R, Zbinden R, et al. Extended-spectrum β-lactamase producing gramnegative pathogens in community-acquired urinary tract infections: an increasing challenge for antimicrobial therapy. *Infection.* 2011;39:333. doi:10.1007/s15010-011-0132-6
3. Askew K. Urinary tract infections and hematuria. In: Tintinalli JE, Stapczynski J, Ma O, et al., eds. *Tintinalli's Emergency Medicine: A Comprehensive Study Guide.* 8th ed. New York, NY: McGraw-Hill; 2016:589–596.
4. Dielubanza EJ, Schaeffer AJ. Urinary tract infections in women. *Med Clin N Am.* 2011;95:27. doi:10.1016/j.mcna.2010.08.023
5. Grabe M, Bartoletti R, Bjerkland Johansen TE, et al. Guidelines on urological infections. Arnhem, Netherlands: European Association of Urology; 2015. https://uroweb.org/wp-content/uploads/19-Urological-infections_LR2.pdf

ALTERED MENTAL STATUS

DIABETIC KETOACIDOSIS

Etiology

Diabetic ketoacidosis (DKA) is a life-threatening emergency and a complication of diabetes mellitus (DM) characterized by hyperglycemia, excess ketone bodies, and resultant metabolic acidosis. Factors that lead to the development of DKA include noncompliance with insulin, new onset of DM, infection, pregnancy, stroke, acute myocardial infarction (MI) or pulmonary embolism (PE), major trauma, or surgery.

> **CLINICAL PEARL:** DKA should be in the differential diagnosis of any patient who presents with altered mental status acutely. A quick fasting blood glucose test at bedside can facilitate immediate diagnosis and intervention.

Epidemiology

DKA primarily occurs in individuals with type 1/insulin-dependent patients but 10% to 30% of new-onset cases occur in type 2 patients.[1] Between 1993 and 2003, the yearly rate of U.S. ED visits for DKA was 64 per 10,000 with a trend toward an increased rate of visits among the African American population compared with the Caucasian population.[1]

> **CLINICAL PEARL:** DKA can be the first presentation in a patient not known to have DM.

Clinical Presentation

The clinical presentation of DKA can vary from polydipsia, polyuria, and lethargy, to abdominal pain, vomiting, and altered mental status. Patients will display any physical exam findings consistent with dehydration such as skin turgor, dry mucous membranes, tachycardia, and/or hypotension. Hypothermia may also be noted due to decreased peripheral circulation. The manifestations of electrolyte disturbances due to DKA can manifest as abdominal pain, vomiting, EKG changes (i.e., flattened T waves with hypokalemia), subjective dyspnea, and altered mental status.

Diagnosis

The diagnosis of DKA requires all of the following:[1]

- Blood glucose >250 mg/dL
- Anion gap >10 mEq/L
- Bicarbonate level <15 mEq/L
- pH <7.3
- (+) moderate ketones noted in the blood or serum

Check serum ketones; venous or arterial pH; BMP (with particular attention to potassium and bicarbonate levels); serum anion gap; and urinalysis, including ketones. Obtain an EKG to check for signs of electrolyte disturbance. If the patient has DKA secondary to an infectious insult, send blood cultures and urine cultures as well.

> **CLINICAL PEARL:** As DKA is often precipitated by an infectious or metabolic insult, be sure to search for a potential cause.

Management

These patients should receive, at minimum, two large-bore IV lines if not central access. Without waiting for laboratory results, obtain a fast bedside blood glucose level and, if noted to be elevated, initiate aggressive fluid hydration. Goals of treatment in DKA include

- Improvement of circulatory volume and tissue perfusion, reduction of serum glucose and osmolality, correction of electrolyte abnormalities, and resolution of ketosis.
- Patients with DKA have a profound fluid deficit. They should receive 1 to 1.5 L during the first hour using either normal saline (NS) or ½ NS. After 2 hours, change fluid based on hydration, electrolytes, and urine output. Change to 0.45% NS 150 to 300 mL/hour until glucose is less than 250 mg/dL.
- Insulin should be given as a 0.1 unit/kg bolus IV then a continuous infusion at 0.1 unit/kg/hr. A decrease in glucose of 50 to 70 mg/hr should be targeted. Decreasing glucose too fast can precipitate the accumulation of cerebral edema, which has been documented more frequently in children than adults. When glucose reaches 200 mg/dL, fluid should be changed to D5 ½ NS and insulin decreased.
- Insulin should not be started until potassium is greater than 3.3 mEq/L, as insulin administration can drive potassium into the cell. In the setting of hyperkalemia, fluid and insulin alone should allow for serum potassium to normalize as it will migrate back into the intracellular space. Correct the potassium derangement carefully because the rapid change can lead to hypokalemia, which is an acute concern during this treatment course. IV KCl 20 mEq can be added to each liter of IV fluid and continued until K+ >4. Maintain K+ at less than 5 mEq/L.
- Check glucose every hour and BMP every 1 to 2 hours until stable, then q4 x 24h.
- DKA is resolved when glucose ≤200 mg/dL, bicarbonate ≥18 mmol/L, anion gap is ≤12, and venous pH ≥7.3.[1]
- Giving bicarbonate is not required in treating DKA as the goal is to treat the underlying insult.

REFERENCE

1. Nyce AL, Lubkin CL, Chansky ME. Diabetic ketoacidosis. In: Tintinalli JE, Stapczynski J, Ma O, et al., eds. *Tintinalli's Emergency Medicine: A Comprehensive Study Guide.* 8th ed. New York, NY: McGraw-Hill; 2016:1457–1463. http://accessmedicine.mhmedical.com/content.aspx?bookid=1658&sectionid=109443771

HEPATIC ENCEPHALOPATHY

Etiology

Encephalopathy, a general term for brain dysfunction, is the hallmark of liver disease.[1] The etiology can be varied, related to infection, liver failure, or cirrhosis, but the pathology is not completely understood. The symptoms of mental-status change occur in part due to the accumulation of neurotoxic agents that bypass the liver, such as ammonia.

Epidemiology

Hepatic encephalopathy is most common in those with advanced liver disease, particularly those with cirrhosis. Hepatic encephalopathy occurs more often in patients with chronic hepatitis, history of transfusions, positive HIV status, frequent use of pain medications (as they are liver metabolized), type 2 diabetes mellitus, and hyperlipidemia (as they are related to nonalcoholic steatohepatitis [NASH]).[1] Additional potential causes include alcohol, infections, exposure to the hepatitis virus variants, and use of certain medications that are liver metabolized such as isoniazid, phenytoin, and acetaminophen.

Clinical Presentation

Signs and symptoms involve cognition, behavior, and neuromuscular function. Historical findings range from impaired concentration and confusion, to drowsiness, somnolence, and ultimately coma. Neuromuscular impairment starts with tremor and apraxia, and progresses to dysarthria, asterixis, hyper- or hyporeflexia, and ultimately decerebrate posturing.

When a patient presents with altered mental status in addition to jaundice, nausea, vomiting, evidence of coagulopathy, (excess bruising or bleeding) consider liver disease as a possible etiology.

Diagnosis

Because liver disease can manifest in nearly every system, the physical exam findings that can facilitate diagnosis are many:

General: Patients may appear cachectic

Skin: Look for jaundice due to elevated bilirubin or evidence of easy bruising due to coagulopathy and forcutaneous spider nevi

Head, eyes, ears, nose, and throat (HEENT): Look for scleral icterus due to jaundice

Cardiovascular/pulmonary: Increased jugular venous distention due to portal hypertension (HTN)

Abdomen: Ascites, a fluid-wave shift, shifting dullness, or increased abdominal girth can be found, in addition to caput medusa

Extremities: Muscle atrophy in the extremities; palmar erythema; lower extremity edema

Neuro: Altered mental status due to encephalopathy; asterixis

LABS

- CBC, comprehensive metabolic panel (CMP), prothrombin time (PT)/ international normalized ratio (INR), and serum ammonia levels
  - ○ In patients with cirrhosis, encephalopathy is often found as a result of precipitating events. These can include infection, increased dietary protein, electrolyte disturbances, and hypokalemia. Ammonia levels are increased due to decreased hepatic clearance.

> **CLINICAL PEARL:** Elevated ammonia levels respond well to administration of lactulose.

DIAGNOSTIC IMAGING

- Patients with hepatic encephalopathy are at risk for cerebral edema and increased intracranial pressure (ICP) when in fulminant liver failure. When a patient presents with altered mental status and hepatic encephalopathy is being considered, a CT of the brain should be ordered.

Management

The treatment of hepatic encephalopathy is primarily aimed at treating the underlying cause. Hepatic encephalopathy is a clinical diagnosis, and one of exclusion. Evaluate for and treat hypoglycemia, as this is common. Nutritional deficits, such as thiamine deficiency. should be managed with parenteral thiamine 100 mg. Lactulose at an initial dose of 30 mL q2–4h should be administered, which results in colonic acidification and catharsis. Ascites can be treated with diuretics. If patients develop evidence of multiorgan disease, including renal deficits, they may require transient dialysis or antibiotic administration if sepsis is an underlying etiology.

REFERENCE

1. O'Mara SR, Gebreyes K. Hepatic disorders. In: Tintinalli JE, Stapczynski J, Ma O, et al., eds. *Tintinalli's Emergency Medicine: A Comprehensive Study Guide.* 8th ed .New York, NY: McGraw-Hill; 2016:525–531. http://accessmedicine .mhmedical.com/content.aspx?bookid=1658&sectionid=109430616

HYPOGLYCEMIA

Etiology/Epidemiology

Hypoglycemia occurs when glucose is low, generally less than 50 to 70 mg/dL, in the setting of symptoms such as sweating, tachycardia, and shakiness, altered mental status and stroke-like complaints.

> **CLINICAL PEARL:** Patients with long-standing diabetes tend to exhibit fewer symptoms of hypoglycemia.

Hypoglycemia presenting to the ED is usually seen in two types of patients:
- Patients with type 1 DM who have taken their insulin but had minimal PO intake.
- Patients with type 2 DM who are on oral hypoglycemic agents that have been newly initiated or have limited PO intake as well.

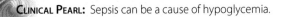

CLINICAL PEARL: Sepsis can be a cause of hypoglycemia.

Clinical Presentation

The clinical presentation of hypoglycemia can range from fatigue and drowsiness to altered mental status (AMS). The altered mental status can vary from the patient being disoriented to being unaware of one's surroundings. It may initially be difficult to distinguish features of hypoglycemia from a patient suffering from a stroke, therefore obtaining an immediate blood-sugar level is relevant.

Diagnosis

The diagnosis of hypoglycemia can be made immediately with a stat fingerstick blood glucose. In general, hypoglycemia is diagnosed in the presence of symptoms and a glucose level less than 70 mg/dL in a patient with DM, or less than 50 mg/dL in a nondiabetic patient.

Management

- Treat hypoglycemia with parenteral glucose in the form of IV dextrose or glucagon if a patient is not alert, awake, and oriented. If you suspect a patient may be unable to maintain a swallowing mechanism, administer medications parenterally. If patients are found to be hypoglycemic but are able to ingest PO, an oral glucose dose in the form of orange juice or a formulated liquid is sufficient, followed by a regular meal.
- Patients who are hypoglycemic secondary to ingestion of oral hypoglycemics (such as sulfonylureas), should be admitted for continued evaluation and treatment as these agents take up to 72 hours to metabolize, and patients may become hypoglycemic again.
- Consider prolonged observation for patients who are taking long-acting insulin.

SEIZURE

Etiology

A seizure is an episode of abnormal neurological function. This is caused by inappropriate electrical discharge of brain neurons, leading to excessive excitatory activity as demonstrated by clinical attacks of abnormal movements.[1] The term *epilepsy* refers to the chronicity of repeat seizure attacks. Seizures are further classified into types based on etiology and movement disorders demonstrated.

Epidemiology

Because seizure disorders have such a broad differential diagnosis and there are so many classifications for seizures, the epidemiological data are multifactorial.

Clinical Presentation

There are many conditions that mimic seizure-like movements, and therefore obtaining specific details about the episode is vital to determining the diagnosis.

- Ask emergency medical services (EMS) about the scene to which they arrived, and ask bystanders or family members to describe what they witnessed, if they were present.
- Inquire about prodromal symptoms. What behaviors did the patient display prior to onset of symptoms? Patients may have what is referred to as an *aura* demonstrated by a headache, tinnitus, scotoma, or other symptoms beforehand.
- These patients are at particular risk for injury to the oral cavity, in particular, the tongue.
- Patients can sustain head or extremity injuries during the seizure.
- Ask about and look for evidence of incontinence to bowel or bladder.
- Inquire about a postictal period.

CLINICAL PEARL: Be sure to differentiate between syncope and seizure. Syncope can cause a secondary hypoxic seizure. In the setting of a true seizure, a postictal period will occur, which is not present in syncope.

Obtaining a thorough history surrounding the events of seizure activity will facilitate the diagnosis. Also inquire about recent alterations in medication type, dose adjustments, and medication compliance in patients with a seizure disorder. It is also relevant to ask about recent stressors that may have induced the seizure, including sleep deprivation, emotional stress, increased strenuous activity, GI symptoms leading to electrolyte disturbances, and alcohol and/or drug use and withdrawal. These factors are relevant because the treatment differs.

To facilitate classification, seizures are divided into subtypes:

- Generalized seizures occur when the patient becomes rigid and falls to the ground with rhythmic clonic movements. Therefore, generalized seizures are known as *grand mal* or *tonic–clonic* seizures. They may have vomiting, incontinence to bowel or bladder, and deep, rapid breathing.
- Petit mal or absence seizures present with the sudden onset of altered mental status with no change in postural tone. This is associated with confusion, withdrawal from interacting with the individuals around them, and sudden cessation of the attack with no awareness that anything has happened.

- Partial seizures occur when the patient has no altered consciousness or mentation but there is focality to the seizure.
- Complex partial seizures occur when there is impact of consciousness or mentation yet the seizure still remains partial. These patients may have memory disturbance or hallucinations as well.

Diagnosis

Obtaining a thorough history surrounding the events of seizure activity will facilitate the diagnosis.

LABS

When sending blood work, the differential diagnosis remains broad as does the diagnostic approach:

- CBC, CMP, magnesium, phosphorus, alcohol level, urinalysis, urine drug screen to evaluate for metabolic cause of symptoms, or concomitant infection
- Serum salicylate and acetaminophen level should be ordered if the history supports a possibility of ingestion of these agents
- Many of the antiepileptic medications can be monitored for compliance through blood work

DIAGNOSTIC IMAGING

- In the presence of hypoxia, diminished breath sounds, or vomiting, a chest x-ray (CXR) should be obtained to evaluate for aspiration pneumonia.
- If the seizure onset is new, there is suspicion of head injury or intracranial bleeding, or with a history of anticoagulant use, a head CT should be obtained.
- A lumbar puncture in the setting of an acute seizure is only indicated if the patient is immunocompromised, febrile, or if there is suspicion of a subarachnoid hemorrhage in the setting of a normal brain CT (a patient on anticoagulants).

> **CLINICAL PEARL:** Any patient taking oral anticoagulants who presents with seizure or altered mental status should undergo a brain CT to rule out bleeding.

- An EEG is not typically done in the ED setting but rather by neurology for patients who are admitted for critical care assessment. This may also be deferred to the outpatient setting.

Management

The treatment approach depends on whether or not a patient has a known history of seizure disorder.

- One of the most common reasons for seizure in patients with a history of epilepsy is medication adjustment or lack of compliance. As a result, a neurology consult should be obtained and a loading dose of the appropriate agent should be initiated. If the patient remains postictal, and not yet alert and oriented × three (person, place, and time), then some of these medications can be administered parenterally. If the patient returns to baseline functioning, he or she may be discharged home with a reliable family member or friend, with outpatient neurology follow-up. If noncompliance is the cause of seizures or the patient ran out of medication, he or she can receive a prescription for a short supply with close outpatient follow-up arranged.
- Patients with new-onset unprovoked seizures should be admitted for further evaluation if a cause has not been identified.
- There is no one antiepileptic that works for all patients. Agents, such as valproate, phenytoin, carbazepine, oxcarbazepine, topiramate, and levetiracetam, are options for adults.
- Patients should be instructed to minimize injury risk to themselves and others by avoiding driving, avoiding consumption of alcohol or illicit substances, operating heavy machinery, working at heights, and swimming.[1] In many states, it is illegal for patients with new-onset seizures to operate motor vehicles; this should be discussed with the patient and documented.
- There are some special populations to consider in treating a seizure.
- If a woman is pregnant beyond 20 weeks' gestation and presents with hypertension, edema, proteinuria, and seizure, this is defined as *eclampsia* and should be treated with magnesium sulfate. Eclampsia can develop in the postpartum period, therefore recent pregnancies should be inquired of in the history.
- The treatment for patients with a history of alcohol abuse who suffer from seizures secondary to withdrawal is a benzodiazepine.[2]
- Patients who are in status epilepticus, which is a sustained single seizure lasting longer than 5 minutes without recovery of consciousness is considered a neurological emergency and requires emergent treatment with airway maintenance and immediate control of the seizure to prevent anoxic brain injury.[1] IV lorazepam is considered the initial agent of choice.[1]

REFERENCES

1. Ginde AA, Camargo CA, Pelletier AJ. National study of U.S. emergency department visits with diabetic ketoacidosis, 1993–2003. *Diabetes Care.* 2006;29:9. doi:10.2337/dc06-0627
2. Kornegay JG. Seizures. In: Tintinalli JE, Stapczynski J, Ma O, et al., eds. *Tintinalli's Emergency Medicine: A Comprehensive Study Guide.* 8th ed. New York, NY: McGraw-Hill; 2016:1173–1177. http://accessmedicine.mhmedical.com/content.aspx?bookid=1658&sectionid=109413404
3. Greene S. General management of poisoned patients. In: Tintinalli JE, Stapczynski J, Ma O, et al., eds. *Tintinalli's Emergency Medicine: A Comprehensive Study Guide.* 8th ed. New York, NY: McGraw-Hill; 2016:1207–1212. http://accessmedicine.mhmedical.com/content.aspx?bookid=1658&sectionid=109437481

Chest Pain

ACUTE CORONARY SYNDROME

Etiology

Acute coronary syndrome (ACS) encompasses ST-elevation myocardial infarction (STEMI), non–ST-elevation myocardial infarction (NSTEMI), and unstable angina; it is caused by an imbalance of blood supply to the myocardium and oxygen demand. This imbalance causes myocardial ischemia in cases of unstable angina, and myocardial necrosis in the case of myocardial infarction (MI). Atherosclerosis causes narrowing of the vessel lumen over time and is accelerated by smoking, hypertension, hyperlipidemia, diabetes, and other patient characteristics and genetic factors. Atherosclerotic plaque rupture or thrombus formation can occlude coronary arteries leading to ischemia and infarction.

Epidemiology

Heart disease remains the leading cause of death in the United States and is responsible for at least one third of deaths in people over the age of 35 in developed countries.[1-3] Risk factors include age, male gender, family history of heart disease, hypertension, diabetes, hyperlipidemia, smoking tobacco, obesity, and sedentary lifestyle.

Clinical Presentation

Clinical presentation typically includes gradual onset of chest pain that increases with exertion. Stable angina symptoms usually involve chest pain that is worse with physical exertion that is relieved with rest or nitrates, in a generally predictable pattern. Unstable angina may involve pain at rest, pain unrelieved by medication, or other changes in previously stable/predictable symptoms.

Acute MI may present with more abrupt onset of pain or pain that is higher in intensity or that lasts longer than previous episodes. Pain is generally described as pressure or tightness located in the mid- to left sternal chest region and may radiate to the left shoulder, jaw, neck, or back. Chest pain from ACS is typically episodic, lasting 20 to 30 minutes, but may last longer in the setting of an acute MI.[4] Elderly, female, and diabetic patients may present in an atypical fashion with vague symptoms such as dyspnea or weakness.

Diagnosis

Diagnosis of ACS is made with EKG and serial measurement of cardiac biomarkers (e.g., troponin I). The American College of Cardiology and American Heart Association guidelines recommend obtaining and interpreting EKG within 10 minutes of ED arrival for any patient with suspected ACS.[5]

- Troponin
  - Troponin I will be elevated within 3 hours of an acute MI, an initial set of negative cardiac biomarkers is not sufficient to rule out ACS. Typically, serial assays will be taken at 0-, 3-, and 6-hour intervals during evaluation.
- EKG findings
  - STEMI
    - New ST elevation of at least 1 mm in two contiguous leads (in all leads other than V2 and V3) with or without reciprocal ST depressions[6] (see Chapter 1, Common Presentations in Emergency Medicine, Figure 1.1)
  - NSTEMI/Unstable angina
    - Horizontal or down-sloping ST depression of at least 0.5 mm in two contiguous leads (see Chapter 1, Common Presentations in Emergency Medicine, Figure 1.2); T wave inversion of 1 mm in two contiguous leads (see Chapter 1, Common Presentations in Emergency Medicine, Figure 1.3)[6]
  - New left bundle branch block (LBBB)
  - Arrhythmias: Ventricular tachycardia or ventricular fibrillation due to cardiac ischemia
- Exercise and nuclear stress testing may be used in patients with non-diagnostic EKG and serial cardiac biomarkers in the setting of an observation unit
- Scoring systems
  - Thrombolysis in myocardial infarction (TIMI; www.mdcalc.com/timi-risk-score-ua-nstemi and www.mdcalc.com/timi-risk-score-stemi) and history, EKG, age, risk factors, and troponin (HEART; www.mdcalc.com/heart-score-major-cardiac-events) scoring systems may be used to further stratify risk and to manage patients with suspected ACS

Management

Immediate intervention for hemodynamic instability, airway compromise, treatment of life-threatening arrhythmias, or other general decompensation takes precedence over any other diagnostic or therapeutic intervention.

- ACS
  - STEMI
    - Antiplatelet therapy with aspirin (ASA) 325 mg should be given as soon as the diagnosis is made, in addition to a P2Y12 inhibitor such as clopidogrel, prasugrel, or ticagrelor.
    - Anticoagulant therapy is needed for patients with planned percutaneous coronary intervention (PCI) with unfractionated heparin or bivalirudin.
    - Relief of pain with nitrates given as sublingual nitroglycerin approximately 5 minutes apart × 3 doses, followed by (IV nitroglycerin for

those patients with persistent chest pain. IV morphine is reserved for patients with severe pain as it may worsen outcomes.

CLINICAL PEARL: Nitroglycerin should be avoided in patients with hypotension, suspected inferior wall or right ventricular infarction, severe aortic stenosis, or patients who have taken phosphodiesterase inhibitors for erectile dysfunction within 24 hours to avoid precipitating severe hypotension or hemodynamic decompensation.

- Oxygen is needed for patients with arterial saturation less than 90%, respiratory distress, underlying comorbidities predisposing to hypoxia (e.g., chronic obstructive pulmonary disease [COPD], congestive heart failure [CHF]).
- PCI needed within 90 minutes of diagnosis.
- Fibrinolytic therapy is needed for patients with onset of symptoms within 12 hours who are unable to receive PCI within 120 minutes of diagnosis.
- Beta-blocker therapy needed except for those with heart failure, bradycardia, heart block, significant COPD/asthma, or other risk for cardiogenic shock.
- Administer IV fluids for patients with hypotension secondary to right ventricular (RV) or inferior MI.

CLINICAL PEARL: IV fluids should be avoided in patients with left ventricular (LV) failure as it can exacerbate pulmonary edema.

- ○ NSTEMI/Unstable angina:
  - Same therapies are needed as for STEMI, except fibrinolytic therapy should be avoided in all patients.
  - Glycoprotein IIb/IIIa inhibitors may be added to antiplatelet therapy (aspirin + clopidogrel, prasugrel, or ticagrelor) for patients with ongoing ischemia.
  - PCI/cardiac catheterization generally takes place within 24 hours except for patients with severe heart failure, persistent rest angina, new or worsening mitral regurgitation or new ventricular septal defect, or sustained ventricular arrhythmias. Such patients should receive immediate cardiac catheterization.[7]

REFERENCES

1. Nichols M, Townsend N, Scarborough P, Rayner M. Cardiovascular disease in Europe 2014: epidemiological update. *Eur Heart J.* 2014;35(42):2950. doi:10.1093/eurheartj/ehu299
2. Benjamin EJ, Blaha MJ, Chiuve SE, et al. Heart diseases and stroke statistics-2017 update: a report from the American Heart Association [published corrections appears in Circulation. 2017;135(10):e646. doi:10.1161/CIR.0000000000000491]. *Circulation.* 2017;135(10):e146–e603. doi:10.1161/CIR.0000000000000485

3. Heron M. Deaths: leading causes for 2017. *Natl Vital Stat Rep.* 2019;68(6):1–77. https://www.cdc.gov/nchs/data/nvsr/nvsr68/nvsr68_06-508.pdf

4. Yelland MJ. Outpatient evaluation of the adult with chest pain. In: Aronson MD, ed. *UpToDate.* https://www.uptodate.com/contents/outpatient-evaluation-of-the-adult-with-chest-pain. Updated June 25, 2019.

5. Kamel H, Navi BB, Sriram N, et al. Risk of a thrombotic event after the 6-week postpartum period. *N Engl J Med.* 2014;370(14):1307–1315. doi:10.1056/NEJMoa1311485

6. Thygesen K, Alpert JS, Jaffe AS, et al. Third universal definition of myocardial infarction. *Circulation.* 2012;126(16):2020–2035. doi:10.1161/CIR.0b013e31826e1058

7. Aroesty JM, Simons M, Breall JA. Overview of the acute management of non-ST elevation acute coronary syndromes. In: Cannon CP, Hoekstra J, Cutlip D, eds. UpToDate. https://www.uptodate.com/contents/overview-of-the-acute-management-of-non-st-elevation-acute-coronary-syndromes. Updated December 31, 2018.

AORTIC DISSECTION

Etiology

Aortic dissection occurs when a tear in the aortic intima allows for the passage of blood into the media causing a separation and creating a false lumen. Dissection occurs with rupture and hemorrhage of this process and is most often due to chronic hypertension, atherosclerosis, connective tissue disease, or trauma. Type A dissections involve the ascending aorta; type B dissections involve the descending aorta.

Epidemiology

The incidence of aortic dissection is rare, occurring in 2.6 to 3.5 per 100,000 person-years.[1] Aortic dissection is more common in men over the age of 60. Risk factors include hypertension, connective tissue disease (Marfan syndrome, Ehlers–Danlos syndrome), congenital aorta and aortic valve abnormalities, trauma, pregnancy, and recent instrumentation (cardiac surgery, catheterization).

Clinical Presentation

Aortic dissection typically presents with abrupt onset of constant, severe, tearing chest pain (back pain may be the presenting complaint in cases of abdominal aortic dissection). Pain may radiate to back or arms and be associated with coolness, pulse discrepancy, numbness, tingling, or weakness of the extremities. Although hypertension is more common in patients with descending aortic dissection, hypotension associated with syncope or shock is more common with ascending aortic dissection.[2]

CLINICAL PEARL: Aortic dissection is life-threatening and must be recognized immediately.

Diagnosis

Widened mediastinum on CXR is concerning for thoracic aortic dissection. D-dimer levels of less than 500 ng/mL have been shown to have high sensitivity and negative predictive value for patients in screening for aortic dissection. If normal, this may be useful in ruling out aortic dissection. Patients who are hemodynamically unstable may have bedside transesophageal echocardiography (TEE) or transthoracic echocardiography (TTE) to confirm diagnosis. Stable patients may undergo computed tomography angiography (CTA) of the chest/abdomen/pelvis that demonstrates a true and false lumen with or without intimal flap or thrombus.

High suspicion for aortic dissection should be present when evaluating a patient with the triad of severe chest or abdominal pain, pulse discrepancies/abnormalities, and widened mediastinum on CXR. Such patients should be evaluated in close consultation with cardiac surgery.

Management

- Immediate intervention for hemodynamic instability with prompt cardiac surgery consultation
- Control of pain, heart rate, and hypertension with IV esmolol or labetalol (first-choice agents) with a target heart rate of less than 60 bpm and target systolic BP of less than 100 to 120 mmHg.[3]
- Type A (involving the ascending aorta): **Immediate** cardiac surgical intervention
- Type B (involving any portion of the descending aorta)
  - Stable, uncomplicated patients may be treated with BP control and monitoring.
  - Unstable patients, patients with severe hypertension or pain, or those with end-organ ischemia should be treated surgically.

REFERENCES

1. Black JH, 3rd, Manning WJ. Clinical features and diagnosis of acute aortic dissection. In: Joekstra J, Mills JL, Sr, Eidt JF, eds. *UpToDate.* https://www.uptodate.com/contents/clinical-features-and-diagnosis-of-acute-aortic-dissection. Updated April 2, 2019.
2. Nallamothu BK, Mehta RH, Saint S, et al. Syncope in acute aortic dissection: diagnostic, prognostic, and clinical implications. *Am J Med.* 2002;113(6):468–471. doi:10.1016/s0002-9343(02)01254-8
3. Black JH, 3rd, Manning WJ. Management of acute aortic dissection. In: Aldea GS, Verrier E, eds. *UpToDate.* https://www.uptodate.com/contents/management-of-acute-aortic-dissection. Updated June 10, 2019.

MUSCULOSKELETAL CHEST PAIN

Etiology

Musculoskeletal chest pain arises from structures within the chest wall such as muscle, bone, tendons, ligaments, and cartilage. Chest wall or rib trauma, costochondritis/Tietze's syndrome, lower rib pain syndromes, thoracic back pain, chest wall sprain/strain, and pain syndromes involving the sternum and sternoclavicular joints are common causes of musculoskeletal chest pain. Other atraumatic causes of chest wall pain include rheumatic disease (rheumatoid arthritis, systemic lupus erythematosus, fibromyalgia), osteoporosis, osteoarthritis, or neoplasms.

Epidemiology

Studies estimate that approximately 25% of patients in the ED have a musculoskeletal etiology of chest pain (ranging from 10% to 50% depending on study design). This number increases to over 33% of patients in nonemergency ambulatory clinics. Musculoskeletal chest pain is more common in female patients.[1]

Clinical Presentation

Musculoskeletal chest pain is usually insidious or gradual in onset lasting for hours to days. Pain is generally described as sharp or as an "ache" or "soreness" by patients and is worse with palpation, specific movements, or deep breathing. Traumatic causes are usually associated with a fall, heavy lifting, or other injury. Pain may be localized to a specific area or diffuse.

Diagnosis

Diagnosis of musculoskeletal chest pain is largely clinical. A careful history and physical exam can be sufficient in the workup of musculoskeletal chest pain, particularly in young, otherwise healthy individuals with clear mechanisms of injury or a history suggestive of certain inflammatory processes.

- Labs may be helpful in diagnosis underlying systemic inflammation (rheumatoid arthritis, systemic lupus erythematosus) as a potential cause of musculoskeletal chest pain but are generally not needed except to help rule out other important diagnoses.
- Troponin I in ACS, D-dimer in pulmonary embolism or aortic dissection should be considered if the clinical scenario is suggestive.
- Any patient with potential for ACS as a cause of chest pain should have an EKG and further evaluation to rule out ACS based on risk stratification (see ACS section).
- CXR may be helpful in diagnosis of rib fractures or neoplastic lesions.
- CT and MRI can provide detailed information about anatomical processes and lesions (osteoarthritis, masses), pleural processes, and connective tissues and may help to rule out other diseases in the differential diagnosis.

Management

Patients in whom life-threatening disease processes have been ruled out can be reassured and treated with monitoring and close follow-up with a primary care provider.

- Patients with overuse or sprain/strain injuries should be instructed on rest and avoidance of heavy lifting. Icing may also provide relief in cases of chest wall injury. Pain should be treated with topical agents (capsaicin cream, topical lidocaine, topical NSAIDs), acetaminophen, or NSAIDs. NSAIDs are particularly helpful for underlying inflammatory processes. Rib fractures may require opioid pain medication for adequate pain control.
- Patients should be given an incentive spirometer with instructions on deep-breathing exercises for prevention of pneumonia.
- Muscle relaxants (e.g., cyclobenzaprine) may be helpful in patients with muscle spasm of the chest wall.
- Patients with underlying inflammatory processes who do not respond to measures previously described may be referred for follow-up with orthopedics, rheumatology, or pain management for localized glucocorticoid injections.

REFERENCE

1. Wise CM. Major causes of musculoskeletal chest pain in adults. In: Goldenberg DL, ed. *UpToDate*. https://www.uptodate.com/contents/major-causes-of-musculoskeletal-chest-pain-in-adults. Updated July 18, 2019.

PERICARDITIS

Etiology

Pericarditis develops when there is inflammation of the pericardial sac due to infection, trauma, radiation/drugs/toxins, malignancy, metabolic disorders (uremia), systemic inflammatory disease (systemic lupus erythematosus), and following cardiac injury (MI, Dressler syndrome, iatrogenic). Pericarditis can result in pericardial effusion and cardiac tamponade.

Epidemiology

Acute pericarditis accounts for approximately 5% of patients with nonischemic chest pain in the ED and 0.2% of hospital admissions and is more common in male patients.[1] The majority of these cases are presumed to be of viral etiology (80%–90%).[2]

Clinical Presentation

Acute pericarditis typically presents with chest pain that is constant, sharp, and worsened with deep breathing or lying supine. Pain is usually relieved with sitting up or leaning forward. The patient may have a history of recent viral illness, malignancy, cardiac injury, trauma, or underlying inflammatory disease. A pericardial friction rub may be present.

CLINICAL PEARL: Although the pericardial friction rub is the hallmark of pericarditis, it can be subtle and difficult to appreciate on physical exam.

Dyspnea, tachycardia, and fever may also be present. It is important to look for signs of cardiac tamponade, including severe dyspnea or tachycardia, hypotension, distended neck veins, or muffled heart sounds, as this requires immediate intervention.

Diagnosis

Elevated troponin levels indicate involvement of the myocardium (myopericarditis). Inflammatory markers, such as leukocytosis, elevated erythrocyte sedimentation rate, and C-reactive protein levels, may be present.

Although EKG abnormalities in pericarditis can be variable, the classic findings include diffuse ST elevations with PR depressions. Pericarditis with effusion may demonstrate low voltage on EKG, enlarged cardiac silhouette on CXR (if >200–300 mL present) and increased pericardial fluid on bedside echocardiography. Cardiac tamponade may demonstrate electrical alternans on EKG; RV collapse will be present on bedside echocardiography.

Management

Patients at high risk for complications with acute pericarditis include those with advanced age, comorbid disease, and history of cardiac disease. These patients should be admitted to the hospital for continued monitoring and further evaluation and treatment as needed. Consultation with cardiology and cardiac surgery may be required. Patients with suspected cardiac tamponade require immediate percutaneous pericardiocentesis or cardiac surgical consultation for a pericardial window procedure.

High-risk features that require hospitalization include[3]

- Fever
- Immunosuppression
- Large pericardial effusion or tamponade
- Anticoagulation therapy
- Trauma
- Elevated troponin/myocardial involvement

Low-risk patients can be managed on an outpatient basis with close follow-up by a primary care provider or cardiology. Treatment includes[3]

- Avoidance of rigorous physical activity until asymptomatic
- Colchicine: 0.6 to 1.2 mg PO QD × 1 day followed by 0.6 mg QD–BID for 3 months PLUS
- NSAIDs: Ibuprofen 600 to 800 mg PO TID; ASA 650 to 1,000 mg PO TID; or indomethacin 25 to 50 mg PO TID for 2 to 4 weeks
- Steroids may be used for patients who fail the therapies just described or who have contraindications to NSAIDs with dosing of 0.25 to 0.5 mg/kg/day of prednisone with taper over 2 to 4 weeks as the preferred regimen.

REFERENCES

1. Kytö V, Sipilä J, Rautava P. Clinical profile and influences on outcomes in patients hospitalized for acute pericarditis. *Circulation*. 2014;130(18):1601–1606. doi:10.1161/CIRCULATIONAHA.114.010376 li

2. Imazio M, Gaita F, LeWinter M. Evaluation and treatment of pericarditis: a systematic review. *JAMA*. 2015;314(14):1498–1506. doi:10.1001/jama.2015.12763

3. Imazio M. Acute pericarditis: Clinical presentation and diagnostic evaluation. In: LeWinter MM, ed. *UpToDate*. https://www.uptodate.com/contents/acute-pericarditis-clinical-presentation-and-diagnostic-evaluation. Updated July 11, 2019.

PNEUMOTHORAX

Etiology

Pneumothorax develops when air enters the pleural space between the visceral and parietal pleura leading to chest pain, dyspnea, and collapse of part or all of the affected lung. A primary spontaneous pneumothorax develops from the rupture of a small bleb or trauma, whereas secondary spontaneous pneumothorax can develop from underlying lung disease. Iatrogenic causes (mechanical ventilation, central-line placement) may also lead to the development of pneumothorax. Tension pneumothorax is acutely life-threatening and occurs when a one-way valve effect causes progressive buildup of air in the pleural space leading to lung collapse and compression of the heart and great vessels.

Epidemiology

The incidence of primary spontaneous pneumothorax is estimated to be 7.4 to 37 cases per 100,000 population for males and 1.2 to 15.4 cases per 100,000 population for females.[1,2] Other risk factors for primary spontaneous pneumothorax include smoking, family history, Marfan syndrome, male gender, and mitral valve prolapse. Peak incidence is between 20 and 30 years of age.

Clinical Presentation

The typical presentation of pneumothorax is sudden onset of dyspnea and pleuritic chest pain, usually worse on the affected side. Severity of symptoms is generally dependent on the size of the pneumothorax. Physical exam may reveal tachypnea, hypoxia, tachycardia, diminished or absent breath sounds on affected side with hyperresonance on percussion. Tension pneumothorax often presents with severe respiratory distress, tachycardia, hypotension, and tracheal deviation.

Diagnosis

Diagnosis is made on clinical exam and with CXR. Upright CXR will demonstrate deviation of the visceral pleural line away from the chest wall and loss of lung markings. Large pneumothorax or tension pneumothorax will demonstrate tracheal deviation. Supine CXR may demonstrate a deep sulcus sign.

> **CLINICAL PEARL:** Suspected tension pneumothorax in an unstable patient should be treated immediately without delay for imaging or other diagnostic testing.

Ultrasound, particularly in the setting of an extended focused assessment with sonography for trauma (eFAST) exam, can demonstrate pneumothorax with absence of normal lung sliding. Pneumothorax is also easily visualized on chest CT; however, this is usually not necessary except in the setting of multiple traumatic injuries or for further investigation of other underlying lung abnormalities.

Management

Initial management of a small primary spontaneous pneumothorax (<20%) is supplemental oxygen (3 L/min via nasal cannula to 10 L/min via nonrebreather mask) to facilitate reabsorption of pleural air and observation for at least 4 hours in the ED. If the patient's symptoms and repeat CXR improve, the patient may be discharged home with close follow-up within 24 hours.[3] Patients with larger pneumothoraces who are stable should be treated with needle aspiration or chest tube placement. Tension pneumothorax is acutely life-threatening and requires immediate intervention with needle thoracostomy and chest tube placement.

REFERENCES

1. Gupta D, Hansell A, Nichols T, et al. Epidemiology of pneumothorax in England. *Thorax.* 2000;55:666–671. doi:10.1136/thorax.55.8.666
2. Light RW. Pneumothorax in adults: epidemiology and etiology. In: Broaddus VC, ed. *UpToDate.* https://www.uptodate.com/contents/pneumothorax-in-adults-epidemiology-and-etiology. Updated July 24, 2019.
3. Nicks BA, Manthey D. Pneumothorax. In: Tintinalli JE, Stapczynski J, Ma O, et al., eds. *Tintinalli's Emergency Medicine: A Comprehensive Study Guide.* 8th ed. New York, NY: McGraw-Hill; 2016:464–467. http://accessmedicine.mhmedical.com/content.aspx?bookid=1658&sectionid=109429615

PULMONARY EMBOLISM

Etiology

Pulmonary embolism (PE) develops when a blood clot, often from a deep vein thrombosis (DVT), travels to the lung and obstructs the pulmonary arterial circulation. The most common sites of thrombus formation are the legs, arms, or pelvis. Less often, PE can develop from the jugular vein; inferior vena cava; or from fat, air, or tumor emboli.

Epidemiology

PE is relatively common in the United States with an estimated 200,000 new or recurrent cases diagnosed each year.[1] PE and DVT together affect approximately one in 500 people per year and one in 300 adult ED patients in North America.[2] Incidence increases with age and is more common in females. Other well-known risk factors include malignancy, pregnancy, recent prolonged immobility, surgery, trauma, oral contraceptives and other exogenous estrogen therapy, hereditary hypercoagulability, and smoking.

Clinical Presentation

The clinical presentation of PE is notoriously variable, ranging from asymptomatic to sudden death. It is common for PE to present with dyspnea and pleuritic chest pain. Chest pain and dyspnea generally worsen with exertion. Patients may have associated lower extremity edema, pain, or other symptoms of DVT. Other less common associated symptoms are fever, hemoptysis, or syncope.

On physical exam, patients may have tachycardia, tachypnea, hypoxia, or unilateral extremity edema if DVT is present. Hypoxia or dyspnea with a normal lung exam must be further evaluated. Massive PE with large clot burden may lead to arrhythmias.

> **CLINICAL PEARL:** Many patients with PE will have only subtle physical exam findings or will have a completely normal physical exam so a high index of suspicion is necessary for diagnosis.

Diagnosis

Pulmonary embolism rule-out criteria (PERC) rule (www.mdcalc.com/perc -rule-pulmonary-embolism) and Wells criteria (www.mdcalc.com/wells -criteria-pulmonary-embolism) are scoring systems that can be used to stratify risk for patients and determine appropriate diagnostic testing. Stable patients with normal vital signs and low probability (<2% chance of PE based on PERC or Wells score) do not require further testing. Patients with one or more risk factors for PE based on history or physical exam should have D-dimer testing.

> **CLINICAL PEARL:** Patients with high risk or strong clinical suspicion for PE may undergo computed tomography angiography (CTA) testing without prior D-dimer to avoid delays in diagnosis and treatment.

Patients with D-dimer less than 500 ng/mL do not require further testing (sensitivity ranges from 94%–98%); patients with D-dimer greater than 500 ng/mL require further testing with CT angiography of the chest.[2,3] CTA of the chest will demonstrate a filling defect in the pulmonary artery at the site of the thrombus. Patients who cannot undergo CTA imaging should have ventilation/perfusion (V/Q) scanning done.

Pregnant patients with suspected PE should have CXR to rule out alternative diagnoses and to facilitate interpretation of V/Q scan. D-dimer levels are difficult to interpret in pregnant patients and are of limited use. V/Q scan is the preferred diagnostic modality for pregnant patients with normal CXR; CTA is preferred for patients with abnormal CXR and may be indicated if V/Q results are indeterminate.[4]

> **CLINICAL PEARL:** It is always important to weigh the risks and benefits of diagnostic testing in the evaluation of PE in pregnant patients given the potential risk of radiation to the mother and the fetus. In patients for whom suspicion is high, clear discussion and shared decision-making with the patient are important as PE is the leading cause of mortality (20%–30% of maternal deaths) in pregnancy and the postpartum period.[4]

Hemodynamically unstable patients may undergo bedside echocardiography to look for signs of RV failure, dilatation, or signs of pulmonary artery hypertension prior to empiric thrombolytic treatment. CXR and EKG may show nonspecific findings but are generally nondiagnostic in the evaluation of PE. CXR may demonstrate Westermark's sign, Hampton's hump, focal atelectasis, or pleural effusion. EKG findings may include sinus tachycardia, S1Q3T3, or nonspecific ST–T wave abnormalities. Venous duplex sonography of the extremities can be used to diagnose DVT.

> **CLINICAL PEARL:** Patients with new-onset of atrial fibrillation on EKG may have PE as etiology.

Management

Many patients diagnosed with PE will require admission to the hospital for monitoring, initiation of anticoagulation therapy, and possible further workup to investigate the etiology of thrombosis. Some stable, low-risk patients who are able to comply with treatment and monitoring may be managed in the outpatient setting. Prognostic models, such as the Pulmonary Embolism Severity Index (PESI), can be useful tools in evaluating a patient's mortality risk; however, such decisions should be weighed carefully and clear discussions with patients regarding risks and benefits of specific management plans should take place. Some patients may require immediate intervention for hemodynamic instability, airway compromise, or life-threatening arrhythmias.

- Treatment of PE: Stable patients
  - Initiation of anticoagulation therapy with low-molecular-weight heparin, unfractionated heparin, fondaparinux, or direct factor Xa and thrombin inhibitors with continuation of anticoagulation therapy for 3 to 12 months, or indefinitely in certain patients.
    - Factor Xa inhibitors (rivaroxaban, apixaban, edoxaban) and direct thrombin inhibitors (dabigatran) are preferred agents for nonpregnant patients without renal insufficiency or active cancer.[5]

- Warfarin is preferred for patients with severe renal insufficiency, those who require monitoring (poor compliance), or those who require an agent that can be reversed with an antidote.[5]
- Low-molecular-weight heparin is preferred for pregnant patients and patients with active malignancy.[5]

- Treatment of PE: Unstable patients
  - If suspicion for PE is high and no absolute contraindications exist (recent surgery, hemorrhagic stroke, active bleeding), may start empiric unfractionated heparin prior to diagnostic imaging.
  - If the patient is persistently hemodynamically unstable, may do bedside echocardiography to evaluate for RV dysfunction and start empiric thrombolytic therapy.

REFERENCES

1. Goldhaber SZ. Venous thromboembolism: epidemiology and the magnitude of the problem. *Best Pract Res Clin Haematol.* 2012;25:235-242. doi:10.1016/j.beha.2012.06.007.
2. Kline JA. Venous thromboembolism. In: Tintinalli JE, Stapczynski J, Ma O, et al., eds. *Tintinalli's Emergency Medicine: A Comprehensive Study Guide.* 8th ed. New York, NY: McGraw-Hill; 2016:388–398. http://accessmedicine.mhmedical.com/content.aspx?bookid=1658&sectionid=109429015
3. Thompson BT, Kabrhel CK. Overview of acute pulmonary embolism in adults. In: Mandel J, ed. *UpToDate.* https://www.uptodate.com/contents/overview-of-acute-pulmonary-embolism-in-adults. Updated August 21, 2018.
4. Malhotra A, Weinberger SE. Pulmonary embolism in pregnancy: epidemiology, pathogenesis, and diagnosis. In: Leung LLK, Mandel J, Lockwood CJ, eds. *UpToDate.* https://www.uptodate.com/contents/pulmonary-embolism-in-pregnancy-epidemiology-pathogenesis-and-diagnosis. Updated March 25, 2019.
5. Hull RD, Lip GYH. Venous thromboembolism: Anticoagulation after initial management. In: Mandel J, Leung LLK, eds. *UpToDate.* https://www.uptodate.com/contents/venous-thromboembolism-anticoagulation-after-initial-management. Updated July 26, 2019.

DYSPNEA

ASTHMA

Etiology

Asthma is a chronic inflammatory disorder characterized by increased responsiveness of the airways to multiple stimuli.[1] Asthma occurs due to an accumulation of mast cells, eosinophils, and macrophages in airways with resultant airway diameter reduction, increased secretions, and bronchial wall edema.[1]

Epidemiology

Approximately 8% of the U.S. population suffers from asthma.[1] It frequently presents in the pediatric population as nearly 50% of cases present under the age of 10.[1]

Clinical Presentation

Patients with asthma may present with coughing, wheezing, and dyspnea. They may note a trigger such as a URI, exposure to cold weather, or exposure to an allergen/pollen such as thick carpeting or animal dander. Asthma presentation is further divided into severity of clinical presentation:[2]

- Mild: Dyspnea only with activity
- Moderate: Dyspnea interferes with or limits usual activity
- Severe: Dyspnea at rest that interferes with conversation
- Subset: Life-threatening, too dyspneic to speak, diaphoretic

   Physical exam findings include an increased respiratory rate greater than 12. In patients with progressively worsening symptoms, there may be evidence of supraclavicular or subcostal retractions as the chest wall muscles begin to fatigue. Patients may also have notable end-expiratory wheezing on chest auscultation. The appearance of paradoxical respiration, which is chest deflation and abdominal protrusion during inspiration followed by chest expansion and abdominal deflation during expiration, is a sign of impending ventilatory failure.[3]

CLINICAL PEARL: If the pulmonary examination is abnormal with rales or crackles, consider a CXR to rule out an infiltrate.

Diagnosis

A bedside spirometry provides a rapid assessment. The forced expiratory volume (FEV_1) and peak expiratory flow rate (PEFR) provide direct measurement of the degree of airway obstruction. One method of trending a patient's response to therapy is to perform an initial and subsequent peak flow measurement after a series of breathing treatments. If there is improvement in the patient's peak flow measurements (which are predetermined by height and weight), this means he or she is responding to treatment. For chronic asthma patients, asking them what their baseline peak flow values are is also helpful.

CLINICAL PEARL: If a 70-kg male states his peak flow on a normal day is 600 L and he presents with 300-L capacity during an asthma attack, this is an objective assessment of a subjective presentation.

   Pulse oximetry is another modality that can be used in evaluating an asthmatic's response to treatment and can facilitate the disposition. If a patient's respiratory rate, symptoms, and pulmonary examination have improved, place a pulse ox on a finger while the patient ambulates. Ambulatory pulse oximetry that is normal can be another positive indicator that the patient may be discharged.

Management

- Beta-agonists are the preferred first-line treatment for patients with acute asthma due to their rapid onset and mechanism of stimulating bronchodilation.[1] The most common side effect is skeletal muscle tremor. Several beta-agonists are available, including albuterol and levalbuterol. These are typically administered through a spacing device attached to the wall oxygen unit.

- Corticosteroids are the cornerstone of asthma treatment.[1] Steroids reduce inflammation and restore beta-adrenergic response. The peak effect does not occur for up to 4 to 8 hours after administration so the route of administration can be either PO or IV. Options include prednisone or methylprednisone.

- When used with beta-agonists, anticholinergics can facilitate dilation of the larger airways. The most commonly used type is ipratropium bromide.

- It is not uncommon for ED providers to administer a combination of beta-agonist and anticholinergic up to six to seven doses before assessing a patient's status for admission versus discharge.

- When discharged home, patients may require several prescriptions, including a nebulizer.

- Patients should be discharged home with a prescription for steroids.

- If they do not have an inhaler to use at home, patients should receive one for breakthrough shortness of breath.

- If an asthmatic has a history of tobacco smoking, smoking-cessation education should be provided and the patient can receive a prescription for nicotine patches.

- If a CXR indicates the existence of an infection, patients should receive antibiotics to adequately treat pneumonia.

- Avoidance of potential triggers is advised.

REFERENCES

1. Cydulka RK. Acute asthma. In: Tintinalli JE, Stapczynski J, Ma O, et al., eds. *Tintinalli's Emergency Medicine: A Comprehensive Study Guide*. 8th ed. New York, NY: McGraw-Hill; 2016:468–474.

2. National Heart, Lung, and Blood Institute; National Institutes of Health; U.S. Department of Health and Human Services. National Asthma Education and Prevention Program Coordinating Team, Third Expert Panel on the Management of Asthma. *Guidelines for the Diagnosis and Management of Asthma*. Washington, DC: U.S. Department of Health and Human Services; 2007. https://www.nhlbi.nih.gov/files/docs/guidelines/asthsumm.pdf.

3. Sarko J, Stapczynski J. Respiratory distress. In: Tintinalli JE, Stapczynski J, Ma O, et al., eds. *Tintinalli's Emergency Medicine: A Comprehensive Study Guide*. 8th ed. New York, NY: McGraw-Hill; 2016:427–235. http://accessmedicine .mhmedical.com/content.aspx?bookid=1658&sectionid=109439081

CHRONIC OBSTRUCTIVE PULMONARY DISEASE (ACUTE EXACERBATION)

Etiology

COPD refers to an obstructive process within the lungs that limits airflow. Typically, this is due to repeated exposure to irritants, resulting in a breakdown of lung tissue. It is a progressive disease characterized by persistent airflow limitation.[1] COPD exacerbation is characterized by bacterial (most common) or viral infections of the lung parenchyma.[2]

Epidemiology

COPD accounted for over 700,000 hospitalizations in the United States in 2010 with an estimated cost of nearly $50 billion.[1] Men and women are affected roughly equally; however, there has been an increased prevalence in women.[1] Major risk factors include cigarette smoking, air pollution, and occupational exposures such as coal mining and construction.

Clinical Presentation

Chronic bronchitis and emphysema are the two types of COPD. *Chronic bronchitis* refers to the presence of a chronic productive cough for 3 months for 2 consecutive years. Emphysema occurs as a result of alveolar and bronchial wall destruction. Symptoms of both include sputum production, cough, and dyspnea. Chest tightness may be present as a result of repeated coughing.[1]

Patients are defined as having an exacerbation of either of these processes when the symptoms negatively impact and prevent day-to-day activities. Triggers are similar to those for asthma, including viral or bacterial infection, cold weather, opiate use, and beta-blocker use.

Physical examination often reveals increased work of breathing, cyanosis, tachycardia, and a fever. In order to compensate for the hypoxia related to COPD, sometimes patients may sit in a tripod position, upright and leaning forward. Chest auscultation often reveals crackles. The skin may have a bluish appearance. Patients may demonstrate pulsus paradoxus manifested by a drop of more than 10 mmHg in blood pressure during respiration cycles. Impending clinical signs of respiratory failure include altered mental status, cyanosis, and respiratory acidosis on arterial blood gas (ABG) results.

Diagnosis

The diagnosis of COPD is based on the patient's history of the disease, physical examination findings, and pulse oximetry. Inquiring about triggers and sputum changes is helpful.

- ABG analysis is the best tool in evaluating the patient's gas exchange capability and compensation. If the patient has a pH less than 7.35, this may be an indication of acute and uncompensated respiratory or metabolic acidosis.[1]
- If there is a suspicion of infectious etiology, diagnostics should include a CBC and CXR.

- If there is a possibility of metabolic derangement associated with respiratory acidosis, a BMP) is warranted.
- CXR findings are often consistent with COPD and include a flattened diaphragm and large lung fields. Existence of an infiltrate can rule in pneumonia and existence of Kerley B lines and pulmonary congestion adds heart failure to the differential diagnosis.
- Respiratory failure is characterized by a PaO_2 less than 60 mmHg or an arterial oxygen saturation less than 90%.[1] This can also include patients with ventilation failure and critically elevated carbon dioxide levels.
- Sometimes hypoxia can lead to an acuteMI or an acute MI can be an exacerbating factor. An EKG may be included in the workup if cardiac compromise is suspected.

Management

- The patient's O_2 saturation should remain above 90%.
- Beta-agonists and anticholinergics are the first line of therapy in managing COPD patients with acute exacerbation.[1]
- Ipratropium or glycopyrrolate can be given.
- The use of steroids helps to improve lung function and reduce hypoxemia.[1]
- If there is an associated pulmonary infiltrate noted, patients should receive antibiotic coverage specifically for *Streptococcus pneumoniae, Haemophilus influenza, and Moraxella catarrhalis.*[1] Antibiotics include azithromycin, tetracycline, doxycycline, or amoxicillin with clavulanic acid.
- Some providers also give methylxanthines, such as theophylline and aminophylline, to impose an anti-inflammatory effect and improve mechanisms of breathing.
- Positive pressure airway in the form of bilevel positive airway pressure (BiPAP) has allowed for many COPD exacerbation patients to be managed without the invasive procedure of endotracheal intubation.
- Mechanical assisted ventilation is indicated if the patient develops unrelenting respiratory muscle fatigue, deteriorating altered mental status, or refractory hypoxia despite previous interventions.
- Patients with acute or chronic COPD exacerbation frequently require admission to the hospital for further management.

REFERENCES

1. Cydulka RK, Bates CG. Chronic obstructive pulmonary disease. In: Tintinalli JE, Stapczynski J, Ma O, et al., eds. *Tintinalli's Emergency Medicine: A Comprehensive Study Guide.* 8th ed. New York, NY: McGraw-Hill; 2016:475–480.
2. Ma I, Lucey CR. Dyspnea. In: Henderson MC, Tierney LM, Jr, Smetana GW, eds. Section V: Respiratory system. In: Henderson MC, Tierney LM, Smetana GW, eds. *The Patient History: An Evidence-Based Approach to Differential Diagnosis.* 2nd ed. New York, NY: McGraw-Hill; 2012: chap 25, 241–250.

Heart Failure

Etiology

Heart failure results when cardiac function is not able to meet the physiologic demands of the body due to diastolic or systolic dysfunction.

- Heart failure with preserved ejection fraction (HFpEF) occurs when left ventricular filling is abnormal or filling pressures are elevated due to stiffness, but left ventricular ejection fraction is normal (EF>50%).
- Heart failure with reduced ejection fraction (HFrEF) occurs when impaired cardiac contractile function leads to dilatation and remodeling in the setting of a reduced ejection fraction (EF>40%).

Decompensation of previously stable heart failure patients often occurs as a result of medication noncompliance or failure, increased sodium intake, physical activity, or underlying illness/physiologic stressor (infection, arrhythmia).

Epidemiology

The American Heart Association (AHA) data from 2017 estimates that 6.5 million Americans aged 20 and older are affected by heart failure. Given increased survival rates from MI and an aging population, the AHA projects 8 million Americans aged 18 and older to will be living with the disease by 2030. Heart failure is the leading cause of hospitalization in the elderly and accounts for 309,000 deaths in America per year. An estimated 960,000 new cases of heart failure are diagnosed annually.[1] Risk factors for heart failure include

- Cardiomyopathy, prior MI or coronary artery disease, valvular heart disease, hypertension, diabetes, alcohol use, dyslipidemia, chemotherapy, or radiation to the chest

Clinical Presentation

Patients with acute heart failure or an acute exacerbation of chronic underlying disease classically present with exertional dyspnea, orthopnea, paroxysmal nocturnal dyspnea, chest pain or pressure, palpitations, or lower extremity edema. Other more nonspecific symptoms include fatigue, weakness, nocturia, weight gain or bloating, anxiety, nausea, anorexia, or confusion. Patients may report recent medication or dietary noncompliance or increasing difficulty tolerating physical activity.

Physical exam findings include abnormal vital signs such as hypoxia, tachycardia, and tachypnea. The patient may appear diaphoretic, cyanotic, or pale and may demonstrate signs of fluid overload such as jugular venous distention, increased hepatojugular reflex, lower extremity edema, ascites, or bilateral rales or wheezing on lung examination. An S_3 gallop is common in patients with significant heart failure. New York Heart Association (NYHA) Functional Classification of heart failure can be found at www.heart.org/en/health-topics/heart-failure/what-is-heart-failure/classes-of-heart-failure.

Diagnosis

Diagnostic evaluation of patients with suspected heart failure involves laboratory analysis, EKG, chest x-ray, and echocardiography.

LABS

- CBC may indicate leukocytosis in underlying infection or anemia.
- CMP: Patients with severe heart failure may have dilutional hyponatremia, increased BUN/creatinine levels, decreased glomerular filtration rate (GFR), or increased liver enzymes.
- B-type natriuretic peptide levels higher than 100 pg/mL are highly sensitive for acute heart failure, whereas levels less than 50 pg/mL have a high negative predictive value.
- Troponin levels may be increased if myocardial ischemia or infarction are the cause of heart failure.
- ABG may demonstrate hypercarbia in severe decompensated heart failure but is rarely indicated.

DIAGNOSTIC IMAGING

- EKG may suggest left atrial or left ventricular enlargement, arrhythmia, or myocardial ischemia or infarction.
- Chest x-ray may demonstrate cardiomegaly, pleural effusions, or pulmonary vascular congestion.
- Echocardiography may be used to determine chamber size, left ventricular systolic and diastolic function, ejection fraction, pulmonary artery and ventricular filling pressures, and valvular abnormalities.

Management

Patients with acute decompensated heart failure may require immediate intervention for any of the following:

- Cardiogenic shock/hemodynamic instability, acute myocardial ischemia/infarction, treatment of life-threatening arrhythmias, airway compromise, or altered mental status due to hypoxia or hypercarbia.
- Patients with severe respiratory distress may require endotracheal intubation. Moderate respiratory distress may be treated with noninvasive ventilation with continuous positive airway pressure (CPAP) or bilevel positive airway pressure (BiPAP) via facemask. Mild respiratory distress may be treated with supplemental oxygen via nasal cannula as needed.

Patients with hypotensive heart failure should be assessed for STEMI with EKG and started on dobutamine or dopamine witha systolic BP goal of at least 90 to 100 mmHg. Patients with hypertension and pulmonary edema should be treated with sublingual or IV nitroglycerin:[2]

- 0.4 mg sublingual nitroglycerin up to 1 per minuteor
- 0.5 to 0.7g/kg/min IV nitroglycerin titrated up to 200 g/min or higher until blood pressure decreases and symptoms improve

- IV nitroprusside may be used if no response to IV nitroglycerin; 0.3 g/kg/min IV nitroprusside titrated up every 5 to 10 minutes to 10 g/kg/min until blood pressure decreases and symptoms improve

Volume overload should be treated with IV diuretics:[2]

- 40 mg IV furosemide if no prior diuretic use or give patient's usual PO dose as IV bolus or
- 1 to 3 mg IV bumetanide or
- 10 to 20 mg IV torsemide

> **CLINICAL PEARL:** Nitrates should be administered before diuretics; diuretics administered without vasodilators can increase mortality.[2]

Acute heart failure patients should be admitted to ICU/cardiac/coronary care unit (CCU) or heart failure observation unit for further stabilization.

REFERENCES

1. Benjamin EJ, Blaha MJ, Chiuve SE, et al. Heart disease and stroke statistics—2017 update: a report from the American Heart Association [published corrections appears in *Circulation*. 2017;135(10):e646. doi:10.1161/CIR.0000000000000491]. *Circulation*. 2017;135(10):e146–e603. doi:10.1161/CIR.0000000000000485
2. Collins SP, Storrow AB. Acute heart failure. In: Tintinalli JE, Stapczynski J, Ma O, et al., eds. *Tintinalli's Emergency Medicine: A Comprehensive Study Guide*. 8th ed. New York, NY: McGraw-Hill; 2016:366–372.

ELECTRONIC RESOURCES

NYHA Classification of heart failure: www.heart.org/en/health-topics/heart-failure/what-is-heart-failure/classes-of-heart-failure

PNEUMONIA

Etiology

Pneumonia is an infection of the lower respiratory tract caused by bacteria, viruses, or fungi. Bacterial pneumonia can be classified as community-acquired pneumonia (CAP) or nosocomial (hospital-acquired or ventilator-associated) pneumonia. CAP can further be classified as "typical" or "atypical" in reference to the pathogen causing the infection.

- "Typical" CAP is caused most commonly by: *Streptococcus pneumoniae, Haemophilus influenzae, Moraxella catarrhalis, Staphylococcus aureus* (particularly following influenza) and group A *Streptococci*
- "Atypical" CAP is caused most commonly by *Mycoplasma pneumoniae, Chlamydia pneumoniae,* and *Legionella*

Nosocomial pneumonia develops within 48 to 72 hours of hospitalization or intubation and is caused most commonly by *Staphylococcus aureus, Pseudomonas aeruginosa, Klebsiella pneumoniae,* or other Gram-negative aerobes. Nosocomial pneumonia can be complicated by drug-resistant pathogens such as methicillin-resistant *Staphylococcus aureus* (MRSA) and polymicrobial infections. This section will focus primarily on the diagnosis and treatment of CAP.

Epidemiology

CAP is a relatively common disease entity, particularly in the elderly and during the winter months. It is estimated that in the United States, CAP is responsible for 1.5 million adult hospitalizations annually and 100,000 deaths during hospitalization. Approximately one third of hospitalized patients will die within 1 year.[1] Coupled with influenza, pneumonia is the eighth leading cause of death in the United States.[2]

Clinical Presentation

Patients with "typical" CAP will present with fever, chills, rigors, productive cough, dyspnea, and pleuritic chest pain. On physical exam, patients will have productive cough, fever, and rales over the affected lung field(s). You may also appreciate tactile fremitus and egophony. Patients with underlying comorbidities, severe or late disease may present with respiratory distress, hypotension, tachycardia, or other signs of septic shock.

Patients with "atypical" CAP are typically younger (school-aged children, college students) and have malaise; headache; low-grade fever; and persistent, dry cough. Chest wall pain or soreness may develop from incessant coughing. Patients will often complain of disrupted sleep secondary to persistent coughing. Associated symptoms may include sore throat, rhinorrhea, and ear pain. Physical exam may demonstrate mild pharyngeal erythema, nasal congestion, or tympanic membrane erythema. Lung sounds are typically normal, but some patients may develop wheezes, scattered rales, and rhonchi.

Bordetella pertussis (whooping cough) is an important pathogen to keep in mind for patients with particularly persistent cough (>2–3 weeks) as immunity from vaccination is not lifelong and symptoms can be hard to distinguish from other common upper respiratory infections.

Diagnosis

Labs

- CBC may demonstrate leukocytosis in "typical" CAP, but is normal in the majority of "atypical" CAP.
- Blood and sputum cultures may be helpful in directing antibiotic therapy but should only be obtained in cases of severe illness, outpatient antibiotic failure, or when specific organisms, such as *Legionella*, are suspected.

Diagnostic Imaging

- A CXR should be ordered for all patients with suspected CAP in the setting of clinical features described earlier. "Typical" pneumonia classically appears as a lobar consolidation but may also take on a patchy infiltrate appearance. "Atypical" pneumonia will generally have interstitial infiltrates; peribronchial cuffing and localized atelectasis may also be present.

- In some cases where clinical suspicion for CAP is high and CXR is negative, CT scan may aid in diagnosis, but is not recommended for routine use.

Management

Patients with significant comorbidities, increased severity of disease (SPO_2 <92% on room air), advanced age, concern for medication adherence, or with multilobar infection will require admission to the hospital for monitoring and IV antibiotic therapy. Clinical scoring tools, such as the Pneumonia Severity Index (www.mdcalc.com/psi-port-score -pneumonia-severity-index-cap) and CURB-65 (www.mdcalc.com/curb -65-score-pneumonia-severity), may aid in determining the appropriate disposition of your patient. Patients with septic shock or respiratory failure require admission to the ICU and often require initiation of fluid bolus or vasopressors, IV antibiotics (within 1 hour), and supplemental oxygen or intubation in the ED.

> **CLINICAL PEARL:** Ideally, patients requiring blood or sputum cultures should have specimens taken before initiation of IV antibiotic therapy; however, DO NOT delay initiation of antibiotic therapy to obtain specimens for culture.

Patients requiring hospital admission for CAP with no risk factors for antibiotic resistance or *Pseudomonas* infection should be treated with the following regimen:[3]

- Ceftriaxone 1 to 2 g IV qd OR cefotaxime 1 to 2 g IV q8h OR ceftaroline 600 mg IV q12h OR ertapenem 1g IV qd OR ampicillin–sulbactam 1.5 to 3 g IV q6h **PLUS** azithromycin 500 mg IV or PO qd OR clarithromycin 500 mg PO BID OR clarithromycin XL 1000 mg PO qd OR doxycycline 100 mg PO or IV BID
- Levofloxacin 750 mg IV or PO qd OR moxifloxacin 400 mg IV or PO qd OR gemifloxacin 320 mg PO qd
- Patients with penicillin or cephalosporin allergies may be treated with respiratory fluoroquinolone as indicated **PLUS** aztreonam 500 mg IV q8–12h

Patients requiring hospital admission for CAP with risk factors for antibiotic resistance or *Pseudomonas* infection should be treated with the following regimen:[3]

- Piperacillin–tazobactam 4.5 gm IV q6h OR imipenem 500 mg IV q6h OR meropenem 1 gm IV q8h OR cefepime 2 g IV q8h or ceftazidime 2 gm IV q8h **PLUS** ciprofloxacin 400 mg IV or PO q8h or levofloxacin 750 mg IV or PO qd
- Patients with penicillin or cephalosporin allergies may be treated with respiratory fluoroquinolone as indicated previously **PLUS** aztreonam 500 mg IV q8–12h **PLUS** aminoglycoside (e.g., gentamicin, amikacin)

Patients at risk of MRSA infection should be treated with the addition of [3]

- Vancomycin 15 mg/kg IV q12h OR linezolid 500 mg IV q12h
- Alternatives include clindamycin 600 mg q8h OR ceftaroline 600 mg q12h (**not** Food and Drug Administration [FDA] approved for MRSA pneumonia)

Patients with **no** comorbidities or recent antibiotic use, in regions with **low** rates of macrolide-resistant *Streptococcus pneumoniae* (<25%) should be treated with one of the following:[4]

- Azithromycin 500 mg PO qd × 1 d + 250 mg PO qd × 4 d (Z-pak)
- Clarithromycin 500 mg PO BID × 5 d or clarithromycin XL 1,000 mg PO qd × 5 d

Patients with **no** comorbidities or recent antibiotic use, in regions with **high** rates of macrolide-resistant *Streptococcus pneumoniae* (>25%) should be treated with the following:[4]

- Doxycycline 100 mg PO BID × 5–7 d
  or
- Amoxicillin 1 g PO TID × 5 d OR amoxicillin–clavulanate XR 2 g PO BID × 5 d OR cefpodoxime 200 mg PO BID × 5 d OR cefuroxime 500 mg PO BID **PLUS** Azithromycin 500 mg PO QD × 1 d + 250 mg PO QD × 4 d (Z-pak) OR Clarithromycin 500 mg PO BID × 5 d OR Clarithromycin XL 1,000 mg PO QD × 5 d
  or
- Levofloxacin 750 mg PO qd × 5 d OR moxifloxacin 400 mg PO qd × 5 d OR gemifloxacin 320 mg PO qd × 5 d

Patients discharged home from the ED should receive follow-up with a primary care provider within 24 to 48 hours for reevaluation and should be advised to have repeat CXR in 7 to 12 weeks.

REFERENCES

1. Ramirez JA, Wiemken WL, Peyrani P, et al. Adults hospitalized with pneumonia in the United States: incidence, epidemiology, and mortality. *Clin Infect Dis.* 2017;65(11):1806–1812. doi: 10.1093/cid/cix647
2. Heron M. Death: leading causes for 2017. *Natl Vital Stat Rep.* 2019;1(6):1–77. https://www.cdc.gov/nchs/data/nvsr/nvsr68/nvsr68_06-508.pdf
3. File TM, Jr. Treatment of community-acquired pneumonia in adults who require hospitalization. In: Bartlett JG, Ramirez JA, eds . *UpToDate.* https://www.uptodate.com/contents/treatment-of-community-acquired-pneumonia-in-adults-who-require-hospitalization. Updated August 8, 2019.
4. File TM, Jr. Treatment of community-acquired pneumonia in adults in the outpatient setting. In: Bartlett JG, Ramirez JA, eds. *UpToDate.* https://www.uptodate.com/contents/treatment-of-community-acquired-pneumonia-in-adults-in-the-outpatient-setting. Updated May 2, 2019.

PULMONARY EDEMA

Etiology

The etiology of pulmonary edema can be broad, including systemic hypertensive pulmonary edema, CHF complications, immersion edema secondary to diving, and high-altitude pulmonary edema. The focus of this discussion is acute hypertensive pulmonary edema related to systemic hypertension. The underlying pathophysiology can be varied and includes transient LV failure, diastolic dysfunction, or ischemic mitral regurgitation. The left ventricular ejection fraction (LVEF) may also be normal as the myocardial capacity adapts to changes. In cardiogenic pulmonary edema such as this, there is abnormal fluid movement as a result of an elevation in pulmonary capillary pressure.

Epidemiology

Acute heart failure is one of the most common reasons for patients older than 65 years to be hospitalized, and these patients represent a significant mortality risk in the months after discharge. Pulmonary edema is common in patients who present with acute heart failure. A systematic review of 23 acute heart failure trials determined the prevalence of pulmonary edema to range from 75% to 83%.[1] Individual risk factors for pulmonary edema are the same as those for the underlying disease, in this case, hypertensive heart disease and heart failure.

Clinical Presentation

The clinical presentation of pulmonary edema is similar to CHF. Patients may present with dyspnea, wheezing, bilateral rales, inspiratory crackles, and low oxygen saturation. For patients who have increased respiratory compromise, there may be evidence of accessory muscle use and tripod positioning. The cardiovascular exam may demonstrate signs of RV failure with jugular venous distention and peripheral edema. An S3 gallop and/or S4 are commonly appreciated.

Diagnosis

For patients presenting with hypertensive pulmonary edema, the diagnosis can be made by using several modalities.

LABS
- Troponin level may be elevated.
- B-type natriuretic peptide (BNP) is elevated in heart failure.

DIAGNOSTIC IMAGING
- An EKG should be obtained to evaluate the presence of acute myocardial injury or infarction.
- A CXR may demonstrate evidence of pulmonary edema within the lung fields, with Kerley B lines and cardiomegaly.

- A bedside ultrasound of the lungs can be used to identify pleural effusions, cardiac tamponade, or pneumothorax, if physical exam findings suggest their presence.

Management

- The mainstay of treatment for hypertensive pulmonary edema is vasodilators and IV diuretics.[2] The goal is to maintain a PaO_2 greater than 60 mmHg and SaO_2 greater than 90%.
- Patients can also receive nitrates to reduce BP and improve blood flow to the coronary arteries.
- Diuretics provide quick symptomatic relief.
- If hypertensive pulmonary edema is secondary to ACS or atrial fibrillation with rapid ventricular response, patients may receive beta-blockers.
- If secondary to sympathetic crisis from cocaine or amphetamines, patients should receive benzodiazepines, such as lorazepam or diazepam, to decrease adrenergic stimulation.[2]
- If a patient becomes severely hypoxic, develops altered mental status, demonstrates respiratory fatigue, administer supplemental oxygen and BiPAP. If there is no improvement, proceed to intubation and assisted mechanical ventilation.

REFERENCES

1. Platz E, Jhund PS, Campbell RT, McMurray JJ. Assessment and prevalence of pulmonary oedema in contemporary acute heart failure trials: a systematic review. *Eur J Heart Fail*. 2015;17(9):906–916. doi: 10.1002/ejhf.321
2. Baumann BM. Systemic hypertension. In: Tintinalli JE, Stapczynski J, Ma O, et al., eds. *Tintinalli's Emergency Medicine: A Comprehensive Study Guide*. 8th ed. New York, NY: McGraw-Hill; 2016:399–408.

HEADACHE

ACUTE ANGLE-CLOSURE GLAUCOMA

Etiology

Acute angle-closure glaucoma develops when there is a rapid increase in intraocular pressure due to an obstruction of aqueous humor outflow. Blockage typically occurs when the lens or peripheral iris obstructs the trabecular meshwork and is more common in people with shallow anterior chambers.

Epidemiology

Acute angle-closure glaucoma is relatively rare. Incidence varies depending on race. It more commonly affects patients of Inuit and Asian descent, women, and people over the age of 50.[1] Incidence is particularly high in the Inuit populations.

Clinical Presentation

The classic presentation of acute angle-closure glaucoma is abrupt onset of eye pain or unilateral frontal/periorbital headache associated with blurry vision, nausea, and vomiting. Patients may report visual halos around lights. Physical exam reveals a fixed, mid-dilated pupil with a cloudy cornea. There is usually conjunctival injection and the globe will feel very firm on palpation.

Diagnosis

Thorough examination of the eye, including visual acuity, pupil exam, tonometry, slit-lamp exam, visual field testing, and undilated fundoscopy exam should be performed

> **CLINICAL PEARL:** Do NOT dilate the pupil on exam as this may cause worsening symptoms and further damage.

Visual acuity is usually decreased in the affected eye and intraocular pressure will be greater than 20 mmHg, typically markedly elevated. Slit-lamp examination will demonstrate a shallow anterior chamber.

Management

Acute angle-closure glaucoma is an ophthalmologic emergency and requires immediate consultation with ophthalmology. Treatment to lower the intraocular pressure is initiated in the ED in consultation with ophthalmology and may include

- IV acetazolamide (500 mg IV or PO), IV mannitol (1–2 g/kg IV)
- Topical beta-blocker (0.5% timolol), topical alpha-2 agonist (1% apraclonidine), topical pilocarpine (1%–2% pilocarpine)[2]

  Definitive treatment is laser iridectomy by ophthalmology.

REFERENCES

1. Freedman J. Acute angle-closure glaucoma in emergency medicine. In: Dronen SC, ed. *Medscape.* https://emedicine.medscape.com/article/798811-treatment. Updated November 19, 2018.
2. Walker RA, Adhikari S. Eye emergencies. In: Tintinalli JE, Stapczynski J, Ma O, eds. *Tintinalli's Emergency Medicine: A Comprehensive Study Guide.* 8th ed. New York, NY: McGraw-Hill; 2016:1543–1578. http://accessmedicine.mhmedical.com/content.aspx?bookid=1658&sectionid=109444274

CEREBROVASCULAR ACCIDENT

Etiology

Cerebrovascular accident (CVA), or stroke, is defined as brain tissue necrosis due to arterial occlusion or hemorrhage. CVA results in focal neurologic deficits corresponding to the area of brain that is affected.

- Ischemic CVA is the most common type. It develops from thrombotic disease that causes reduction of blood flow through large or small (lacunar infarcts) cerebral vessels, due to atherosclerosis or thromboembolic fragments. Ischemia may also develop from embolism that develops in another part of the body and travels to the brain (e.g., cardiac) or as a result of systemic hypoperfusion (e.g., cardiogenic shock).
- Hemorrhagic CVA is caused by intracerebral hemorrhage (ICH) or subarachnoid hemorrhage (SAH) that can arise from hypertension, aneurysmal rupture, vascular malformations, trauma, bleeding diathesis, or illicit drug use.
- Transient ischemic attack (TIA) is a temporary focal neurologic deficit caused by ischemia, but not infarction, that resolves without clinical or diagnostic evidence of permanent injury (e.g., symptoms resolve over time without evidence of infarction on neuroimaging).[1]

Epidemiology

Stroke is the fifth leading cause of death in the United States with an incidence of both new and recurring stroke of 795,000 per year.[2] Ischemic strokes account for 87% of CVAs, whereasICH accounts for 10%, and SAH accounts for 3%.[3] Some of the most common risk factors for ischemic stroke are hypertension, diabetes, smoking, hyperlipidemia, increasing age, atrial fibrillation (embolic stroke), coronary artery disease, and carotid artery stenosis. Risk factors for hemorrhagic stroke include hypertension, increasing age, bleeding diathesis, anticoagulation therapy, family history, smoking, Black ethnicity, and high alcohol intake.

Clinical Presentation

Persistent focal neurologic deficit (e.g., facial droop, dysarthria, unilateral motor weakness) is the hallmark of ischemic CVA. Focal symptoms may include hemiparesis, hemisensory deficits, unilateral cranial nerve dysfunction, ataxia, or vertigo. Patients may present with more subtle signs and symptoms such as lightheadedness, changes in sensorium, or mild alteration in mental status. Acute ICH and SAH are more likely to present with abrupt onset of severe headache associated with vomiting. Hypertension, pupil asymmetry, fixed unilateral gaze, and altered mental status are also common in ICH/SAH.

Diagnosis

Prompt diagnosis of CVA is of utmost importance as treatment is time sensitive. Immediate consultation with a neurology stroke team and neuroimaging (most commonly CT brain without contrast) is warranted for any patient with suspected CVA. At some stroke centers, stroke alerts may be activated in the field by EMS personnel prior to arrival to the ED to expedite management for patients with suspected CVA. Diagnosis involves a thorough neurologic evaluation, determination of onset of symptoms (e.g., last known well time) for possible administration of tissue plasminogen activator (tPA), and

CT without IV contrast. The initial workup should be carried out in close consultation with neurology.

The National Institutes of Health (NIH) Stroke Scale (www.mdcalc .com/nih-stroke-scale-score-nihss) may be used to help determine stroke severity and to predict outcomes. Blood glucose and oxygen saturation levels should be obtained to rule out other etiologies of symptoms. CBC, coagulation studies, and EKG (assess for presence of atrial fibrillation or myocardial infarction [MI]) should be obtained. MRI, MR angiography, CT angiography, and lumbar puncture (LP) may be helpful adjuncts in the diagnosis of CVA.

> **CLINICAL PEARL:** All patients with history or physical exam concerning for SAH/ICH should undergo LP if head CT is negative.[4,5]

Management

Immediate intervention for hemodynamic instability, airway compromise, or other general decompensation takes precedence over any other diagnostic or therapeutic intervention. Severely obtunded patients (e.g., severe hemorrhagic stroke) may require intubation.

- Acute ischemic stroke should be managed in conjunction with immediate neurologic consultation in the ED.
  - Once neuroimaging is obtained and hemorrhagic stroke has been ruled out, patients presenting within **3 to 4.5 hours** of symptom onset should receive IV alteplase (tPA) if inclusion/exclusion criteria (www.mdcalc.com/tpa-contraindications-ischemic-stroke) are met (see Tables 1.15 and 1.16).
  - Patients with large arterial occlusion presenting within 6 hours of onset of symptoms may be candidates for endovascular thrombectomy.
  - The goal is to arrive at a treatment decision within 60 minutes of the patient's arrival to the ED.[6]
- Acute hemorrhagic stroke (SAH/ICH) is also a time-sensitive diagnosis requiring prompt recognition and management. Initial management includes:
  - Prompt neurosurgical consultation/intervention (e.g., clipping or coiling of aneurysm, evacuation of clots, ventriculostomy placement).
  - Control of hyperglycemia, fever, and BP as needed.
    - Systolic BP higher than 200 mmHg or higher than 180 mmHg with evidence of elevated intracranial pressure should be reduced with IV antihypertensive medication.
  - Reverse anticoagulation therapy/bleeding diathesis:
    - Warfarin → vitamin K, prothrombin complex concentrate (PCC)
    - Heparin → protoamine sulfate
    - Thrombocytopenia → platelet transfusion
    - Clotting factor deficiency (e.g., hemophilia) → factor replacement

○ Manage increased ICP.
  ▪ Elevate the head of the bed to 30 degrees
  ▪ Appropriate analgesia/sedation
  ▪ Mannitol

REFERENCES

1. Furie KL, Hakan A. Definition, etiology and clinical manifestations of transient ischemic attack. In: Kasner SE, ed. *UpToDate*. https://www.uptodate.com/contents/definition-etiology-and-clinical-manifestations-of-transient-ischemic-attack. Updated March 23, 2018.
2. Heron M. Death: leading causes for 2017. Natl Vital Stat Rep. 2019;68(6):1–77. https://www.cdc.gov/nchs/data/nvsr/nvsr68/nvsr68_06-508.pdf
3. Benjamin EJ, Blaha MJ, Chiuve SE, et al. Heart disease and stroke statistics-2017 update: a report from the American Heart Association [published corrections appears in *Circulation*. 2017;135(10):e646. doi:10.1161/CIR.0000000000000491]. *Circulation*. 2017;135(10):e146–e603. doi: 10.1161/CIR.0000000000000485
4. Vermeulen M, van Gijn J. The diagnosis of subarachnoid haemorrhage. *J Neurol Neurosurg Psychiatry*. 1990;53(5):365–372. doi: 10.1136/jnnp.53.5.365
5. Connolly ES, Jr, Rabinstein AA, Carhuapoma JR, et al. Guidelines for the management of aneurysmal subarachnoid hemorrhage: a guideline for health-care professionals from the American Heart Association/American Stroke Association. *Stroke*. 2012;43(6):1711–1737. doi: 10.1161/STR.0b013e3182587839
6. Adams HP, Jr, del Zoppo G, Alberts MJ, et al. Guidelines for the early management of adults with ischemic stroke. *Stroke*. 2007;38(4):1655–1711. doi: 10.1161/STROKEAHA.107.181486

MENINGITIS

Etiology

Meningitis is inflammation of the meninges surrounding the brain and spinal cord due to bacterial (e.g., *Streptococcus pneumoniae, Neisseria meningitidis, Borrelia burgdorferi/Lyme meningitis*), viral (e.g., enteroviruses, HSV), or fungal infection (*Cryptococcus neoformans, Coccidioides* spp). Pathogens invade the CSF and meningeal layers via colonization of epithelial layers, transmission into the bloodstream and passage through the blood–brain barrier. This process creates inflammation and injury and can lead to rapid death with certain virulent strains of bacteria (e.g., *N. meningitidis*). Viral meningitis is generally self-limiting and rarely fatal. Fungal meningitis is more common in immunosuppressed patients (e.g., patients with AIDS, transplant patients) and can cause serious, potentially fatal disease. Rarely, parasites can cause an eosinophilic meningitis.

Epidemiology

According to data collected from 2003 to 2007, there were an average of 4,100 cases of bacterial meningitis and 500 deaths in the United States each year.[1] The most common cause of bacterial meningitis in adults in the United States is *S. pneumonia*. CDC data[2] indicate the most common pathogens by age group are

- Newborns (≤30 days): Group B *Streptococcus, S. pneumoniae, Listeria monocytogenes, Escherichia coli*
- Infants (>30 days) and children: *Streptococcus pneumoniae, N. meningitidis, Haemophilus influenzae* type B (more common in unvaccinated children), group B *Streptococcus*
- Teens and young adults: *S. pneumoniae, N. meningitidis*
- Adults: *S. pneumoniae, N. meningitidis, H. influenzae* type B, group B *Streptococcus, L. monocytogenes* (particularly in elderly, immunosuppressed or alcoholic patients)

Viral meningitis is the most common type of meningitis. Enteroviruses (e.g., Coxsackievirus, Echovirus, nonpolioEnterovirus) are the most common cause of viral meningitis, followed by HSV and varicella zoster virus.[3] The most common cause of fungal meningitis is *Cryptococcus*. Other causes include *Histoplasmosis, Blastomyces, and Coccidioides.*

Clinical Presentation

Patients with meningitis may present with the classic triad of fever, nuchal rigidity, and altered mental status, but only about two thirds of patients will have all three symptoms.[4]

> **CLINICAL PEARL:** Patients with meningitis generally have mildly altered mental status (e.g., lethargy, mild confusion). Patients with overtly altered mental status (e.g., altered behavior, personality, speech, or movement) should be considered for possible encephalitis.

Other common symptoms include headache, seizure or focal neurologic deficits (more common in *L. monocytogenes* infections), petechiae, or purpura (more common in *N. meningitidis* infections). The mortality of bacterial meningitis is high; if left untreated or if treatment is initiated late in the course, it is almost always fatal. Even with appropriate antibiotic use, the bacterial meningitis mortality rate in adults was 16.4% according to a surveillance study from 1998 to 2007.[1]

Although patients with viral meningitis will have a clinical presentation similar to bacterial meningitis, it is generally self-limiting and rarely fatal. Fungal meningitis generally presents in a more insidious fashion, generally over weeks. Patients typically present with fever, headache, malaise with or without altered mental status. Patients may also have other signs or symptoms of disseminated fungal infection (e.g., cough, dyspnea, rash).

Diagnosis

Laboratory analyses that may be helpful in the diagnosis of meningitis include CBC with differential, coagulation studies (if concern for disseminated intravascular coagulation [DIC]), and blood cultures. All patients with suspected meningitis should undergo LP; patients with increased risk for herniation should have a CT of the head prior to an LP. It is ideal to obtain LP and blood cultures prior to the administration of empiric antibiotic therapy; however, treatment should not be delayed if an LP cannot be done expeditiously.

Opening pressure will be elevated in bacterial meningitis with mean opening pressures of 350 mm H_2O (normal = 200 mm H_2O)[5] and with *Cryptococcal* meningitis. Opening pressure in viral meningitis is generally normal. Gram stain will be positive for the causative agent in bacterial meningitis. Gram stain will be negative in viral meningitis. India ink staining will demonstrate encapsulated yeast organisms and *Cryptococcal* antigen (CrAg) will be positive in patients with *Cryptococcal* meningitis.

Cultures should be sent to confirm diagnosis and further direct antimicrobial therapy. Polymerase chain reaction (PCR) is available for certain strains of bacteria (e.g., *N. meningitidis, S. pneumoniae, H. influenzae* type b) and can make a definitive diagnosis in viral meningitis (e.g., HSV). CSF antibodies to *B. burgdorferi* may be present in Lyme meningitis. CSF analysis findings are discussed in Chapter 1, Common Presentations in Emergency Medicine, "Headache, Diagnostic Plan."

Management

- Bacterial meningitis: Empiric antibiotic therapy should be started immediately after CSF is obtained or prior to obtaining CSF if suspicion is high and LP will be delayed.
  - Empiric antibiotic therapy:
    - Immunocompetent patients: *S. pneumoniae,N. meningitidis, H. influenza,* group B *Streptococcus* → ceftriaxone (2 g IV q12h) *or* cefotaxime (2 g IV q12h) *plus* vancomycin (15–20 mg/kg IV q8–12h)
      - Add ampicillin to cover *L. monocytogenes* in adults older than 50 years (2 g IV q4h)
    - Immunocompromised patients/impaired cellular immunity: *S. pneumoniae, L. monocytogenes* and Gram-negative bacilli (*Pseudomonas aeruginosa*)[6] → vancomycin (15–20 mg/kg IV q8–12h) *plus* ampicillin (2 g IV q4h) *plus* cefepime (2 g IV q8h) *or* meropenem (2 g IV q8h)*

      *NOTE: May substitute moxifloxacin (400 mg IV qd) for beta-lactam-allergic patients and trimethoprim–sulfamethoxazole (5 mg/kg of trimethoprim IV q6h) for penicillin- allergic patients.

    - Head trauma/neurosurgical patients/ventricular drains: Gram-positive and gGram-negative pathogens (e.g., *Klebsiella pneumonia* and *P. aeruginosa*)[7,8] → vancomycin (15–20 mg/kg IV q8–12h *plus* ceftaizidime (2 g IV q8h) *or* cefepime (2 g IV q8h) *or* meropenem (2 g IV q8h)
    - Lyme meningitis: Ceftriaxone (2 g IV daily)[9]

- Therapy will be further guided once Gram stain, culture, and susceptibility results are back
- IV dexamethasone (0.15 mg/kg q6h) therapy is recommended initially as adjunctive therapy with antibiotics, and should be continued in patients with pneumococcal meningitis[10]
- Aseptic meningitis
  - Treatment can involve observation, starting empiric antibiotic therapy as suggested earlier until routine bacterial sources are ruled out, and treating the causative agent.
    - In suspected cases of HSV meningitis may begin empiric treatment with IV acyclovir (10 mg/kg q8h)

REFERENCES

1. Thigpen MC, Whitney CG, Messonnier NE, et al. Bacterial meningitis in the United States, 1998-2007. *N Engl J Med.* 2011;364(21):2016–2025. doi: 10.1056/NEJMoa1005384
2. Thigpen MC, Whitney CG, Messonnier NE, et al. Emerging Infections Programs Network. Bacterial meningitis in the United States, 1998-2007. *N Engl J Med.* 2011;364:2016-2025.
3. Kuplia L, Vuorinen T, Vainionpää R, et al. Etiology of aseptic meningitis and encephalitis in an adult population. *Neurology.* 2006;66(1):75–80. doi: 10.1212/01.wnl.0000191407.81333.00
4. Durand ML, Calderwood SB, Weber DJ, et al. Acute bacterial meningitis in adults—a review of 493 episodes. *N Engl J Med.* 1993;328(1):21–28. doi: 10.1056/NEJM199301073280104
5. de Gans J, van de Beek D. Dexamethasone in adults with bacterial meningitis. *N Engl J Med.* 2002;347(20):1549–1556. doi: 10.1056/NEJMoa021334
6. Quagliarello VJ, Scheld WM. Treatment of bacterial meningitis. *N Engl J Med.* 1997;336(10):708–716. doi: 10.1056/NEJM199703063361007
7. van de Beek D, Drake JM, Tunkel AR. Nosocomial bacterial meningitis. *N Engl J Med.* 2010;362(2):146–154. doi: 10.1056/NEJMra0804573
8. Tunkel AR, Hasbun R, Bhimraj A, et al. 2017 Infectious Disease Society of America's clinical practice guidelines for healthcare-associated ventriculitis and meningitis. *Clin Infect Dis.* 2017;64(6):e34–e65. doi: 10.1093/cid/ciw861
9. Halperin JJ. Nervous system Lyme disease. In: Steere AC, Shefner JM, eds. *UpToDate.* https://www.uptodate.com/contents/nervous-system-lyme-disease. Updated April 13, 2017.
10. Tunkel AR, Hartman BJ, Kaplan SL, et al. Practice guidelines for the management of bacterial meningitis. *Clin Infect Dis.* 2004;39(9):1267–1284. doi: 10.1086/425368

MIGRAINE HEADACHE

Etiology

Although the etiology of migraine headaches is not fully understood, it is thought that they develop due to dysfunction in neuronal depolarization, trigeminal nerve activation, and abnormal serotonin function. Migraine headaches arise when dysfunction in the neuronal system causes abnormal depolarization across the cerebral cortex, activating the trigeminal nerve.

This abnormal depolarization is thought to lead to the aura that precedes migraine headaches in some patients. Activation of the trigeminovascular system leads to sensitization of neurons, which contributes to symptoms of the unilateral, throbbing pain that is common in migraines.

Epidemiology

Migraine headaches are very common and affect up to 12% of the population in the United States.[1] They are more common in women and the peak incidence occurs between ages 30 and 40 years of age, with a gradual decline after age 40. Migraine without aura is the most common type, accounting for approximately 75% of cases.[2] There appears to be a genetic component as most patients with migraine headaches have family members with migraines.

Clinical Presentation

Migraine headaches are typically unilateral, gradually increasing in severity, and last hours to days. Patients may have a preceding aura such as visual changes, tinnitus, or other sensory or motor abnormalities. The pain is usually characterized as throbbing or pulsatile, mild to moderate in severity, and worse with physical activity. Photophobia, phonophobia, nausea, and vomiting are common associated symptoms. Patients with a history of migraine headaches or with chronic migraines will typically report similar symptoms in the past. Common migraine triggers are changes in sleeping patterns, chocolate, emotional stress, menstruation, alcohol, and not eating.

> **CLINICAL PEARL:** It is important to establish whether your patient has a history of similar prior headache symptoms. First-time migraines or changes in patients' typical migraine symptoms may require further workup and investigation.

Diagnosis

The diagnosis of migraine is primarily a clinical one and can be made with a careful history and thorough physical exam, including a detailed neurologic exam. Oftentimes patients will report a history of similar headaches and associated symptoms in the past. Patients without a history of migraines, particularly those over the age of 50, with new or different symptoms, unexplained neurologic abnormalities, or abrupt onset of severe pain may require neuroimaging or consultation with neurology in the ED. Other red-flag symptoms for headaches are discussed in the "Headache" section of Chapter 1, Common Presentations in Emergency Medicine. A CT of the head without contrast is the study of choice for most patients who require further workup. MRI, magnetic resonance angiography (MRA), or magnetic resonance venography (MRV) may be helpful for further evaluation for mass or posterior fossa lesion, vascular lesion, or sinus venous thrombosis.

Management

Treatment of migraine headache is centered around pain control and alleviating associated symptoms (e.g., nausea, vomiting). Most patients presenting to the ED with migraine headache will have moderate to severe pain that is unrelieved with their typical medications used for treatment.

- Mild to moderate pain may be treated with sumatriptan (6 mg subcutaneous injection), dihydroergotamine (1 mg IV) *with* metoclopramide (10 mg IV), ketorolac (15–30 mg IV).
  - Note: avoid dihydroergotamine, sumatriptan in patients with ischemic vascular disease.
- Pain associated with nausea and vomiting may be treated with metoclopramide (10 mg IV), prochlorperazine (10 mg IV or IM), chlorpromazine (0.1 mg/kg up to 25 mg IV).

> **CLINICAL PEARL:** Diphenhydramine (12.5–25 mg q1h × up to 2 doses) may be given in addition to metoclopramide, prochlorperazine, or chlorpromazine to avoid dystonic reactions. These medications also may be given as a slow IV push or mixed in with saline as a drip infusion to avoid dystonic reactions.

- IV dexamethasone (10–25 mg IV or IM) may be given to prevent headache recurrence.
- Opioids should be used sparingly and only as a last resort.
- Patients who are unresponsive to typical treatments may require admission to the hospital for status migrainosus and consultation with neurology.
- Patients who are discharged home should have close follow-up with a primary care provider or neurology.

REFERENCES

1. Lipton RB, Stewart WF, Diamond S, et al. Prevalence and burden of migraine in the United States: data from the American Migraine Study II. *Headache.* 2001;41(7):646–657. doi: 10.1046/j.1526-4610.2001.041007646.x
2. Cultrer FM, Bajwa ZH. Pathophysiology, clinical manifestations, and diagnosis of migraine in adults. In: Swanson JW, ed. *UpToDate.* https://www.uptodate.com/contents/pathophysiology-clinical-manifestations-and-diagnosis-of-migraine-in-adults. Updated November 17, 2018.

TEMPORAL ARTERITIS

Etiology

Temporal arteritis (giant cell arteritis) is a rheumatologic disease involving inflammation of the wall of the arteries branching from the carotid. It can affect the large, medium, and small intracranial and extracranial arteries, but most often affects the small and medium superficial vessels of the temporal artery.

Epidemiology

Temporal arteritis is rare before the age of 50; the mean age of onset is 71 years. It is more common in females and in patients of northern European descent. The incidence is 15 to 25 per 100,000 persons over the age of 50.[1] It is associated with polymyalgia rheumatica (PMR).

Clinical Presentation

Patients with temporal arteritis typically present with unilateral headache, transient monocular vision loss, jaw claudication, fever, malaise, and other constitutional symptoms. Fatigue and proximal muscle weakness may be present in patients with PMR. Physical exam may demonstrate tenderness overlying the temporal artery and vision abnormalities on the affected side.

Diagnosis

The diagnosis of temporal arteritis is based on clinical presentation and elevated erythrocyte sedimentation rate (ESR). Definitive diagnosis is made with temporal artery biopsy. The American College of Rheumatology criteria for the diagnosis of temporal arteritis are listed as follows:[2]

- Age of onset 50 years
- New headache, typically unilateral or jaw claudication
- Temporal artery abnormality: Tenderness overlying the temporal artery on exam or decreased pulsation of temporal arteries
- ESR of 50 mm/hr (Westergren method)
- Abnormal artery biopsy results: Vasculitis, mononuclear cell predominant infiltration or granulomatous inflammation, multinucleated giant cells

Management

Treatment of temporal arteritis should be initiated as soon as possible to avoid irreversible blindness. General principles of treatment are

- High-dose steroids: Methylprednisolone (1,000 mg daily IV) if vision loss is present at diagnosis, prednisone (40–60 mg daily for 2–4 weeks followed by taper) if no visual change
- Treat as soon as the diagnosis is suspected, do not wait for temporal artery biopsy results to initiate treatment
- Patients should have close follow-up with rheumatology

REFERENCES

1. Flood TA, Veinot JP. Temporal arteritis pathology. In: Burke AP, ed. *Medscape.* https://emedicine.medscape.com/article/1612591-overview. Updated August 10, 2018.
2. Hunder GG, Bloch DA, Michel BA, et al. The American College of Rheumatology 1990 criteria for the classification of giant cell arteritis. *Arthritis Rheum.* 1990;33(8):1122–1128. https://www.rheumatology.org/Portals/0/Files/Giant%20Cell%20(Temporal)%20Arteritis%20-%201990_Completed%20Article.pdf

TENSION-TYPE HEADACHE

Etiology

The precise cause of tension-type headache is not known. It is thought that the etiology is complex, multifactorial, and may vary from one patient to another. Headaches may be either episodic (14 days per month) or chronic (15 or more days per month.) Sensitization of myofascial nociceptors and pain pathways in the central nervous system (CNS) appear to contribute to both episodic and chronic tension-type headaches. Increased muscle tension in the scalp, neck, and shoulder muscles is thought to contribute to episodic tension-type headache.[1]

Epidemiology

Tension-type headache is the most common cause of primary headache and is subsequently responsible for high burden of disease and loss of work and productivity. A study in Demark found that the 1-year prevalence of tension-type headache between ages 12 and 41 years was 86%.[2] Another study in the United States found that the 1-year prevalence of episodic tension-typeheadache was 38.3% and chronic tension-type headache was 2.2%[3] Tension-type headache is more common in females.

Clinical Presentation

Tension-type headache typically presents as mild to moderate, bilateral headache. Pain is usually gradual in onset and nonpulsatile. Patients describe the pain as a dullpressure, fullness, and vice- or bandlike in nature. Pain may be precipitated by physical or emotional stress. Scalp, neck, and shoulder muscles may be tender on exam. Neurologic exam will be normal in patients with tension-type headache.

Diagnosis

Tension-type headache is diagnosed based on history and physical exam. There are no specific laboratory or imaging studies for the diagnosis of tension-type headache; these studies, if obtained, will yield negative results.

CLINICAL PEARL: Given the relatively normal and benign clinical presentation of tension-type headache, any neurologic abnormalities on physical exam and/or unexpected/unexplained abnormalities on laboratory or imaging studies must be further evaluated to rule out other etiology of headache.

Management

The majority of tension-type headaches will be successfully treated with the following measures:

- Over-the-counter analgesics such as acetaminophen, ibuprofen, aspirin, naproxen, or caffeine-containing combination medications
  - NSAIDs are generally the safest, mosteffective medication with lowest potential for medicationoveruse headache
- Nonpharmacologic measures, such as heat, ice, acupuncture, massage therapy, and rest, may be helpful adjuncts
- Moderate to severe headaches may be treated with chlorpromazine, metoclopramide, or ketorolac

REFERENCES

1. Taylor FR. Tension-type headache in adults: pathophysiology, clinical features, and diagnosis. In: Swanson JW, ed. *UpToDate*. https://www.uptodate.com/contents/tension-type-headache-in-adults-pathophysiology-clinical-features-and-diagnosis. Updated November 17, 2018.
2. Russel MB, Levi N, Šaltytė-Benth J, Fenger K. Tension-type headache in adolescents and adults: a population based study of 33,764 twins. *Eur J Epidemiol.* 2006;21(2):153–160. doi: 10.1007/s10654-005-6031-3
3. Schwartz BS, Stewart WF, Simon D, Lipton RB. Epidemiology of tension-type headache. *JAMA*. 1998;279(5):381–383. doi: 10.1001/jama.279.5.381

TRAUMATIC BRAIN INJURY

Etiology

Traumatic brain injury (TBI) occurs when an external force (e.g., fall, motor vehicle collisions [MVC], sports-related injury) causes transient or permanent altered mental status; neurologic deficits; physical, cognitive, or psychosocial dysfunction. TBI is a broad spectrum of injury ranging from mild concussive symptoms to permanent brain injury or death. Examples of such injuries include skull fracture, penetrating head injury, ICH, subdural hematoma (SDH), epidural hematoma, and concussion/postconcussive syndrome.

Pathophysiology of TBI depends on the mechanism of injury but generally includes direct trauma to the skull, dura, brain tissue, blood vessels, or transmitted forces involving tissue compression, shearing, or stretching of intracranial structures.

Epidemiology

Data from 2003 estimated the overall incidence of TBI to be approximately 538.2 per 100,000 people with about 1.5 million new cases per year.[1] TBI accounts for 40% of deaths related to acute injury in the United States and approximately 52,000 deaths per year; an estimated 200,000 patients per year require hospitalization.[2] TBI is more common in males with the highest rates occurring between 0 to 4 years, 15 to 24 years, and older than 65 years of age.[1] The most common mechanisms of injury are falls, MVCs, and sports-related injuries. It is estimated that 3.2 to 5.3 million people (1%–2% of the population) have long-term disability secondary to TBI in the United States.[3,4]

Clinical Presentation

The clinical presentation of TBI varies depending on the severity of injury. Patients will have a history of head trauma with or without loss of consciousness. Patients or witnesses may report amnesia leading up to (retrograde), during, or after (anterograde) the traumatic event or altered mental status ranging from mild cognitive impairment to overt behavioral changes or unresponsiveness. Patients may complain of headache, nausea, vomiting, dizziness, photophobia, or fatigue.

Physical exam should include a thorough neurologic evaluation. Patients may have altered mental status, decreased Glasgow Coma Scale (GCS) score, cranial nerve dysfunction or other focal neurologic deficits, ataxia or other motor dysfunction, CSF leak, otorrhea or rhinorrhea, nausea, vomiting, and external signs of trauma (abrasions, lacerations, contusions to scalp or face). Acute hearing loss, battle's sign, hemotympanum, and periorbital ecchymosis may be present in basilar skull fractures. Patients with ICH may have severe hypertension. Patients with mild injury may have a normal physical exam. Any significant neurologic abnormality on exam requires further evaluation for possible intracranial injury.

Diagnosis

Diagnosis of mild TBI is typically clinical and based on thorough history and physical exam. Laboratory analysis is generally not helpful in the evaluation of TBI. Blood glucose levels may be checked to rule out other causes of altered mental status, CBC, or coagulation studies may be obtained in patients with a history of coagulopathy or anticoagulant therapy. The following scenarios represent an indication for head CT without IV contrast:

- Patients with significant mechanism of injury, concerning historical features (e.g., prolonged loss of consciousness, anticoagulant therapy, persistent vomiting, elderly, unwitnessed injury, or inability for patient to give reliable history), or abnormal physical exam. Skull fractures, ICH, subdural hematoma (SDH), and epidural hematoma can all be detected with head CT.

Canadian CT Head Injury/Trauma Rule (www.mdcalc.com/canadian-ct-head-injury-trauma-rule), New Orleans/Charity Head Trauma/Injury Rule (www.mdcalc.com/new-orleans-charity-head-trauma-injury-rule), and Nexus II scoring systems can be used to determine the need for CT imaging in the setting of head trauma.

CTA may be useful in the diagnosis of traumatic carotid or vertebral artery dissection. MRI may also be helpful in further evaluation of TBI if CT is negative, but is generally not useful in the ED setting.

Management

Management of the critically ill patient with severe TBI should begin with evaluation of airway, breathing, and circulation. Immediate intervention is required for unstable patients or those with life-threatening injuries. Coordination of care with trauma surgery or neurosurgery prior to or upon arrival of patients with severe traumatic injury to the ED can facilitate immediate surgical intervention.

- Traumatic ICH is a time-sensitive diagnosis requiring prompt diagnosis and management. Initial management is similar to that of hemorrhagic stroke and was discussed previously in the section "Cerebrovascular Accident."
- SDH, epidural hematoma, ICH:
  - Immediate neurosurgical consultation to evaluate for appropriateness of operative versus nonoperative management.
- Skull fractures
  - Linear skull fractures without evidence of underlying brain injury or other associated injury may be discharged home with clear instructions to patients and family members or household contacts to return to the ED for severe headache, vomiting, or altered mental status.
  - Basilar skull fractures require admission for observation and consultation with neurosurgery and otolaryngology (for patients with hemotympanum, CSF leak or hearing loss).
  - Depressed skull fractures and penetrating injury require neurosurgical consultation.
    - Tetanus should be updated as needed.
    - Antibiotic prophylaxis should be given.
    - Anticonvulsant prophylaxis may be started in consultation with neurosurgery.
  - Patients on anticoagulant therapy with skull fractures should be admitted for observation.
- Concussion/postconcussion syndrome
  - Provide symptomatic treatment of pain and nausea.
  - Close monitoring with careful discharge instructions on signs/symptoms of severe head injury are needed.
  - Physical and cognitive rest is required until symptom free prior to reevaluation for clearance to work/sports activities.
  - Follow up with primary care provider or neurology.

REFERENCES

1. Rutland-Brown W, Langlois JA, Thomas EK, Xi YL. Incidence of traumatic brain injury in the United States, 2003. *J Head Trauma Rehabil.* 2006;21(6):544–548. https://journals.lww.com/headtraumarehab/Abstract/2006/11000/Incidence_of_Traumatic_Brain_Injury_in_the_United.9.aspx

2. Dawodu ST. Traumatic brain injury (TBI)—definition, epidemiology, pathophysiology. In: Kishner S, ed. *Medscape.* https://emedicine.medscape.com/article/326510-overview#a2. Updated June 27, 2019.

3. Thurman D, Alverson C, Dunn KA, et al. Traumatic brain injury in the United States: a public health perspective. *J Head Trauma Rehabil.* 1999;14(6):602–615. http://journals.lww.com/headtraumarehab/Citation/1999/12000/Traumatic_Brain_Injury_in_the_United_States__A.9.aspx

4. Zaloshnja E, Miller T, Langlois JA, et al. Prevalence of long-term disability from traumatic brain injury in the civilian population of the United States, 2005. *J Head Trauma Rehabil.* 2008;23(6):394–400. doi: 10.1097/01.HTR.0000341435.52004.ac

Low-Back Pain

Abdominal Aortic Aneurysm (Symptomatic)

Etiology

For young healthy patients, the abdominal aorta measures approximately 2 cm. When the diameter exceeds 3 cm, it is considered aneurysmal. The risk of rupture increases significantly once the diameter exceeds 5 cm.[1] The underlying pathophysiology is related in part to inflammatory processes, extracellular matrix degradation, and oxidative stress. Atherosclerosis accelerates aneurysm growth.

Epidemiology

Most patients who develop abdominal aortic aneurysm (AAA) are male, older than 60 years of age, and have associated cardiovascular risk factors, such as hypertension, hyperlipidemia, or established atherosclerotic cardiovascular disease. Smoking is a substantial risk factor. AAA is found in 2% of men over 55 years old with a male:female ratio of 4:1.[1]

Clinical Presentation

Symptoms may include sudden onset of abdominal pain radiating directly to the back described as a "ripping" or "tearing" pain.[2] It may present with syncope or near syncopal episodes as the aneurysm size progresses and cerebral perfusion decreases. Most AAAs are asymptomatic until they rupture, which can lead to hypotension and shock.

Physical examination findings may be limited. Palpate the abdomen to estimate aneurysmal width. This may be difficult in the obese patient. Assess the lower extremity pulses, including femoral, popliteal, dorsalis pedis, and posterior tibialis. In the setting of acute rupture, you may note a Cullen's sign (periumbilical ecchymosis) or Grey Turner's sign (flank ecchymosis).[2]

Diagnosis

Labs

- A CBC should be ordered to evaluate for anemia secondary to blood loss in the setting of rupture.

- EKG should be performed to rule out an associated acute MI.
- Plain films can be performed and may demonstrate abdominal aortic calcification with bulging aortic contour.[2]
- If a bedside ultrasound is readily available, it should be done to assess size of the aorta in preparation for emergent consultation with a vascular surgeon.
- CTA allows for a detailed anatomical view and can be done if a patient is stable. An aortic diameter of less than 3.0 cm excludes acute aneurysmal disease.[2]

Management

Management is dependent on aneurysm size and patient presentation. All patients with symptomatic AAA require emergent consultation with a surgeon or transfer to a center that has the capability to perform vascular surgery. In the ED, the patient should be managed by following advanced cardiac life support (ACLS) protocols, including fluids and blood products, if needed.[2] One-time screening for AAA by ultrasound in men aged 65 to 75 years is associated with reduced risk of AAA-related mortality. Women do not appear to benefit from screening.[3]

References

1. Gasper WJ, Rapp JH, Johnson MD. Blood vessel & lymphatic disorders. In: Papadakis MA, McPhee SJ, Rabow MW, eds. *Current Medical Diagnosis & Treatment.* 57th ed. New York, NY: McGraw-Hill; 2018:479–506. http://accessmedicine.mhmedical.com/content.aspx?bookid=2192&sectionid=168192658
2. Prince LA, Johnson GA. Aneurysmal disease. In: Tintinalli JE, Stapczynski J, Ma O, eds. *Tintinalli's Emergency Medicine: A Comprehensive Study Guide.* 8th ed. New York, NY: McGraw-Hill; 2016:416–419. http://accessmedicine.mhmedical.com/content.aspx?bookid=1658&sectionid=109388462
3. Pignone M, Salazar R. Disease prevention & health promotion. In: Papadakis MA, McPhee SJ, Rabow MW, eds. *Current Medical Diagnosis & Treatment* 57th ed. New York, NY: McGraw-Hill; 2018:1–18. http://accessmedicine.mhmedical.com/content.aspx?bookid=2192&sectionid=168005867

Compression Fractures: Vertebral Body (Due to Osteoporosis)

Etiology

Osteoporosis is a skeletal disorder characterized by a loss of bone osteoid, which reduces bone integrity and bone strength. This predisposes one to an increased risk of fracture, with vertebral fractures being the most common.[1] Thoracic and lumbar spine fractures account for almost half of all osteoporotic fractures in the elderly, with the most common site being T12-L1 and T7-T8 levels.[2] The most common type of fractures are anterior wedge compression fractures.

Epidemiology

Contributing factors for the development of osteoporosis include advanced age, alcoholism, smoking, chronic use of PPIs, and chronic use of high-dose glucocorticoid use. Men who use antiandrogen therapy for prostate cancer are also at risk.[1] It is more common to see a vertebral body compression fracture at the thoracolumbar site for the elderly patient versus a young patient who sustains a compression fracture due to direct trauma or axial loading. For the purpose of following epidemiological prevalence, the discussion of compression fractures here is limited to that of the elderly population who suffer from osteoporosis.

Clinical Presentation

The back pain associated with vertebral body compression fractures can vary. Some patients have sudden onset of pain due to a spontaneous (atraumatic) fracture or collapse of the vertebra. It is common for these patients to have a loss of height as well. The most important clinical assessment includes a thorough neurological exam to rule out cord compression, specifically evaluating for lower extremity paralysis, saddle anesthesia, and loss of rectal tone.

Diagnosis

LABS

- There is rarely a need for laboratory testing in the setting of vertebral body compression fractures for the elderly patient in the ED.
- If the differential diagnosis includes any infectious etiology, or there is bleeding in or around the affected region then a CBC with differential may be ordered to look for leukocytosis and anemia.
- If the patient is on anticoagulants, coagulation studies, including PT/INR may be helpful for the team that executes inpatient management.
- If there is suspicion of a urinary etiology of the back pain, a BMP for renal function and electrolytes and a urine analysis with culture should be done.

DIAGNOSTIC IMAGING

- It is sometimes difficult to discern whether a compression fracture is acute or chronic and plain films tend to have low sensitivity. CT scan of the thoracolumbar spine without contrast is the first-line imaging modality for adults.[2] This will also reveal any retropulsion of fracture fragments that may impinge the spinal cord.

Management

In general, ED providers have a low threshold for admission when it comes to geriatric patients. Due to the complexity and chronicity of the diseases concomitant with advanced aging, any elderly patient with the potential to become further injured, who has a lack of support or care at home, or with associated dementia should be admitted for management.

Preventive management includes

- Guidance on smoking and alcohol cessation
- Enhanced exercise, including strength training
- Patient education on fall-prevention modalities
- Vitamin D and calcium supplementation, along with bisphosphonates
- Patients can initially have pain managed on a conservative basis similar to that of low back pain; aback brace for support may be helpful
- Percutaneous vertebroplasty or kyphoplasty may be considered for patients with vertebral compression fractures who fail conservative pain management[1]

REFERENCES

1. Fitzgerald PA. Endocrine disorders. In: Papadakis MA, McPhee SJ, Rabow MW, eds. *Current Medical Diagnosis & Treatment*. 57th ed.. New York, NY: McGraw-Hill; 2018:1117–1221. http://accessmedicine.mhmedical.com/content.aspx?bookid=2192&sectionid=167996562
2. Fleischman RJ, Ma O. Trauma in the elderly. In: Tintinalli JE, Stapczynski J, Ma O, et al., eds. *Tintinalli's Emergency Medicine: A Comprehensive Study Guide*. 8th ed. New York, NY: McGraw-Hill; 2016:1688–1691. http://accessmedicine.mhmedical.com/content.aspx?.bookid=1658&sectionid=109445304

EPIDURAL ABSCESS

Etiology

A spinal epidural abscess is an uncommon but potentially life-threatening cause of low-back pain resulting from an accumulation of pus or infectious material in the epidural space. Most spinal abscess cases are secondary to *Staphylococcus aureus*. With the development of resistant organisms, MRSA is an important consideration to keep in mind.

CLINICAL PEARL: Consider Pott's disease for patients who may be traveling to/from the United States from a developing country. This should also be considered in patients with a history of tuberculosis (TB) exposure and/or weight loss.

Epidemiology

Risk factors for spinal epidural abscess include diabetes mellitus, renal failure, injection drug use, immunocompromised status (e.g., HIV), alcohol abuse, recent spinal procedure, history of diabetes, chronic use of an indwelling catheter, and fever of unknown origin.[1]

Clinical Presentation

The patient may present with low-back pain combined with constitutional symptoms, fever, chills, and night sweats, along with spinal pain. There may be progressive limb weakness as well. Patients can present with symptoms for several weeks to several months. The classic triad of symptoms suggesting spinal epidural abscess is severe back pain, fever, and neurological deficits.[1] On physical exam, these patients are often febrile, tachycardic, and toxic appearing. A thorough neurological assessment should be performed. Because epidural abscesses occur in close proximity to the brain and spinal cord, neurologic defects and/or paralysis can occur.

Diagnosis

Labs

- Blood cultures with sensitivity
- CBC often reveals leukocytosis
- ESR is typically greater than 20 mm/hr
- Urinalysis with culture and sensitivity
- LP with CSF for Gram staining and culture: may be considered in order to exclude meningitis

> **Clinical Pearl:** LP is relatively contraindicated in epidural abscess due to the potential for seeding the infection into the subarachnoid space.

Diagnostic Imaging

- For all spinal infections, the gold standard imaging study is a contrast MRI [1]
- CXR is needed to rule out pneumonia.

Management

Epidural abscess treatment includes pharmacologic and interventional methods. Patients should receive antipyretics and be placed in a negative pressure isolation room if there is suspicion of a pathogen with a high degree of contagion (e.g., TB). Begin hydration with IV fluids. Antibiotic treatment for epidural abscess should be continued for up to 6 to 8 weeks parenterally. Agents include coverage piperacillintazobactam 3.375 g and vancomycin 1 g IV. Broad-spectrum coverage is key. Abscess drainage may be performed by neurosurgery or interventional radiology, but that decision should be made by an interdisciplinary team based on the patient's response to treatment.

Reference

1. Della-Giustina D, Dubin JS, Frohna W. Neck and back pain. In: Tintinalli JE, Stapczynski J, Ma O, et al., eds. *Tintinalli's Emergency Medicine: A Comprehensive Study Guide.* 8th ed. New York, NY: McGraw-Hill; 2016:1887–1893.

NEOPLASM

Etiology

Tumors may lead to spinal cord dysfunction by direct cord compression, ischemia by obstructing an artery or venous structure, or by invasive infiltration.[1]

Epidemiology

Approximately 10% of spinal tumors are intramedullary.[1] In the case of metastasis, the more common primary neoplasms that metastasize to the spine include cancer of the prostate, breast, lung, and kidney.

> **CLINICAL PEARL:** Because prostate cancer is more prevalent in Black men, if a patient with a history of prostate cancer presents with back pain, neoplasm should be at the top of the differential diagnosis.

Clinical Presentation

The majority of patients with back pain from a neoplasm develop symptoms gradually over time. Back pain may be worse with coughing or straining. Radicular symptoms may be present and suggest nerve root involvement. Pain typically precedes specific neurological symptoms of spinal cord compression from epidural metastases by several months.[1] Red flags include lower extremity paresthesia or paralysis, saddle anesthesia, loss of rectal tone, or complaints of incontinence to bowel or bladder.

Diagnosis

The imaging modality of choice, if available, is an MRI with contrast or CT myelography to identify and locate the lesion.[1]

Management

If the neoplasm is intramedullary, treatment is aimed at surgical excision followed by radiation therapy. Treatment of epidural spinal metastasis consists of radiation. Patients may also receive dexamethasone 10 to 100 mg parenterally in the ED to reduce local swelling and minimize the potential for cord compression, followed by 16–96 mg/day in divided doses over the next several days. Surgical decompression is part of the long-term management of spinal neoplasm that does not respond to radiation, that is associated with evidence of neurological instability, or in patients who have an uncertain diagnosis.

REFERENCE

1. Aminoff MJ, Douglas VC. Nervous system disorders. In: Papadakis MA, McPhee SJ, Rabow MW, eds. *Current Medical Diagnosis & Treatment.* 57th ed. New York, NY: McGraw-Hill; 2018:986–1058. http://accessmedicine.mhmedical.com/content.aspx?bookid=2192&sectionid=168019736

SCIATICA

Etiology

The most common cause of symptomatic low-back pain presenting with sciatica is a herniated disk.[1] Keep in mind that anything that causes compression or impingement of the spinal nerve roots can present in a similar fashion, including cauda equina syndrome.[1] The majority of herniated disks occur at the L4-L5 or L5-S1 nerve root.

Epidemiology

Although sciatica only affects a small proportion of all patients with back pain, it is present in the vast majority of patients with a symptomatic herniated disk. Therefore, sciatica is a relatively common condition in the adult population.

Clinical Presentation

Sciatica often presents as an acute episode in a chronic degenerative process. Patients may present with pain following sneezing or lifting. Due to the common anatomical location of herniated disks, patients most often present with radicular back pain extending below the knee that follows a dermatomal distribution of that nerve root. The physical exam may include a positive straight leg on the ipsilateral side and a positive straight leg on the contralateral side as a crossed straight leg. Be sure to document areas of pain, paresthesia, diminished reflexes, and any muscle weakness. These particular history and physical exam findings are important, as they will help you differentiate between a lumbosacral strain and sciatica.

Piriformis syndrome includes symptoms of sciatic radiculopathy associated with tenderness in the prirformis muscle region in the absence of MRI evidence of herniated lumbar disc protrusion.[2] This results in and is the most common complaint of sciatica.[2]

Diagnosis

History and physical examination provide the cornerstones for diagnosis, including radicular pain that extends below the knee and a positive straight leg and crossed-leg raise test. In the setting of suspected trauma, infection, malignancy, or cauda equina syndrome, plain films or possibly CT scan are indicated. Otherwise, no further testing is required.

> **CLINICAL PEARL:** Be cognizant of signs and symptoms of cauda equina syndrome, including loss of bowel or bladder function and saddle anesthesia, in addition to low-back pain and pain that radiates below the knee, as this is a surgical emergency.

Management

Treatment is similar to that of lumbosacral strain. NSAIDs are the pharmacologic treatment of choice for sciatica. Continuation of activities of daily living is recommended and bed rest should be avoided. Physical therapy may be useful if symptoms do not resolve with initial conservative therapy.

For acute, severe sciatica, consider epidural steroid injections. Consider spinal decompression for patients with disabling sciatica due to neurological deficits or for patients with chronic symptoms despite optimal medical management. Most patients recover in 1 to 2 months with conservative therapy.

REFERENCES

1. Della-Giustina D, Dubin JS, Frohna W. Neck and back pain. In: Tintinalli JE, Stapczynski J, Ma O, et al., eds. *Tintinalli's Emergency Medicine: A Comprehensive Study Guide.* 8th ed. New York, NY: McGraw-Hill; 2016:1887–1893.
2. Borenstein D, Calin A. *Fast Facts: Low Back Pain.* 2nd ed. Abingdon, UK: Health Press; 2012.

THORACIC/LUMBAR STRAIN

Etiology

Mechanical disorders of the lumbar spine are related to injury, overuse, or deformity of a spinal structure, which can lead to spasms of the paravertebral muscles of either the midback, lower back, or both.[1] Injury occurs when the load being lifted cannot be supported by the paraspinal muscles. The thoracic spine is a more rigid segment compared to the cervical spine above it. As a result, not only is injury to the thoracic spine less common than either the cervical or lumbar regions, but this also means the presence of a thoracic vertebral injury in a young patient is the result of severe traumatic forces.[2] This distinction is important to keep in mind when obtaining the history.

Epidemiology

Muscle strain of the lumbar region is the most common cause of back pain in the 20- to 40-year-old age group.[1] Back pain is more likely to be from an infection or a tumor in patients under the age of 18 years, and over the age of 50.[3] Patients over age 50 are also more prone to fractures of the vertebral bodies and spinal stenosis. AAA should be considered in the differential diagnosis, particularly in the presence of cardiovascular risk factors.

Clinical Presentation

Inquire about precise identifiers as to how the pain started. Patients who are younger tend to present with back injury due to heavy lifting, shoveling snow, work-related injuries, or sports-related injuries and may complain of onset of back pain after engaging in these activities. Older patients are more likely to complain of mid-thoracic back pain related to compression fractures.

As a result of injury, the paraspinal muscles are contracted, in part to promote healing. Because of this, many patients may complain of limited range of motion. Patients will often ambulate slowly with a cautious gate. Observe them as they attempt to change into a hospital gown and sit down on the exam table. This information should be documented in the chart. Typically, patients take care not to bend forcefully. Radiculopathy is typically not noted.

Diagnosis

The diagnosis of any back strain is primarily clinically based on history and physical exam findings. The lack of historical "red flags" also facilitates the diagnosis. If a patient sustained a high fall, a blow to the back inflicted by the use of objects (such as a bat or metal pole) or was involved in a motor vehicle crash with substantial extrication time, he or she may require imaging. Imaging should be strongly considered in patients over the age of 55 years, those with a history of IV drug use, or a history of long-term steroid use.

> **CLINICAL PEARL:** "Red flags" to inquire about include a history of fever, chills, constitutional symptoms, history of neoplasm, history of incontinence to bowel or bladder, or lower extremity paresthesia/paralysis.

In the setting of direct trauma, an initial x-ray of the thoracic and lumbar spine is an appropriate choice. If there is any evidence of fractures or asymmetry in spinal alignment, a CT scan can be ordered. CT is generally preferred over MRI in this particular setting because an MRI is not always readily available. CT scans are more sensitive for fractures whereas MRI is better for soft tissue injuries such as the spinal cord or the intervertebral disks.

Management

Treatment for muscle strain is gradual movement, use of NSAIDs, and prescribed muscle relaxants. Acetaminophen is considered the first-line agent for low-back pain.[3] For patients with unrelenting pain, a combination of acetaminophen 650 to 1,000 mg every 4 to 6 hours with ibuprofen 800 mg three times daily or naproxen 250 to 500 mg twice daily can be used. If there is concern for GI bleed, add a PPI such as omeprazole 20 mg a day.[3] The use of opioids should be limited to only 1 week and only if all other modalities have failed. Muscle relaxants are also useful as an adjunct to the medications mentioned previously. Diazepam 5 to 10 mg every 6 to 8 hours and cyclobenzaprine 5 to 10 mg every 6 hours are options for treatment.

> **CLINICAL PEARL:** Patients should not exceed an acetaminophen dose of 4 g in a 24-hour period and prescribers should advise that they are to AVOID taking acetaminophen if receiving an opioid prescription.

Within reason, patients should continue their activities of daily living and avoid limited range of motion. Recommend avoidance of heavy lifting, but indicate that remaining motionless for an extended period of time may delay recovery. Recommend applying ice to the affected area for the first 3 to 4 days after an acute injury to minimize local inflammation. After that, heat can be applied.

Patients should be instructed to return to the ED for any concerning symptoms such as paralysis, sensory or other motor deficits to the lower extremity, worsening condition despite use of conservative treatment, incontinence to bowel or bladder, or difficulty breathing. Patients should follow up with their primary care provider within a week if symptoms do not resolve. If symptoms progress, patients may require an MRI and possibly physical therapy with monitoring for up to 4 to 6 weeks.

REFERENCES

1. Borenstein D, Calin A. *Fast Facts: Low Back Pain.* 2nd ed. Abingdon, UK: Health Press; 2012.
2. Go S. Spine trauma. In: Tintinalli JE, Stapczynski J, Ma O, et al., eds. *Tintinalli's Emergency Medicine: A Comprehensive Study Guide.* 8th ed. New York, NY: McGraw-Hill; 2016:1708–1723. http://accessmedicine.mhmedical.com/content.aspx?bookid=1658&sectionid=109387434
3. Della-Giustina D, Dubin JS, Frohna W. Neck and back pain. In: Tintinalli JE, Stapczynski J, Ma O, et al., eds. *Tintinalli's Emergency Medicine: A Comprehensive Study Guide.* 8th ed. New York, NY: McGraw-Hill; 2016:1887–1893.

TRAUMATIC INJURY

BITE WOUNDS

Etiology

Bite wounds from animals or humans cause various injuries, including abrasions, punctures, lacerations, tissue avulsions, or crush injuries. These injuries often occur to the face or upper extremities. Other injury sites include the neck, trunk, or lower extremities. Bite wounds are a common problem and can cause complications such as deep structure injury, wound infection, and poor cosmetic outcomes. Although rare in the United States in domestic animals, rabies is also a potential complication of wild animal bites.

The most common pathogen found in animal bite wounds is *Pasteurella*, whereas *Eikenella* is the most common pathogen found in human bite wounds.[1] Skin flora (e.g., *Streptococcus, Staphylococcus*) and other anaerobes are other common isolates from infected wounds.

Epidemiology

Bite wounds are a common occurrence with an annual incidence of 2 to 5 million, accounting for approximately 1% of all ED visits.[1] Dog bites are the most common cause of bite wounds (60%–90%) followed by cat bites (5%–20%), human bites (2%–3%), and bites from other animals (e.g., rodents, other wild animals).[1]

Clinical Presentation

Patients will report a history of bite wound from an animal or human and often present with abrasions, avulsions, punctures (more common with cat bites or small dogs), skin tears, or lacerations at the site of injury. Other associated injuries may include contusions, fractures, or joint capsule violation. Patients with boxer's fractures and associated abrasion or laceration (generally overlying the dorsal aspect of the third or fourth metacarpophalangeal joint) should be questioned about contact with another person's tooth or so-called "fight bite." Delayed presentation (>24–72 hours) in seeking medical care is often associated with wound infection. These patients may present with erythema, fluctuance, purulent drainage, swelling, lymphangitis, or fever.

Careful physical examination of the affected area should be performed with particular attention to skin, deeper tissues, neurovascular and musculoskeletal systems. Evaluate the wound, affected area, and areas distal to injury for evidence of tendon, muscle, bone or neurovascular injury, and the presence of foreign body such as a tooth.

Diagnosis

Diagnosis of bite wounds is predominantly clinical and is made by history and physical exam.

Labs

- Laboratory studies are generally unhelpful, except for cases of wound infection.
- Patients with wound infection complications such as cellulitis, joint infection, osteomyelitis, or sepsis may have elevated WBC, ESR, CRP levels.
- Wound cultures may be obtained for infected wounds to direct antibiotic therapy but are not helpful in uninfected wounds.

Diagnostic Imaging

- Associated injuries, such as fracture, foreign-body contamination, and joint capsule involvement, may be diagnosed with x-ray or CT imaging.

Management

Initial management involves thorough inspection and irrigation of the wound. Meticulous wound care at the time of initial injury is important to reduce the risk of infection. In cases of severe injury, controlling hemorrhage and stabilizing fractures or joint injuries may be necessary. Debride devitalized tissue and debris from the wound. Although it is preferable to leave bite wounds open, wounds with active bleeding, gaping wounds, or wounds with potential for poor cosmetic outcomes (e.g., facial wounds) should be loosely approximated with suture or staple repair.

> **Clinical Pearl:** All wounds requiring closure should be given antibiotic prophylaxis.

Orthopedic surgery consultation may be necessary for wounds that penetrate bones, joints, tendons, neurovascular structures, or other deep, complex wounds. Plastic surgery consultation may be necessary for complex facial lacerations.

Update tetanus vaccinations as needed. Rabies prophylaxis is discussed in further detail in Chapter 4, Patient Education and Counseling in Emergency Medicine,, "Vaccinations." Consider antibiotic prophylaxis for patients at high risk of developing wound infection. High-risk wounds include[1]

- Deep puncture wounds (e.g., cat bites)
- Moderate to severe wounds with associated crush injury
- Wounds in areas of underlying poor venous or lymphatic circulation (e.g., distal lower extremity)
- Facial, hand, or genital wounds
- Wounds involving or in close proximity to bones or joints
- Wounds requiring closure
- Patients with underlying immunocompromise

Patients with bite wounds should be considered for antibiotic prophylaxis. Wounds at high risk for infection may be given an V dose of antibiotics initially, followed by oral antibiotics. Patients with lower risk wounds may be given oral antibiotics. Treatment of choice for IV antibiotic therapy is:[1]

- Ampicillin–sulbactam 3 g IV
- OR (for penicillinallergic patients) ceftriaxone 1 g IV **PLUS** metronidazole 500 mg IV or clindamycin 600 mg IV
- OR (for penicillin-allergic patients) ciprofloxacin 400 mg IV or levofloxacin 750 mg IV **PLUS** metronidazole 500 mg IV or clindamycin 600 mg IV

Treatment of choice for PO antibiotic therapy is:[1]

- Amoxicillin/clavulanate 875 mg/125 mg PO BID for 5 to 7 days
- OR (for penicillin-allergic patients) doxycycline 100 mg PO BID, trimethoprim–sulfamethoxazole 1 DS tab PO BID, ciprofloxacin 500 mg PO BID, or levofloxacin 750 mg PO qd **PLUS** metronidazole 500 mg PO TID or clindamycin 450 mg PO TID

Most patients with bite wounds should have a wound check within 48 to 72 hours, except those with very minor injuries. All patients with bite wounds should be given clear wound-care instructions and instructions to return to the ED for any sign of wound infection such as fever, redness or swelling, worsening pain or tenderness, purulent discharge or lymphangitis.

REFERENCE

1. Baddour LM, Harper M. Clinical manifestations and initial management of bite wounds. *UpToDate.* https://www-uptodate-com.proxy.libraries.rutgers.edu/contents/clinical-manifestations-and-initial-management-of-bite-wounds?search=bite%20wound&source=search_result&selectedTitle=1 150&usage_type=default&display_rank=1. Updated October 13, 2017. Accessed August 3, 2018.

Burns

Etiology

Burns involve damage to the skin, underlying tissues, cardiac function, eyes, or other mucosal membranes due to thermal (e.g., fire, scalding), electrical, or chemical injury. These injuries can lead to local trauma, tissue edema, arrhythmias, shock, disruption of cell membrane function, acid–base disturbances, and electrolyte/fluid imbalances. Severity of injury depends on depth and area of exposure, offending agent, or amount and type of current involved.

Epidemiology

Approximately 486,000 people in the United States are treated in the ED every year for thermal burn injuries; 40,000 of whom require hospitalization.[1] The number of deaths related to fire and smoke inhalation during 2014 was 3,275. Burn patients are more likely to be male and of Caucasian ethnicity. Of patients admitted to burn centers in the United States in 2015, 43% of injuries were due to fire or flame, 34% were due to scald injury, 9% from contact injury, 4% from electrical sources, 3% from chemical burns, and 7% from other causes.[1]

Clinical Presentation

Most patients with mild to moderate burns will report a history of thermal, electrical, or chemical exposure. Patients with severe burn injury may not be able to give a history but may show signs of shock, severe tissue damage, singed nares, or soot in oropharynx, and entry or exit wounds (in electrical burn injuries). Skin may be erythematous or may have blisters, eschar, pallor, or deeper tissue injury. Patients with chemical burns may still have chemical matter on the affected area. Patients with smoke exposure may have vocal hoarseness, singed nares or soot in the nasal passages or oropharynx, oropharyngeal injection or edema, or conjunctival injection and tearing. Likewise, patients with chemical exposure to eyes or mucosal membranes may have conjunctival tearing, photophobia, or nasal/oropharyngeal injection or edema. Patients with electrical injury due to high voltage may have cardiac arrhythmias, transient loss of consciousness or seizure, spinal cord injury, cutaneous burns, intra-abdominal injury, bone or deep muscle injury.

Diagnosis

The diagnosis of burn injury is largely based on clinical exam with careful examination of skin, mucous membranes, and neurovascular systems. Thermal burns are classified as

- Superficial (first degree): Involves only the epidermis
  - Causes erythema to skin without blisters.
- Superficial partial thickness (superficial second degree): Involves epidermis and superficial dermis
  - Causes erythema to skin with blisters.

- Deep partial thickness (deep second degree): Involves epidermis, deep dermis, sweat glands, and hair follicles
  - Causes erythema to skin, hair loss, and blisters; scars with healing.
- Full thickness (third degree): Involves entire epidermis and dermis
  - Causes charred, pale, and fibrous appearance to dermis; scars with healing/may require skin grafting.
- Fourth degree: Involves entire dermis, epidermis, and underlying fat/muscle/bone
  - Causes severe tissue damage and scarring; requires surgery and skin grafting.

Calculation of body surface area for burns in adult patients can be performed using the rule of nines (Figure 2.1):
- Head—9%
- Arms—9% each
- Front of leg—9% each
- Back of leg—9% each
- Anterior chest—9%
- Anterior abdomen—9%
- Upper back—9%
- Lower back—9%
- Groin/genital region—1%

When possible, it is important to determine the type of exposure or materials/chemicals involved, depth and surface area of injury, amount of electrical voltage exposure and whether or not inhalation, mucosal membrane, or eye injury occurred.

Labs
The following labs may be helpful in the diagnosis and management of burn patients:

- ABG: Inhalation injury/burn injury
- Carboxyhemoglobin: Carbon monoxide toxicity/smoke inhalation
- CPK: Rhabdomyolysis in burn, crush, or electrical injuries
- Urine myoglobin: Rhabdomyolysis in burn, crush, or electrical injuries
- Troponin: Cardiac injury sustained in high-voltage electrical injury
- Lactate: Burn injury
- CMP: Electrolyte abnormalities may develop due to large fluid shifts in burn and electrical injury patients; baseline renal function should be established for patients being monitored for potential acute kidney injury (e.g., rhabdomyolysis from severe burn)

Diagnostic Imaging
- EKG and cardiac monitoring should be performed on patients with high-voltage electrical injury.
- Fluorescein staining and pH measurement with litmus paper should be performed for patients with chemical exposure to the eyes.

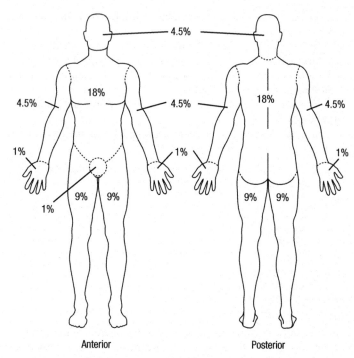

Anterior   Posterior

Figure 2.1 Rule of Nines burn size estimation diagram. For irregularly distributed burns, the palm of the victim's hand represents approximately 1% of the total body surface area.

Source: Veenema TG, ed. *Disaster Nursing and Emergency Preparedness: For Chemical, Biological, and Radiological Terrorism and Other Hazards.* (4th ed). New York, NY: Springer Publishing Company, 2019:432.

Management

- Burn care
  - Mild thermal burns
    - Pain control with cooling measures and oral acetaminophen or NSAIDs
    - Cool the affected area with cool water; do not apply ice
    - Irrigate wound with tap water and soap or normal saline
    - Debride ruptured blisters and nonviable tissue; intact blisters should be left undisturbed after cleansing
    - Superficial first- and second-degree burns do not require topical antibiotic application;patients should be instructed to use moisturizer cream only

- Application of bacitracin or silver sulfadiazine 1% for partial- and full-thickness burns with dry, gauze bandage
- Update tetanus immunization as needed
- Patients should be instructed in wound care and on appropriate topical antibiotic use

○ Moderate and severe thermal burns
  - As previously discussed, patient's airway, breathing, circulation, and any life-threatening conditions should be immediately addressed
    • Patients with suspected significant inhalation injury or respiratory distress should undergo rapid sequence induction (RSI) prior to onset of airway edema
    • High-flow oxygen should be given for cases of carbon monoxide poisoning
  - Initiate fluid resuscitation immediately in cases of severe burns, which can result in large fluid shifts and hypoperfusion
    • The Parkland formula can be used to calculate initial fluid resuscitation needs (www.mdcalc.com/parkland-formula-burns)
    • Body surface area can be calculated using the rule of nines discussed earlier
  - Remove burned clothing, debris, and jewelry
  - Cool the affected area with cool water; do not apply ice
  - Control pain with IV pain medication such as morphine
  - Irrigate wounds with tap water and soap or normal saline
  - Debride ruptured blistered and nonviable tissue; generally, intact blisters should be left undisturbed after cleansing
  - Application of silver sulfadiazine 1% for partial- and full-thickness burns with dry, gauze bandage
  - Update tetanus immunization as needed
  - Patients may need transfer to burn center facility after stabilization; partial- and full-thickness burns should be followed up at burn center to facilitate proper healing and prevent long-term complications
  - Criteria for transfer to burn center include
    • Partial-thickness burns over more than 10% body surface area
    • Burns involving the face, hands, feet, genitalia, perineum, or major joints
    • Third-degree burns for any age group
    • Severe electrical (including lightning injury) or chemical burns
    • Inhalation injury
    • Significant comorbidity or concomitant injury (e.g., fracture) that may complicate management, healing, or increase mortality
    • Hospitals without qualified personnel to care for pediatric patients or patients requiring specific social, emotional, or other rehabilitative services

○ Chemical burns
  - Treatment of injury depends on chemical involved, amount, concentration, and area of exposure

- Guidance for management of specific chemicals can be found in material safety data sheet (MSDS)
- You should thoroughly decontaminate your patient if this has not been done prior to arrival with removal of contaminated clothing and thorough irrigation of infected areas with water or normal saline (further management of chemical burns is discussed in Chapter 1, Common Presentations in Emergency Medicine, "Traumatic Injury")

- Electrical injury
  - Treat all life-threatening cardiopulmonary and neurologic injuries
  - Obtain immediate trauma, neurosurgical, or orthopedic consultation for severe traumatic, limb-threatening, or neurovascular injuries
  - EKG and cardiac monitoring for high-voltage injury
  - Begin aggressive fluid resuscitation for patients with severe soft-tissue or burn injuries
  - Skin wounds should be treated as thermal burns
  - High-voltage injuries should be admitted for observation:
    - Cardiac monitoring
    - Frequent neurovascular assessments to monitor for development of compartment syndrome
    - Lab analysis to monitor for rhabdomyolysis and acute kidney injury

REFERENCES

1. Burn incidence and treatment in the United States: 2016. http://ameriburn.org/who-we-are/media/burn-incidence-fact-sheet

FOREIGN BODY (SOFT TISSUE/SUBCUTANEOUS)

Etiology

Foreign bodies can enter through the skin and become lodged in the soft tissues and subcutaneous space through a number of different mechanisms. It is common for foreign bodies to enter through wound contamination, punctures or splinters of the plantar or palmar surfaces of the extremities, or through piercings in the skin. Retained foreign bodies can cause tissue damage, wound infections, delayed wound healing, and localized inflammation.

Epidemiology

The most common type of puncture wound occurs through the sole of the foot from stepping on an object. The majority of these injuries are from nails, glass, wood, or other metal objects. The most common cause of infections due to foreign bodies are *Staphylococcus aureus*, beta-hemolytic *Streptococci* and *Pseudomonas aeruginosa* (particularly in puncture wounds through the sole of a shoe, water-based injuries, or piercings through ear cartilage).[1] In a study of 185 ED patients with glass-induced lacerations, the rate of retained foreign body was 15%.[2] The risk of retained foreign bodies and puncture wounds increases during warmer weather months due to skin exposure and increased outdoor/recreational activity.

Clinical Presentation

Patients with retained foreign bodies may present with wounds caused by or contaminated with occult foreign material (e.g., glass, needles, wood, or plastic splinters). Patients may also present with the foreign body visibly embedded in soft tissue (e.g., fish hook, nail) in need of removal. Patients may also report an inability to find or remove a foreign body (e.g., piercing or backing of piercing). Patients may report foreign-body sensation in wounds or soft tissues. In cases of occult foreign bodies, wounds may need to be explored or imaged to locate and remove the foreign body.

Diagnosis

The diagnosis of a soft-tissue foreign body is made with direct visualization, wound exploration/debridement, or imaging studies. Radiopaque objects, such as glass or metal, can be visualized on x-ray. In some cases, ultrasound can be used to aid in diagnosis and retrieval of certain foreign bodies.

Management

As with all wounds, appropriate anesthesia should be provided with peripheral nerve block or local infiltration of 1% to 2% lidocaine so that thorough exploration, irrigation (with tap water or saline), and wound debridement can be done. Care should be taken with sharp foreign bodies to avoid further injury to the patient or injury to ED staff. Forceps and needle drivers can be used to grasp and remove foreign bodies that cannot be irrigated out. Skin surrounding embedded foreign bodies may be carefully pared down with a scalpel to facilitate retrieval.

> CLINICAL PEARL: Risk of causing further damage to surrounding tissues versus leaving the foreign body or obtaining surgical consultation should always be considered and discussed with your patient.

Surgical consultation may be required for deep structure involvement or complex wounds. Orthopedic consultation may be necessary if joint capsule violation is suspected. Removal techniques are further discussed in Chapter 6, Common Procedures in Emergency Medicine, "Foreign-Body Removal."

Antibiotic prophylaxis should be considered for patients who are at high risk of wound infection (e.g., delayed presentation, potential for retained foreign body material, immunocompromise). The following regimens may be considered based on patient risk factors and type of wound:

- First-line therapy: First-generation cephalosporin (e.g., cephalexin)
- MRSA risk: Clindamycin, trimethoprim–sulfamethoxazole, or doxycycline
- Pseudomonoas risk (e.g., puncture through the sole of a shoe): Ciprofloxacin

References

1. Baddour LM, Brown AM. Infectious complications of puncture wounds. In: Sexton DJ, ed. *UpToDate*. https://www.uptodate.com/contents/infectious-complications -of-puncture-wounds. Updated June 18, 2018.
2. Steele MT, Tran LV, Watson WA, Muelleman RL. Retained glass foreign bodies in wounds: predictive value of wound characteristics, patient perception, and wound exploration. *Am J Emerg Med*. 1998;16:627–630. doi:10.1016/S0735- 6757(98)90161-9

Fractures

Etiology

Fractures are common injuries for which people seek treatment in the ED. Fractures occur when mechanical force from falls, MVCs, sports-related injuries, bite wounds, and other blunt-force trauma causes injury to bone. Extent and type of injury depends on extrinsic (e.g., mechanism, duration, and direction of mechanical force) and intrinsic (e.g., bone strength, density) factors. Fractures can be identified based on which bone is injured, location of the injury (e.g., metaphyseal, diaphyseal, intra-articular), orientation of the fracture (e.g., transverse, oblique, spiral), description of the fracture (comminuted, displaced, angulated), and whether the fracture is open or closed.

Epidemiology

It is estimated that approximately 5.6 million fractures occur in the United States annually.[1] The most common cause of fracture is fall, with extremity fractures among the most common injuries sustained. Fractures of the metacarpals and phalanges account for approximately 10% of all fractures, whereas clavicle fractures account for approximately 2.6% of all fractures.[2,3] Fractures of the hand and forearm account for 1.5% of all ED visits.[4] The incidence of ankle fractures is increasing and is approximately 187 fractures per 100,000 people per year.[5]

Clinical Presentation

Patients with fractures will generally present with pain and swelling to the site of injury with a history of trauma. Careful head-to-toe evaluation is necessary for trauma patients, particularly in settings of altered mental status, multiple injuries, or distracting injuries. Detailed skin, musculoskeletal, and neurovascular examinations should be done. Ecchymosis, swelling with or without gross deformity, tenderness in the affected area, and localized edema are common findings. Some fractures present subtly with little to no associated signs of trauma (e.g., scaphoid fracture); patients may only complain of pain and have tenderness to the affected area on examination. Pallor, mottled or tented skin, diminished or absent pulses, and open skin wounds or visible bone fragments at fracture sites are concerning findings and may require immediate intervention (e.g., emergent reduction/splinting) and orthopedic consultation.

Diagnosis

Diagnosis of most fractures is made on physical exam and with x-ray. Bone is easily visualized on plain radiography and the majority of fractures can be diagnosed in this manner. CT without IV contrast may be useful in the visualization of skull, facial, spinal, or occult fractures (e.g., tibial plateau). CT imaging can also aid in demonstrating the extent of intra-articular injury (e.g., hip, elbow). MRI can be helpful in the diagnosis of occult fractures (e.g., scaphoid) or stress fractures, but is rarely used in the ED setting.

Management

Management of fractures involves pain control with oral or IV pain medication, stabilization/immobilization of the injured area, elevation, and application of ice. Some patients may benefit from localized pain control using hematoma or peripheral nerve blocks. Immobilization of the fractured bone to support proper healing is the mainstay of fracture management. Immobilization can be achieved using prefabricated Velcro splints or joint immobilizers (e.g., thumb spica, wrist, knee, walking boot, ankle stirrup), fiberglass splitting material with elastic bandages, or slings. Thorough neurovascular examination should be done before and after splinting. Postreduction films are performed to confirm adequate alignment of displaced fracture fragments.

Immediate orthopedic, trauma, oral maxillofacial, spine, or hand surgery consultation may be required for injuries requiring operative care. Such injuries include unstable, open, or grossly displaced fractures or neurovascular injury. Orthopedic consultation may be required for failed attempts to reduce or splint an injury. In addition to surgical consultation, IV antibiotic therapy and thorough irrigation/debridement should be initiated for all open fractures.

Patients being discharged from the ED should be given clear instructions on splint care, weight-bearing or activity restrictions, range–of-motion exercises, precautions about compartment syndrome, and proper follow-up instructions with primary care provider or orthopedics. Crutches and instructions on proper use should be provided as indicated. Management of specific fracture types is discussed in Table 2.2.

TABLE 2.2 Management of Fractures by Location and Type

Fracture Location	Consultation	Treatment/Important Considerations
Skull		
Linear	Assess for associated intracranial injury	May be discharged home with concussion/head injury precautions
Depressed or penetrating	Neurosurgical consultation	Require admission, antibiotics, and anticonvulsants
Basilar	Neurosurgical consultation	Require admission for observation

(continued)

TABLE 2.2 Management of Fractures by Location and Type (*continued*)

Fracture Location	Consultation	Treatment/Important Considerations
Cervical spine	Spine surgery consultation	Most injuries require immediate surgery and hospital admission; minor fractures with no neurologic deficit (e.g., isolated transverse process fracture) may be managed as outpatients in close consultation with spine surgery; cervical spine immobilization collar should be maintained in place until fracture is ruled out
Thoracic and lumbar spine	Spine surgery consultation	Stable fractures may be treated with pain control, rest, braces such as the TLSO and referral for physical therapy; most unstable fractures or those involving neurologic deficit require surgery and hospital admission
Facial bone		
Orbital	Immediate ophthalmology consultation required for globe injury or retrobulbar hematoma. Ophthalmology, OMFS or plastic surgery consultation for extraocular muscle entrap- infraorbital hypesthesia, enophthalmos, or lacrimal apparatus involvement	All patients should follow up with ophthalmology or plastic surgery within 1 week. Oral antibiotics to cover sinus flora should be prescribed, recommend decongestants and avoidance of nose blowing
Zygoma	Consider plastic surgery or OMFS consultation in the ED for displaced fractures, neuromuscular involvement; otherwise may refer patient for outpatient follow-up	Isolated zygoma fractures do not require prophylactic antibiotics unless they involve the maxilla; fractures involving the maxilla should be treated as indicated earlier
Maxilla	Trauma, OMFS, dental or plastic surgery consultation +/- neurosurgery consultation if CSF leak is involved	Generally, result from high force injury (e.g., MVC); can be classified using the LeFort system; carefully evaluate your patient for associated injuries; IV antibiotics
Nasal bone	Outpatient plastic surgery or otolaryngology follow-up	Identify, drain, and pack all septal hematomas to avoid infection or nasal septum necrosis; pack epistaxis; ice and elevation of head

(*continued*)

TABLE 2.2 Management of Fractures by Location and Type (*continued*)

Fracture Location	Consultation	Treatment/Important Considerations
Mandible	Outpatient oral surgeon follow-up for closed fractures; open fractures require admission for operative treatment	Carefully evaluate your patient for second fracture given mandibular anatomy/U-shape, break in the oral mucosa/open fracture, sublingual hematoma, broken or missing teeth, and associated head/neck injuries; open fractures require IV antibiotics such as penicillin or clindamycin
Rib	Trauma or thoracic surgery consultation for associated internal injury, multiple contiguous ribs, displaced fractures; fractures of the first three ribs require further evaluation to rule out intrathoracic or other associated injury	Incentive spirometry and pain control for isolated rib fractures; educate patients about deep-breathing exercises and potential complications (e.g., atelectasis, pneumonia, contusion, pneumothorax)
Clavicle	Outpatient orthopedic follow-up; immediate orthopedic consultation for open fracture, neurovascular compromise	Pain control, ice, immobilization with sling (be sure to give patient proper instructions on ROM of shoulder and elbow to prevent stiffness)
Scapula	Outpatient orthopedic follow-up for isolated, uncomplicated injury	Generally result from high-force injury (e.g., MVC, fall); carefully evaluate your patient for associated injuries, obtain CT chest to rule out associated injury; treatment involves pain control, ice, immobilization with sling (be sure to give patient proper instructions on ROM of shoulder and elbow to prevent stiffness)
Humerus		
Proximal	Outpatient orthopedic follow-up for isolated, uncomplicated injury	Sling with ROM exercises starting at 1–2 weeks
Midshaft	Immediate orthopedic consultation for grossly displaced/unstable fractures or any neurovascular abnormality; outpatient orthopedic follow-up for uncomplicated injury	Coaptation splint
Supracondylar (pediatric)/intercondylar (adult)	Immediate orthopedic consultation for grossly displaced/unstable fractures or any neurovascular injury; outpatient orthopedic follow-up for uncomplicated injury	Posterior long arm splint and sling with proper ROM instructions for shoulder mobility

(continued)

TABLE **2.2** Management of Fractures by Location and Type (*continued*)

Fracture Location	Consultation	Treatment/Important Considerations
Elbow		
Radial head	Immediate orthopedic consultation for fracture/dislocation, grossly displaced fractures or any neurovascular injury; outpatient orthopedic follow-up for uncomplicated injury	Sling with ROM exercises starting at 2–3 days as tolerated
Olecranon process	Immediate orthopedic consultation for grossly displaced fractures or any neurovascular injury; outpatient orthopedic follow-up for uncomplicated injury	Posterior long arm splint and sling with proper ROM instructions for shoulder mobility
Forearm		
Midshaft radius, combined radial/ulnar fractures	Immediate orthopedic consultation for fracture/dislocation any neurovascular injury; outpatient orthopedic follow-up for uncomplicated injury	Double sugar tong splint
Galeazzi, Monteggia	Orthopedic consultation	
Midshaft ulna (night stick fracture)	Immediate orthopedic consultation for fracture/dislocation any neurovascular injury; outpatient orthopedic follow-up for uncomplicated injury	Posterior long arm splint and sling with proper ROM instructions for shoulder mobility
Wrist		
Distal radius, Colles's, Smith's	Immediate orthopedic consultation for fracture/dislocation any neurovascular injury; outpatient orthopedic follow-up for uncomplicated injury	Sugar tong splint
Intra-articular, Barton's, Hutchinson's	Orthopedic consultation	
Hand		
Scaphoid	Outpatient orthopedic follow-up for uncomplicated injury	Thumb spica splint; patients with high suspicion for fracture with negative initial images should be placed in thumb spica and instructed to have follow-up imaging in 7–10 days
Fourth and fifth metacarpal/ boxer's fracture	Immediate orthopedic consultation for open fractures; consider orthopedic consultation for angulation >30 degrees for fourth metacarpal fracture and >30–40 degrees for fifth metacarpal fracture	Ulnar gutter splint

(*continued*)

TABLE 2.2 Management of Fractures by Location and Type (*continued*)

Fracture Location	Consultation	Treatment/Important Considerations
Second and third metacarpal; carpal bones (except trapezium)	Outpatient orthopedic follow-up for uncomplicated injury	Volar splint; thumb spica splint for trapezium fracture
Thumb fractures, including first metacarpal/ Bennet's fracture	Outpatient orthopedic follow-up for uncomplicated injury	Thumb spica
Phalanx	Immediate hand surgery consultation for open fractures outpatient orthopedic follow-up for intra-articular fractures; uncomplicated tuft and phalanx fractures **not** involving MCP, PIP, or DIP joints may follow-up with primary care provider	Aluminum/foam volar or dorsal splint
Hip		
Femoral neck, femoral head, ntertrochanteric	Orthopedic consultation with operative management for most cases	Pain control, admission for surgical or medical management
Trochanteric	Nondisplaced trochanteric fractures, nonambulatory, severely debilitated, or patients with high operative risk may be medically managed	
Femur		
Shaft	Orthopedic consultation with operative management for most cases	Pain control, stabilization/immobilization,admission for surgical management
Distal/condylar	Orthopedic consultation with operative management for most cases	Long leg splint
Knee		
Patellar	Orthopedic consultation for open fracture, severely comminuted or displaced fractures or for associated quadriceps or patellar tendon injury; outpatient orthopedic follow-up for uncomplicated injury	Knee immobilizer
Tibia		
Tibial tuberosity	Orthopedic consultation for large avulsions or grossly displaced fractures, outpatient orthopedic follow-up	Incomplete or small avulsions may be treated with knee immobilizer
Tibial plateau	Orthopedic consultation for displaced or depressed fractures	Knee immobilizer/splint in full knee extension, **strict** non–weight-bearing instructions

(*continued*)

TABLE 2.2 Management of Fractures by Location and Type (*continued*)

Fracture Location	Consultation	Treatment/Important Considerations
Tibial shaft	Outpatient orthopedic follow-up for uncomplicated fractures	Posterior long leg splint, non-weight bearing
Tibial and fibular shaft	Consult orthopedics	Generally caused by high-force injury, carefully evaluate for associated neurovascular injury
Fibula		
Fibular head/ Maisonneuve	Orthopedic consultation	Long leg knee immobilizer, carefully evaluate for associated knee or tibial injury and for peroneal nerve damage
Fibular shaft fracture	Outpatient orthopedic follow-up for isolated fibular injury, orthopedic consultation for associated tibial shaft fracture	If isolated injury may be treated with knee immobilizer (proximal injury), walking boot or stirrup splint (distal injury) with weight-bearing as tolerated
Ankle		
Tibia	Immediate orthopedic consultation for open fracture, fracture/ dislocation, disruption of ankle mortise, or neurovascular injury; outpatient orthopedic follow-up for uncomplicated injury	Posterior short leg splint +/- stirrup splint for mediolateral support, nonweight bearing, stress importance of icing and elevation
Fibula	Isolated, nondisplaced fractures without medial ankle involvement may follow-up as outpatient with primary care provider; outpatient orthopedic follow-up for displaced fracture or concern for deltoid ligament involvement	Stirrup splint or walking boot with weight bearing as tolerated; nonweight bearing if medial ankle injury suspected
Tibial and fibular; bimalleolar and trimalleolar	Orthopedic consultation as these are unstable fractures that will require operative management	Posterior short leg splint +/- stirrup splint for mediolateral support; nonweight bearing; stress importance of icing and elevation
Foot		
Calcaneus	Orthopedic or podiatric consultation for comminuted, intra-articular, or displaced calcaneus fractures, or if associated dislocation injury; outpatient orthopedic or podiatric follow-up for nondisplaced avulsion fracture	Bulky compression dressing with non–weight-bearing instructions, stress importance of icing and elevation
Talus	Orthopedic or podiatric consultation for comminuted, intra-articular, or displaced fractures or associated dislocation; outpatient orthopedic or podiatric follow-up for nondisplaced or small avulsion fractures	Rare; generally results from high-orce injury, assess for associated injury, uncomplicated fractures may be treated with a walking boot

(*continued*)

TABLE 2.2 Management of Fractures by Location and Type (*continued*)

Fracture Location	Consultation	Treatment/Important Considerations
Navicular	Outpatient orthopedic or podiatric follow-up for isolated, nondisplaced fractures	Rare; generally associated with other ligament or tendon injury, may require outpatient advanced imaging (e.g., MRI); nonsurgical fractures are treated with walking boot, short leg posterior splint, or bulky dressing
Cuboid/cuneiform	Outpatient orthopedic or podiatric follow-up for isolated, nondisplaced fractures	Rare; nonsurgical fractures are treated with walking boot, short leg posterior splint, or bulky dressing
Metatarsal	Orthopedic or podiatric consultation for open fractures, multiple metatarsal fractures, displaced or intra-articular fractures (particularly of the first metatarsal) or associated dislocation (Lisfranc injury); outpatient orthopedic or podiatric follow-up for uncomplicated, isolated fractures	Posterior splint, walking boot, or postop shoe; initially non-weight bearing for first week with gradual progression of weight-bearing as tolerated; stress importance of icing and elevation
Fifth metatarsal avulsion/ Dancer's fracture	Outpatient orthopedic or podiatric follow-up for large avulsions or displaced fractures; follow up with primary care provider for uncomplicated fractures	Walking boot or postop shoe, stress importance of icing and elevation
Proximal fifth metatarsal diaphysis fracture/Jones' fracture	Outpatient orthopedic or podiatric follow-up as many cases require outpatient surgery	Posterior splint and strict non–weight-bearing instructions; stress importance of icing and elevation
Great toe	Orthopedic or podiatric consultation for open, displaced, intra-articular, or unstable fractures; associated dislocation; outpatient orthopedic or podiatric consultation for uncomplicated fractures	Buddy taping with supportive footwear or postop shoe, some patients may require walking boot for adequate pain control with weight-bearing; stress importance of icing and elevation
Phalanx	Immediate orthopedic or podiatric consultation for open fractures, grossly contaminated wounds, or neurovascular injury; outpatient orthopedic follow-up for intra-articular fractures; uncomplicated tuft and phalanx fractures **not** involving MTP, PIP, or DIP joints may follow-up with primary care provider	Buddy taping with supportive footwear or postop shoe

DIP, distal interphalangeal; IV, intravenous; MCP, metacarpophalangeal; MVC, motor vehicle collision; OMFS, oral and maxillofacial surgery; PIP, proximal interphalangeal; ROM, range of motion; TLSO, thoracolumbosacral orthoses.

REFERENCES

1. Buckley R, Page JL. General principles of fracture care. In: Poduval M, ed. *Medscape*. https://emedicine.medscape.com/article/1270717-overview#a6. Updated April 9, 2018.

2. Bernstein ML, Chung KC. Hand fractures and their management: an international view. *Injury*. 2006;37(11):1043–1048. doi:10.1016/j.injury.2006.07.020

3. Postacchini F, Gurmina S, De Santis P, Albo F. Epidemiology of clavicle fractures. *J Shoulder Elbow Sur*. 2002:11(5):452–456. doi:10.1067/mse.2002.126613

4. Chung KC, Spilson SV. The frequency and epidemiology of hand and forearm fractures in the United States. *J Hand Surg Am*. 2001;26(5):908–915. doi:10.1053/jhsu.2001.26322

5. Daly PJ, Fitzgerald RH, Melton LJ, Llstrup DM. Epidemiology of ankle fractures in Rochester, Minnesota. *Acta Orthop Scand*. 1987;58(5):539–544. doi:10.3109/17453678709146395

JOINT DISLOCATIONS

Etiology

Joint dislocations occur when external mechanical forces disrupt normal articulation between two or more bones. These injuries generally require significant force and commonly occur in the setting of falls, MVCs, sports-related injuries, and other blunt-force trauma. Sometmes joint dislocations occur spontaneously (e.g., shoulder, prosthetic hip) with little to no trauma. Depending on the force of the injury, significant capsular ligament damage may occur.

Epidemiology

The shoulder joint is the most commonly dislocated joint; shoulder dislocations account for approximately 50% of all major joint dislocation injuries.[1] Of these, anterior dislocations account for 95% to 97%.[1] Phalangeal dislocations are a common cause of small joint dislocations. The second most common major joint dislocation in adults is the elbow with the typical mechanism of injury being a fall onto an outstretched hand.[2] Other major joint dislocations are relatively rare, but can occur at the wrist, hip, knee, and ankle, usually in the setting of significant trauma. MVCs are the most common cause of hip dislocations, of which 90% occur posteriorly.[3] Posterior hip dislocation may occur as a complication of hip arthroplasty. Patients with history of previous joint dislocation are at risk of future dislocation.

Clinical Presentation

Patients with joint dislocations typically present with significant pain, swelling, and inability to move the affected joint. Patients may report hearing or feeling a "pop." Gross deformity is common at the site of injury. On occasion, patients will be able to spontaneously reduce joint dislocations prior to arrival at ED.

A detailed skin, musculoskeletal, and neurovascular exam should be performed to evaluate for associated fractures or neurovascular injury. Pallor, mottled or tented skin, diminished or absent pulses, and open skin wounds or visible bone fragments at fracture sites are concerning findings and may require immediate intervention (e.g., emergent reduction/splinting) and orthopedic consultation. Traumatic hip and knee dislocations are orthopedic emergencies; careful evaluation for associated injuries should be performed, particularly those involving neurovascular structures.

Diagnosis

Diagnosis of the majority of joint dislocations is made on physical exam and with x-ray. CT without IV contrast may be useful in demonstrating the extent of intra-articular injury or associated fractures (e.g., hip, elbow). In general, pre- and postreduction x-rays should be obtained for joint dislocations to rule out associated fracture as significant injury to the patient can be incurred if joint reduction is attempted in this setting. Abnormal neurovascular exam or tented skin may indicate a need for immediate reduction prior to obtaining prereduction films to avoid significant delay in treatment. CTA or arteriography may be useful in the evaluation of knee dislocation as vascular injury is a common complication.

Management

Management of joint dislocations involves reduction of the affected joint. Other measures of care include pain control with oral or IV pain medication, stabilization/immobilization of the injured area, elevation, and application of ice. Some patients may benefit from localized pain control with peripheral nerve blocks (e.g., shoulder). Procedural sedation may be required for large joints (e.g., hip) or difficult reductions (e.g., shoulder with severe muscle spasm). Traumatic hip and knee dislocations are orthopedic emergencies and require urgent consultation. Fracture–dislocation injuries, open dislocations, neurovascular injury, or inability to successfully reduce a joint also require orthopedic consultation in the ED.

Pre- and postreduction x-rays should be obtained to ensure appropriate reduction and rule out traumatic or iatrogenic fractures. Thorough neurovascular examination should be performed pre- and postreduction. Immobilization of the reduced joint is the mainstay of management and can be achieved using sling or splinting.

Patients being discharged from the ED should be given clear instructions on sling/splint care, weight-bearing or activity restrictions, range-of-motion exercises, precautions about compartment syndrome, and proper follow-up instructions with primary care provider or surgeon. Crutches and instructions on proper use should be provided as indicated. Management of specific dislocations is discussed in Table 2.3.

TABLE 2.3 Specific Dislocation Management by Joint

Joint Dislocation	Treatment/Important Considerations
Cervical, thoracic, lumbar spine	Generally, require significant force/mechanism of injury and are often associated with other injuries
	Immediate neurosurgical consultation required
	Almost always present with neurologic findings
Sternoclavicular	Generally, requires significant trauma to chest and may be associated with other injuries, particularly intrathoracic trauma
	Orthopedic consultation for posterior dislocations; should be reduced in the ED with procedural sedation[4]
	Anterior dislocations require reduction by orthopedic surgeon within 12–24 hours[4]
Shoulder	Most patients require pre- and postreduction films
	Patients with history of chronic shoulder dislocation with atraumatic mechanism may not need prereduction x-rays
	Obtain orthopedic consultation for associated fractures
	Most uncomplicated dislocation injuries can be reduced by ED staff without procedural sedation
	Procedural sedation may be required for individuals with large muscle mass/delayed treatment with significant muscle spasm; may consider local administration of lidocaine as an alternative to systemic sedation/analgesia
	Numerous shoulder reduction techniques exist; the following reduction techniques are well-tolerated and have few complications:
	• Scapular manipulation
	• Upright technique
	• Prone technique
	• External rotation technique
	If the preceding maneuvers are unsuccessful, the following techniques may be attempted but carry higher risk of complications:
	• Milch technique
	• Stimson technique
	• Traction–countertraction
	Note: Many other shoulder reduction techniques exist and may be fitting depending on the patient and clinical setting
	Obtain postreduction x-rays to confirm reduction and rule out iatrogenic fracture
	Sling with ROM instructions, pain contro, outpatient follow-up with orthopedics
Elbow	Careful assessment of neurovascular structures of the upper extremity is paramount before and after reduction
	Orthopedic consultation for associated fracture, open dislocation, neurovascular injury; postreduction instability
	May require procedural sedation for pain control and muscle relaxation; may consider local administration of lidocaine as an alternative to systemic sedation/analgesia
	Posterior long arm splint with sling and appropriate ROM instructions, pain control, outpatient follow-up with orthopedics

(continued)

TABLE 2.3 Specific Dislocation Management by Joint (*continued*)

Joint Dislocation	Treatment/Important Considerations
Radius/ulna	Radial head subluxation/"nursemaid's elbow," injuries generally occurs in children <5 years of age
	Management of Galeazzi fracture discussed earlier
	Most distal radius/ulna injuries involving dislocation or that are dissociated with the carpal bones involve associated fractures and require orthopedic consultation
Hand; phalanges *Note:* Carpal bone dislocation/dissociation injuries are discussed in sprain and strain injury section, which follows	Obtain pre- and postreduction x-rays to rule out associated fracture
	Orthopedic or hand surgery consultation for associated fracture, open dislocation, neurovascular injury, postreduction instability, metacarpophalangeal involvement; suspected tendon rupture or inability to reduce
	Will likely need to perform digital block for analgesia prior to reduction
	Some acute (presenting within 1 hour) injuries are quickly and easily reduced without need for analgesia; however, discussion with your patient about preferred technique is warranted
	Splint with volar (metacarpophalangeal injuries), aluminum/foam, or thumb spica splint; pain control, ice, and elevation; outpatient follow-up with orthopedic or hand surgery
Hip	Posterior native hip dislocations involve significant force/mechanism of injury (e.g., MVC); generally require immediate orthopedic consultation and reduction (ideally within 6 hours) with procedural sedation to avoid avascular necrosis of femoral head[5]
	Anterior hip dislocations are rare and require surgical management
	Most prosthetic hip dislocations are posterior and should be reduced under procedural sedation in close consultation with orthopedics
Knee/tibiofemoral	Generally requires significant force and involves associated neurovascular and ligamentous injury
	Immediate orthopedic consultation for reduction and possible surgical management
	Careful assessment of neurovascular status and possible ABI/CTA in cases of spontaneous reduction to rule out vascular injury
Ankle dislocation	Immediate reduction attempt should be made if pulses are absent or tenting of skin prior to obtaining prereduction x-rays
	Prereduction films should be obtained if no concern for neurovascular injury
	Orthopedic consultation for associated fracture or open fracture
	Procedural sedation should be administered prior to reduction
	Posterior splint and nonweight bearing with close follow-up with orthopedics

(continued)

TABLE 2.3 Specific Dislocation Management by Joint (*continued*)

Joint Dislocation	Treatment/Important Considerations
Foot	
Tarsometatarsal joint dislocation/Lisfranc Injury	Orthopedic or podiatric consultation for associated fracture Posterior short leg splint, nonweight bearing, close follow-up with orthopedics or podiatry Pain control; stress icing and elevation
Great toe; phalanges	Orthopedic or podiatric consultation for dislocation of first MTP, open dislocations, associated fractures Uncomplicated interphalangeal dislocations often involve fifth digit and are easily reduced; may follow-up with primary care provider Postreduction buddy tape, pain control; stress icing and elevation

ABI, ankle-brachial index; CTA, computed tomography angiography; MCP, metacarpophalangeal; MTP, metatarsophalangeal; MVC, motor vehicle collision; ROM, range of motion.

REFERENCES

1. Sherman SC. Shoulder dislocation and reduction. In: Wolfson AB, ed. *UpToDate*. https://www.uptodate.com/contents/shoulder-dislocation-and-reduction. Updated June 19, 2019.

2. Halstead ME, Bernhardt DT. Elbow dislocation. In: Young CC, ed. *Medscape*. https://emedicine.medscape.com/article/96758-overview. Updated September 26, 2017.

3. McMillan SR, Doty CI. Hip dislocation in emergency medicine. In: Brenner BE, ed. *Medscape*. https://emedicine.medscape.com/article/823471-overview#a6. Updated April 11, 2016.

4. Legome E. Initial evaluation and management of blunt thoracic trauma in adults. In: Moreira ME, ed. *UpToDate*. https://www.uptodate.com/contents/initial-evaluation-and-management-of-blunt-thoracic-trauma-in-adults. Updated February 11, 2019.

5. Steele M, Stubbs AM. Hip and femur injuries. In: Tintinalli JE, Stapczynski J, Ma O, eds. *Tintinalli's Emergency Medicine: A Comprehensive Study Guide*. 8th ed. New York, NY: McGraw-Hill; 2016:1848–1586.

LACERATIONS (SKIN)

Etiology

Laceration injuries involve damage to layers of the skin and occasionally to underlying structures due to a cut or tear in the tissues, often from traumatic force or a sharp object (e.g., knife, razor, glass). Lacerations typically cause separation of the skin and underlying tissues, whereas abrasion and avulsion wounds involve tissue loss. Deep lacerations have the potential to disrupt fascia, muscle, tendon, galea (scalp wounds), nerves, and blood vessels.

Epidemiology

Lacerations commonly occur on the face, scalp, and extremities, particularly the hands. Laceration to the upper extremities is the eighth most common reason for ED visits in the United States in male patients age 15 to 64 years, accounting for 814,000 visits per year. Open wounds, excluding head injuries, constitute nearly 900,000 ED visits per year in the United States, whereas open wounds of the head account for 870,000 visits per year.[1]

Clinical Presentation

Patients with lacerations to the skin will present with an obvious cut to the affected area with or without active bleeding. Wounds under higher tension tend to gape open and wound edges may be jagged or straight. Patients will generally complain of pain; injuries to the extremities, especially those involving digits and nail tissue are particularly painful. Deeper wounds may have visible defects in or exposed fascia, galea, muscle, tendon, bone, nerves, or blood vessels. Debris within the wound may be visualized.

Diagnosis

Diagnosis is made through clinical examination. Once bleeding is controlled, careful evaluation of wound site, depth, length, and involved structures should be performed. You should note whether or not debris or foreign bodies are within the wound. Such details should be carefully documented in the patient's record. X-ray and CT without contrast may be useful adjuncts for trauma patients or those with potential foreign-body contamination or associated fracture (e.g., distal digit, bite, or crush injuries).

Management

Wound care begins with control of bleeding, thorough wound irrigation, and debridement. Local anesthesia may be instilled to wound borders or as a localized nerve block using 1% lidocaine or 1% lidocaine with epinephrine (1:200,000) prior to irrigation for pain control.

> **CLINICAL PEARL:** Lidocaine with epinephrine should be avoided for all areas with tenuous blood supply, including digits and cartilaginous areas of nose or ears. It is particularly helpful to control bleeding for scalp and intraoral wounds.

It is preferable to close wounds within 4 to 6 hours to decrease risk of wound infection and poor cosmetic outcomes. Closure time may be increased to 18 to 24 hours for clean, uninfected, or facial wounds (up to 48–72 hours for facial wounds in certain low-risk cases). Lacerations of the skin are most often closed with nonabsorbable suture material. Scalp wounds are generally closed with staples. Superficial wounds in areas under low tension, without active bleeding, or in patients with fragile skin may be closed with tissue-adhesive glue or wound-closure strips.

Sutured wounds should be dressed with antibiotic ointment and a nonstick dressing. Patients should be instructed to keep wounds clean and dry for the first 24 hours, followed by gentle washing with warm soapy water. Patients should avoid soaking or fully submerging wounds under water. Patients with potentially retained foreign bodies, other significant wound contamination, delayed wound closure, or those who are immunocompromised should be considered for antibiotic prophylaxis as appropriate. Laceration repairs are discussed in further detail in Chapter 6, Common Procedures in Emergency Medicine, "Wound Repair."

REFERENCES

1. Rui P, Kang K. National Hospital Ambulatory Medical Care Survey: 2014 emergency department summary tables. https://www.cdc.gov/nchs/data/nhamcs/web_tables/ 2014_ed_web_tables.pdf. Updated September 7, 2017.

SPRAINS AND STRAINS

Etiology

A sprain occurs when an injury results in stretching or tearing of a ligament. A strain involves stretching or tearing of muscle or tendon tissue. Both sprains and strains can cause pain, swelling, and difficulty with range of motion at the affected injury site. Strains may lead to muscle spasm development, particularly in neck and back injuries. The mechanism of injury often involves falls, MVCs, or sports-related injuries. Recurrent sprains can lead to chronic joint instability and early degenerative changes.

Epidemiology

Sprains and strains are common injuries. Although many patients will self-treat for such injuries, a significant number will seek medical care in the ED. Studies estimate that approximately 2 million acute ankle sprains occur in the United States each year.[1] It is also estimated that approximately 1 million whiplash injuries occur annually in the United States and that nearly 6.2% of the population in the United States suffer injuries from whiplash syndrome (e.g., cervical strain).[2] The most common back injury is muscle strain, accounting for 60% of back injuries.[3]

Clinical Presentation

Patients with sprain and strain injuries will present with a history of injury and pain to the affected area. Physical exam often demonstrates swelling, ecchymosis, and difficulty with weight bearing or range of motion of the affected area. Diminished or absent range of motion or gross deformity may be present in patients with tendon rupture injuries. Associated neurovascular injuries may present with pale or mottled skin, diminished or absent pulses, weakness, temperature discrepancy, or abnormal sensation to the affected area or areas distal to the injury.

Diagnosis

Diagnosis of sprain and strain injuries is based on history and physical exam. Careful evaluation of skin, musculoskeletal, neurologic, and vascular systems should be performed. Careful evaluation of range of motion and strength should be performed comparing the injured side to the unaffected side, as findings may be subtle.

> **CLINICAL PEARL:** It is important to thoroughly inspect the area of injury free of clothing, blood, or debris, when you examine your patient.

X-ray and CT imaging are often helpful in ruling out fractures and may demonstrate soft-tissue defects in certain ligament and tendon injuries. For definitive diagnosis, some patients may require MRI either in the ED or in an outpatient setting. Specific decision tools, such as the Ottawa Knee Rule (www.mdcalc.com/ottawa-knee-rule) and Ottawa Ankle Rule (www.mdcalc.com/ottawa-ankle-rule), can be helpful in determining which patients need x-rays. Nexus criteria (www.mdcalc.com/nexus-criteria-c-spine-imaging) and Canadian C-spine rules (www.mdcalc.com/canadian-c-spine-rule) can be used to determine which patients may require imaging to rule out cervical injury.

> **CLINICAL PEARL:** Prompt surgical treatment of certain injuries is required (e.g., tendon rupture) to avoid long-term disability or other poor outcomes.

Management

Management of sprains and strains involves pain control, generally with oral pain medication, stabilization/immobilization of the injured area, elevation, and application of ice. Immobilization and compression of the injured ligament, tendon, or muscle to reduce swelling and support proper healing is the mainstay of sprain and strain management. Immobilization can be achieved using prefabricated Velcro splints or joint immobilizers (e.g., thumb spica, volar wrist, knee immobilizer, walking boot, ankle stirrup), fiberglass splitting material with elastic bandages, or slings. Thorough neurovascular examination should be done before and after splinting.

Orthopedic, trauma, spine, or hand surgery consultation may be required in the ED prior to discharging the patient for grossly unstable injuries or injuries that will ultimately require operative care. Immediate consultation should be obtained for any patient with suspected neurovascular injury.

Patients being discharged from the ED should be given clear instructions on splint care, weight-bearing or activity restrictions, range-of-motion exercises, precautions about compartment syndrome, and proper follow-up instructions with primary care provider or surgeon. Crutches and instructions on proper use should be provided as indicated. Management of specific sprain and strain injuries is discussed in Table 2.4.

TABLE 2.4 Specific Sprain/Strain Management

Sprain/Strain Injury	Treatment/Important Considerations
Cervical, thoracic, lumbar spine	Spine surgery consultation for evidence of ligamentous injury on diagnostic imaging or high suspicion based on physical exam (e.g., persistent, severe midline pain)
	If no evidence of fracture or spinal cord/severe ligamentous injury after thorough physical exam with or without diagnostic imaging, patients may be treated with NSAIDs, heat, relative rest with gentle ROM exercise instruction and follow-up with primary care provider or spine surgeon
	Due to potential for adverse reactions and medication abuse, muscle relaxants and opioid pain medications should be avoided except in cases of refractory pain or severe muscle spasm
	In general, the use of soft cervical collar braces should be avoided; potential uses include aiding in support during sleep, persistent midline pain with need for outpatient advanced imaging (e.g., MRI) to rule out ligamentous injury; patients should be instructed to use only 2–3 hours per day for <1–2 weeks[4] with close follow-up with primary care provider or spine surgery
	Patients with lifting or workplace injuries should be instructed on proper lifting technique
Sternoclavicular, chest wall strain	Rest/avoidance of lifting or overuse injury, stretching, administration of NSAIDs or topical pain relievers (e.g., capsaicin, topical lidocaine, topical NSAIDs), muscle relaxants for refractory cases or associated muscle spasm, follow-up with primary care provider
Shoulder	
Acromioclavicular separated shoulder	NSAIDs, res, ice, sling with instructions on proper ROM exercises, outpatient follow-up with orthopedics
	Immediate orthopedics referral for open injury or neurovascular injury
General shoulder sprain or strain, suspected rotator cuff or labral injury, shoulder impingement	NSAIDs, rest, ice, sling with instructions on proper ROM exercises for patients, patients with adequate pain control/joint stability may not need sling, outpatient follow-up with primary care, significant injury or competitive athletes should be referred to orthopedics
Biceps tendon	
Proximal tear/strain	NSAIDs, rest, ice, sling with instructions on proper ROM exercises for patients, outpatient follow-up with primary care or orthopedics
Distal tear/strain	Partial tear/sprain injuries managed as indicated previously
	All complete distal biceps tendon ruptures should be referred for prompt outpatient orthopedic follow-up or have orthopedic follow-up arranged from ED to avoid delay in surgical repair

(continued)

TABLE **2.4** Specific Sprain/Strain Management (*continued*)

Sprain/Strain Injury	Treatment/Important Considerations
Elbow and proximal forearm	
General sprain or strain Distal biceps injury (see previous biceps information)	NSAIDs, rest, ice (taking care not to ice directly over olecranon process/ulnar nerve), ROM exercises, outpatient follow-up with primary care or orthopedics Generally, sling use should be avoided in uncomplicated elbow injuries to preserve ROM
Wrist	NSAIDs, rest, ice, ROM exercises, Velcro/volar splint, outpatient follow-up with primary care
Hand	
Scapholunate dissociation, lunate dislocation, perilunate dislocation, triquetrolunate ligament injury	Injury may be associated with carpal bone fracture NSAIDs, rest, ice, volar short arm splint, elevation Urgent hand surgery follow- up within 2–3 days
Ulnar collateral ligament injury/ gamekeeper's thumb	May have associated avulsion fracture injury Thumb spica, NSAIDs, rest, ice, elevation, follow-up with hand surgery
Extensor tendon injury/mallet finger	Splint if slight hyperextension; follow-up with hand surgery
Phalanx/MCP/IP	NSAIDs, rest, ice, ROM exercises, volar hand/wrist splint for MCP injuries, aluminum/foam volar or dorsal splint for IP injuries, thumb spica for thumb injuries, outpatient follow-up with primary care
Hip	
Groin sprain, hamstring muscle or tendon injury, quadriceps muscle strain	NSAIDs, rest, ice, compression with Ace bandage, avoid stretching in acute healing phase, crutches as needed, follow-up with primary care provider
Knee	
General sprain or strain; suspected ACL/PCL/MCL/LCL injury	NSAIDs, rest, ice, knee immobilizer with ROM instructions, crutches as needed, follow-up with primary care provider or orthopedics; suspected ligament tears should follow-up with orthopedics
Quadriceps tendon injury, patellar tendon injury	NSAIDs; rest, ice, knee immobilizer with ROM instructions, crutches as needed, follow-up with primary care provider or orthopedics **All** complete quadriceps and patellar tendon ruptures should be treated as indicated earlier with non–weight-bearing instructions and referred for prompt outpatient orthopedic follow-up or have orthopedic follow-up arranged from ED to avoid delay in surgical repair; rule out associated avulsion fracture

(*continued*)

TABLE **2.4** Specific Sprain/Strain Management (*continued*)

Sprain/Strain Injury	Treatment/Important Considerations
Gastrocnemius	NSAIDs, rest, ice, avoid stretching in acute healing phase, compression with Ace bandage or walking boot;, crutches as needed, follow-up with primary care provider; patients should be given clear instructions to monitor and return to ED immediately for signs or symptoms of compartment syndrome
Ankle	
Achilles tendon injury	NSAIDs, rest, ice, posterior short leg splint or compression wrap with Ace bandage, crutches as needed. follow-up with primary care provider or orthopedics
	All complete Achilles tendon ruptures should be treated as previously indicated with non–weight-bearing instructions and referred for prompt outpatient orthopedic follow-up or have orthopedic follow-up arranged from ED to avoid delay in surgical repair; rule out associated avulsion fracture injury
Medial ankle/deltoid ligament injury, high ankle sprain/syndesmotic injury	NSAIDs, rest, ice, walking boot or stirrup ankle splint, crutches as needed, ROM exercises, follow-up with primary care provider or orthopedics
Anterior talofibular ligament/lateral ankle injury	NSAIDs, rest, ice, walking boot or stirrup ankle splint, crutches as needed, ROM exercises, follow-up with primary care provider
Foot	
General sprain or strain Lisfranc injury	NSAIDs, rest, ice, compression dressing or postop shoe, crutches as needed, ROM exercises, follow -up with primary care provider
Great toe, phalanges, MTP, IP	NSAIDs, rest, ice, buddy tape or postop shoe, crutches as needed, ROM exercises, follow-up with primary care provider

ACL, anterior cruciate ligament; IP, interphalangeal; LCL, lateral collateral ligament; MCL, medial collateral ligament; MCP, metacarpophalangeal; MTP, metatarsophalangeal; NSAIDs, nonsteroidal anti-inflammatory drugs; PCL, posterior cruciate ligament; ROM, range of motion.

REFERENCES

1. Waterman BR, Owens BD, Davey S, et al. The epidemiology of ankle sprains in the United States. *J Bone Joint Surg Am.* 2010;92(13):2279–2284. doi:10.2106/JBJS.I.01537

2. Freeman MD. Cervical sprain and strain. In: Lorenzo CT, ed. *Medscape.* https://emedicine.medscape.com/article/306176-overview#a6. Updated December 4, 2017.

3. Radebold A. Lumbosacral spine sprain/strain injuries. In: Young CC, ed. *Medscape.* https://emedicine.medscape.com/article/95444-overview#a6. Updated March 11, 2015.

4. Isaac Z. Treatment of neck pain. In: Atlas SJ, ed. *UpToDate.* https://www.uptodate.com/contents/treatment-of-neck-pain. Updated August 29, 2018.

3

Diagnostic Testing in Emergency Medicine

Introduction

Once you have evaluated your patient through history and physical examination, and have developed your differential diagnosis, you will need to develop your diagnostic plan. Diagnostic testing should only be ordered after careful evaluation as it can result in unnecessary cost or harm to your patient, and may uncover extraneous information that can detract from your original workup plan. Results of diagnostic testing can help to confirm or rule out certain diagnoses. This chapter will discuss the most common laboratory tests, imaging studies, and other diagnostic tools you will encounter on your emergency medicine rotation. (Table 3.1)

TABLE 3.1 Common Laboratory Tests in Emergency Medicine

Name	Normal Reference Range	Indication	Interpretation
Ammonia (serum)	Adults: 15–45 mcg/dL	Altered mental status Hepatic encephalopathy	Elevated in patients with hepatic encephalopathy, hepatic failure
Anion gap	9–14 mEq/L	For patients with lactic acidosis, altered mental status	Elevated in lactic acidosis, DKA, alcoholic starvation, ingestion of toxins

(continued)

TABLE 3.1 Common Laboratory Tests in Emergency Medicine (*continued*)

Name	Normal Reference Range	Indication	Interpretation
ABG	Bicarbonate (HCO_3): 21–27 mEq/L Oxygen saturation (SaO_2): 95%–100% pH: 7.35–7.45 Partial pressure of oxygen (PaO_2): 80–100 mmHg Partial pressure of carbon dioxide ($PaCO_2$): 35–45 mmHg	Acid–base disturbance (e.g., DKA), chest trauma, inhalation injury, burn injury, hemorrhagic shock	↓HCO_3: metabolic acidosis, ↑HCO_3: compensation for respiratory acidosis ↓ SaO_2, PaO_2: Hypoxemia; ↑ SaO_2, PaO_2: Hyperoxia/oxygen toxicity ↓pH: Respiratory or metabolic acidosis; ↑pH: respiratory or metabolic alkalosis ↑$PaCO_2$: Hypercarbia/hypercapnia, respiratory acidosis; ↓ $PaCO_2$: respiratory alkalosis, hyperventilation
BNP	<50–100 pg/mL	Suspected heart failure	400 pg/mL: Heart failure 100–400 pg/mL: Intermediate <100 pg/mL: Normal
β-HCG	<5 mIU/mL (serum quantitative) <5–10 mIU/mL (serum qualitative) 20–50 mIU/mL (urine qualitative)	Pregnancy, suspected pregnancy, suspected ectopic pregnancy, confirmation of intrauterine pregnancy (serial measurements)	Values greater than those listed in left column indicate pregnancy >2,000 mIU/mL: Discriminatory zone for detection of intrauterine pregnancy on transvaginal ultrasound
Basic metabolic panel	Sodium (Na): 135–145 mEq/L Chloride (Cl): 96–106 mEq/L Potassium (K): 3.5–5.0 mEq/L Calcium (Ca): 8.5–10.2 mg/dL Glucose: 70–130 mg/dL Bicarbonate (HCO_3): 22–30 mEq/L BUN: 7–20 mg/dL Creatinine (Cr): 0.6–1.2 mg/dL	Altered mental status, suspected hyper- or hyponatremia, suspected hyper- or hypokalemia, suspected hyper- or hypocalcemia, arrhythmia, hyper- or hypoglycemia, DKA; HHNS, metabolic acidosis or alkalosis, renal failure (acute or chronic), severe dehydration, acute renal failure/acute kidney injury, severe preeclampsia	↑Na: Hypernatremia, ↓Na: hyponatremia ↑K: Hyperkalemia, ↓K: hypokalemia ↑Ca: Hypercalcemia, ↓Ca: hypocalcemia ↑Glucose: Hyperglycemia, DKA, HHNS; ↓glucose: hypoglycemia ↑HCO_3: Metabolic alkalosis or compensation for respiratory acidosis, ↓HCO_3: metabolic acidosis or compensation for respiratory alkalosis ↑BUN/↑creatinine: Dehydration, renal failure (acute or chronic), acute kidney injury, urinary obstruction, severe preeclampsia, rhabdomyolysis, medication induced

(*continued*)

TABLE 3.1 Common Laboratory Tests in Emergency Medicine (*continued*)

Name	Normal Reference Range	Indication	Interpretation
Blood type and screen	Type O Type A Type B Type AB Rhesus D (Rh): positive or negative	Severe blood loss, severe anemia, pregnancy with vaginal bleeding or significant trauma	Blood should be properly typed and cross-matched prior to administration of blood transfusion Rh D-negative pregnant women with potentially Rh D-positive fetus should be administered anti-D immune globulin (Rhogam) if risk of fetomaternal hemorrhage
CRP	<1 mg/dL	CRP levels are valuable in the clinical assessment of chronic conditions such as rheumatoid arthritis and systemic lupus erythematosus; some orthopedists use it in the acute care setting to address joint infections as a trending pattern	Elevated in osteomyelitis, cellulitis, infections of the joint
Carbamazepine (Tegretol) serum levels	Normal therapeutic range: 4–12 mcg/mL	To monitor for patients with seizure disorder	For patients who present with acute seizure and the medication reconciliation indicates they should be on carbamazepine, check for medication adherence
Carboxyhemoglobin	Nonsmokers: 0%–3% Smokers: 10%–15% Carbon monoxide poisoning: >15%	Suspected carbon monoxide poisoning	>15%: Carbon monoxide toxicity
CSF	CSF ranges discussed in Chapter 1, Common Presentations in Emergency Medicine, Table 1.13	Suspected meningitis, suspected SAH	CSF analysis discussed in Chapter 1, Common Presentations in Emergency Medicine, Table 1.13

(*continued*)

TABLE 3.1 Common Laboratory Tests in Emergency Medicine (*continued*)

Name	Normal Reference Range	Indication	Interpretation
Coagulation studies	aPTT: 25–35 sec PT/INR: 11–13 sec/<1.1 TT: 14–19 seconds	Patients on anti-coagulation therapy, baseline prior to starting or for monitoring anticoagulation therapy	↑aPTT: With unfractionated heparin therapy ↑PT/INR: With warfarin therapy ↑TT: With unfractionated heparin, low-molecular-weight heparin, direct thrombin inhibitors
CBC	WBC count : 4.4–11/μL Hemoglobin: 14.0–17.5 g/dL (men), 11.5–15.3 g/dL (women) Hematocrit: 42%–50% (men), 36%–45% (women) Platelet count: 150,000–450,000/μL	Suspected infection, concern for leukopenia (chemotherapy induced), anemia, blood loss (acute blood loss not reflected until 6 hours), increased risk of bleeding (thrombocytopenia), severe preeclampsia; malignancy	↑WBC: Infection, malignancy; ↓WBC: leukopenia/neutropenia (chemotherapy induced), viral infection, malignancy ↓Hematocrit/hemoglobin: Anemia, blood loss, malignancy; ↑hemoglobin/hematocrit: polycythemia vera ↓Platelets: Idiopathic thrombocytopenia, medication induced; severe preeclampsia; malignancy; increased risk of ICH or SAH ↓WBC/↓hemoglobin/↓platelets (pancytopenia): Medication induced, hematologic malignancy
CPK	22–198 U/L	Suspected rhabdomyolysis; burn, crush, or electrical injury; compartment syndrome	>5× the normal range (generally 1,500–100,000 units/L) in rhabdomyolysis, burn, crush, or electrical injuries and compartment syndrome
D-Dimer	<500 ng/mL	Suspected DVT or PE, suspected aortic dissection, CVT	<500 ng/mL has high sensitivity in patients with low pretest probability for PE; high sensitivity and negative predictive value for screening patients for aortic dissection >500 ng/mL indicates further workup needed to rule out PE (CT angiography chest); may also be elevated in elderly or pregnant patients or in cases of malignancy, sepsis, recent trauma, or surgery >500 ng/mL may occur in CVT but normal level does not exclude CVT

(*continued*)

TABLE **3.1** Common Laboratory Tests in Emergency Medicine (*continued*)

Name	Normal Reference Range	Indication	Interpretation
Dilantin (phenytoin)	Normal therapeutic range: 10–20 mcg/mL	Monitor adherence	For patients who present with seizure activity and the medication reconciliation indicates they should be on phenytoin, levels can be checked for adherence
ESR	<22 mm/hr (men) <29 mm/hr (women)	Inflammatory process (pericarditis, myocarditis), suspected temporal arteritis	May be elevated in inflammatory process (nonspecific marker) ≥50 mm/hr in temporal arteritis
Ethanol alcohol	0 mg/dL	Altered mental status, suspected alcohol intoxication	>80 mg/dL is considered positive for driving under the influence >300–400 mg/dL can cause life-threatening respiratory depression (unlikely in tolerant individuals)
Glucose	70–130 mg/dL	Altered mental status, suspected hyper- or hypoglycemia	<70 mg/dL: Hypoglycemia; >130 mg/dL: diabetes mellitus, hyperglycemia, DKA, HHNS
INR	In healthy people, INR of 1.1 or below is considered normal; for patients on anticoagulant therapy, reference range of expected INR is 2–3	Trend patients on anticoagulants that are measured by the INR level	2–3 is the recommended range for patients on anticoagulants for the following conditions: proximal DVT, PE, TIA, and atrial fibrillation 2.5–3.5 is the recommended range for patients on anticoagulants for the following conditions: Mechanical prosthetic valves and recurrent venous thromboembolisms
Lactate	0.5–1 mmol/L	Sepsis, metabolic acidosis, shock (hypovolemic, cardiogenic, septic), metformin toxicity, liver impairment	<2 mmol/L (critically ill) >4 mmol/L lactic acidosis
Lipase	Normal range: 0–160 U/L	Pancreatitis	Elevated in patients with suspected acute pancreatitis, PUD, bowel infarction

(*continued*)

TABLE 3.1 Common Laboratory Tests in Emergency Medicine (*continued*)

Name	Normal Reference Range	Indication	Interpretation
Liver function test	ALT: 7–56 U/L AST: 10–40 U/L Albumin: 3.5–5.5 g/DL Bilirubin: 0.1–1.2 mg/dL (total), <0.3 mg/dL(direct) Alkaline phosphatase: 44–147 IU/L Protein: 6–8 g/dL	Liver function, acute liver injury, chronic liver disease (e.g., alcohol abuse), liver failure, hepatitis, severe preeclampsia,nutritional status	↑ ALT/AST: Hepatitis (acute or chronic), acute liver injury, liver failure, medication induced; severe preeclampsia ↓Albumin: Malnutrition, liver disease, nephrotic syndrome ↑Bilirubin: Hemolytic anemia, congestive heart failure, liver disease; ↑Direct bilirubin: liver disease or injury (infectious, drug- or alcohol induced), cirrhosis, gallstones
Magnesium	1.5–2.5 mEq/L	Arrhythmia, suspected hyper- or hypomagnesemia	↑Mg: Hypermagnesemia, ↓Mg: hypomagnesemia
STI testing	Negative	Suspected PID, sexual assault, dysuria, vaginitis	Generally not available for immediate results in ED
			May be positive for chlamydia, gonorrhea, trichomonas, HIV, herpes simplex virus (type 1 or type 2)
Troponin I	<0.04 ng/mL	Suspected MI/ACS, myocarditis, high-voltage electrical injury	>0.04 ng/mL within 3 hr of acute MI, cardiac injury Typically, serial assays taken at 0-, 3-, and 6-hr intervals
Type and screen			
Urinalysis	Color (yellow) Clarity/turbidity pH: 4.5–8 Specific gravity: 1.001–1.025 Glucose: <130 mg/dL Ketones: Negative Nitrites: Negative Bilirubin: Negative Urobilinogen: <0.5–1 mg/dL Blood: <3 RBCs Protein: <150 mg/dL RBCs: <2 RBCs/hpf	Suspected UTI, pyelonephritis, renal colic, renal injury, cervicitis,vaginitis, prostatitis, urethritis, dehydration, diabetes mellitus/DKA, rhabdomyolysis	Dark amber, red, brown: UTI, dehydration, renal colic, kidney disease or injury, pyelonephritis Cloudy/turbid: UTI; STI ↑Specific gravity: Dehydration, UTI; ↓specific gravity: SIADH, renal failure, diabetes insipidus, kidney disease, pyelonephritis ↑Glucose: Diabetes mellitus, DKA Ketones: Dehydration, DKA, alcoholic ketoacidosis Nitrites: UTI, pyelonephritis Bilirubin: Liver disease, gallbladder disease ↑Urobilinogen: Liver disease

(*continued*)

TABLE **3.1** Common Laboratory Tests in Emergency Medicine (*continued*)

Name	Normal Reference Range	Indication	Interpretation
	WBCs: <2–5 WBCs/hpf Squamous epithelial cells: <15–20 cells/hpf Casts: 0–5 hyaline cases/hpf Crystals: 0-occasionally Bacteria, yeast: None		>3+ on urine dipstick or >5 g/24-hour collection: Severe preecclampsia; ↑protein: diabetes mellitus, kidney disease, hypertension, medication induced Blood/↑RBCs: Renal colic, kidney disease, urinary tract or kidney injury, UTI, pyelonephritis, STI, benign prostatic hyperplasia, prostatitis, renal, bladder or prostate malignancy ↑WBCs: UTI, pyelonephritis, STI, renal colic ↑Hyaline casts: Dehydration, vigorous exercise, rhabdomyolysis Crystals: Renal colic Bacteria: UTI, pyelonephritis, prostatitis, cervicitis, vaginitis, urethritis Yeast: Candidiasis
Urine drug screen	Negative	Altered mental status, suspected drug intoxication	May be positive for amphetamines, barbiturates, benzodiazepines, cannabinoids, cocaine, methadone, opiates, PCP, propoxyphene (Darvon)
Urine myoglobin	0–1 mg/L	Rhabdomyolysis	>1–15 mg/L: Vigorous exercise, mild rhabdomyolysis, MI >15 mg/L: At risk for acute renal failure >100–300 mg/dL produces urine color change

ABG, arterial blood gas; ACS, acute coronary syndrome; ALT, alanine aminotransferase; aPTT, activated partial thromboplastin time; AST, aspartate aminotransferase; β-HCG, human chorionic gonadotropin; BNP, brain natriuretic peptide; BUN, blood urea nitrogen; CBC, complete blood count; CPK, creatine phosphokinase; CRP, C-reactive protein; CSF, cerebrospinal fluid; CVT, central venous thrombosis; DKA, diabetic ketoacidosis; DVT, deep vein thrombosis; ESR, erythrocyte sedimentation rate; HHNS, hyperosmolar hyperglycemic nonketotic syndrome; ICH, intracranial hemorrhage; INR, international normalized ratio; MI, myocardial infarction; PCP, phencyclidine; PE, pulmonary embolism; PID, pelvic inflammatory disease; PT, prothrombin time; PUD, peptic ulcer disease; RBC, red blood cell; SAH, subarachnoid hemorrhage; SIADH, syndrome of inappropriate antidiuretic hormone; STI, sexually transmitted infection; TIA, transient ischemic attack; TT, thrombin time; UTI, urinary tract infection; WBC, white blood cell.

Source: From Ferri FF, Ferri FF. *Ferri's Best Test: A Practical Guide to Clinical Laboratory Medicine and Diagnostic Imaging.* 4th ed. Elsevier; 2019.[1]

LABS

Keep in mind that normal reference ranges are lab dependent and may vary based on your location.

DIAGNOSTIC IMAGING STUDIES

CT

Head/Facial Bones

- CT without intravenous (IV) contrast: Suspected cerebrovascular accident (CVA), subarachnoid hemorrhage (SAH), intracranial hemorrhage (ICH), hypertensive emergency with severe headache or neurologic abnormality, and for suspected traumatic injury/intracranial trauma, suspected facial bone fracture
  - Pertinent findings
    - CVA: Visualization of intravascular thrombus/embolus, loss of gray–white matter differentiation, cortical hypodensity, and effacement of sulci
    - SAH/ICH: Blood in the meninges in SAH or into the brain parenchyma in ICH
    - Clotted blood can be seen on 92% of SAH if CT is done within 24 hours of bleed[2]
    - Subdural hematoma will appear as blood accumulation in the subdural spaces, generally with a crescent or concave shape
    - Epidural hematoma will appear as blood accumulation in a convex pattern between the skull and outermost layer of the dura
    - Skull or facial bone fracture: Linear, depressed, or basilar skull fracture pattern; affected facial bone and fracture pattern
- Computed tomography angiography (CTA) with IV contrast for suspected carotid or vertebral artery dissection
  - Pertinent findings
    - Enlargement of the affected artery, narrowed lumen with surrounding crescent-shaped mural thrombus and thin annular enhancement, intimal flap

Neck/Cervical Spine

- CT cervical spine without IV contrast is imaging study of choice for suspected cervical spine injury
  - Pertinent findings: Vertebral fracture pattern or dislocated vertebra(e)

- CTA is imaging study of choice for suspected vertebral artery dissection as indicated previously
  - Pertinent findings: Enlargement of the affected artery, narrowed lumen with surrounding crescent-shaped mural thrombus and thin annular enhancement, intimal flap

Chest

- CT with IV contrast for chest trauma evaluation
  - Pertinent findings
    - Rib fractures, sternal fracture, scapular fracture: Fracture pattern, number and location of affected ribs, flail chest injury
    - Pneumothorax/hemothorax: Air (pneumothorax) or blood (hemothorax) in the pleural space between the visceral and pleural linings (more sensitive than chest x-ray [CXR] for small pneumothoraces)
    - Pulmonary contusion: Focal parenchymal opacification, generally located peripherally
    - Mediastinal/esophageal injury: Extraluminal gas appears as linear lucencies within the mediastinum, oral contrast may demonstrate site of extravasation in esophageal rupture
- CTA chest with IV contrast for pulmonary embolism (PE)
  - Pertinent findings
    - PE: Filling defect within the pulmonary vasculature
- CTA with and without IV contrast chest/abdomen/pelvis for aortic dissection
  - Pertinent findings: Intimal flap, double lumen, dilated aorta, or intramural hematoma

Abdomen

> **CLINICAL PEARL:** For the most part, CT scans of the abdomen are ordered in conjunction with the pelvis (i.e., CT abdomen and pelvis)

- CT with IV contrast for suspected intra-abdominal trauma
  - Pertinent findings
    - Liver and splenic injuries: Lacerations appear as areas of linear hypoattenuation, may see active extravasation into the parenchyma; hematomas appear as areas of hypodensity within the parenchyma or between the liver or spleen and its capsule
    - Intestinal injury: Extraluminal gas/free air, hemoperitoneum, extravasation of oral contrast in intestinal perforation
- CTA with and without IV contrast chest/abdomen/pelvis with IV contrast for aortic dissection
  - Pertinent findings: intimal flap, double lumen, dilated aorta, or intramural hematoma

- CT scan with IV and per os (PO) contrast to rule out a colonic pathology such as diverticulitis, colitis, large bowel obstruction, or colonic mass
  - Findings may be consistent with diverticular pockets with thickening of the colonic wall/microperforations/diverticular abscess; findings associated with bowel obstruction may demonstrate evidence of stool proximal to the site of obstruction with colonic wall edema

Pelvis

- May see incidental findings of bladder injury on CT with IV contrast in trauma scan; should follow up with CT cystography in stable patients
  - Pertinent findings: Extravasation of contrast in cystography
- CTA with and without IV contrast chest/abdomen/pelvis for aortic dissection
  - Pertinent findings: Intimal flap, double lumen, dilated aorta, or intramural hematoma

Musculoskeletal

- CT cervical, thoracic, and lumbar spine without contrast for patients with significant mechanism of traumatic injury or with high suspicion for spinal injury
  - Pertinent findings: Fracture pattern in affected vertebra(e)
- Indication:
  - Improved delineation of fractures not easily visualized on x-ray (e.g., cervical, thoracic, or lumbar vertebrae; ribs; sternum; subtle hip fracture patterns)
  - Improved delineation of complex, intra-articular fractures or improved delineation of fractures for which surgical management is necessary (e.g., shoulder, elbow, hip, knee)
    - Pertinent findings: Fracture pattern in affected area; associated dislocation injuries

MRI

Brain

- MRI without IV contrast indications:
  - Suspected mass, lesion, or malignancy, pituitary apoplexy
    - Pertinent findings: Delineation and grading of mass, distinguish primary tumors from metastatic lesions
    - Pituitary mass with hemorrhagic or nonhemorrhagic necrosis
  - Can also be used in cases of CVA or trauma to further delineate areas of injury, but length of time of study and immediate availability generally limit use in ED setting
    - Pertinent findings: Early CVA findings include increased diffusion weighted imaging (DWI) signal, cortical contrast enhancement in the infarcted parenchyma

- MRI with IV contrast: Brain abscess
  - Pertinent findings: Ring-enhancing lesion
- Magnetic resonance angiography (MRA): Further enhance imaging in cases of vertebral or carotid artery dissection
  - Pertinent findings: Crescent-shaped hyperintensity in the wall of the affected vessel
- Magnetic resonance venography (MRV): Central venous thrombosis (CVT)
  - Pertinent findings: Lack of flow in area of thrombosis, parenchymal edema and ischemia

Neck/Cervical Spine/Thoracic Spine/Lumbar Spine

- MRA: Further enhances imaging in cases of vertebral or carotid artery dissection
  - Pertinent findings: Crescent-shaped hyperintensity in the wall of the affected vessel
- MRI without contrast: Spinal injury
  - Acute spinal cord injury
    - Pertinent findings: Spinal cord edema, contusion, intramedullary hemorrhage, spinal cord transection
  - Epidural hematoma
    - Pertinent findings: Hyperintense epidural mass
  - Intervertebral disc or ligamentous injury of the spine
    - Pertinent findings: Disc extrusion with or without nerve root compression

Abdomen/Pelvis Indication

- In patients who require CT scan imaging but may be pregnant, an MRI is also an option as it does not emit ionizing radiation
  - Pertinent findings: Evidence of appendicitis such as periappendiceal swelling, fecalith, or periappendiceal fluid

Musculoskeletal Indications

- Occult fractures (e.g., hip) for which fracture is suspected and x-ray is negative
  - Pertinent findings: Fracture pattern (e.g., intertrochanteric fracture) with or without soft-tissue injury (e.g., labral tear) or edema
- Further delineation of occult fracture (e.g., scaphoid), ligament or tendon injury
  - More likely to be used for subsequent imaging and not in the acute ED setting
- Osteomyelitis
  - Pertinent finding: Shows clearance of any tracer administered from the soft tissues with progressive uptake in the bone on a skeletal phase

ULTRASOUND

◼ FORMAL ULTRASOUND

Abdomen Indications

- Right upper quadrant (RUQ) pain
  - ○ Pertinent finding: Mobile calculi noted within the gallbladder lumen indicating gallstones or sludge with possible gallbladder wall thickening and pericholecystic fluid
- Right lower quadrant (RLQ) pain in a pregnant female
  - ○ Pertinent finding: If suspecting appendicitis in a pregnant female for whom an MRI is not available, one may be able to distinguish periappendiceal thickening and a fecalith in the form of a distal calculus with posterior shadowing

> CLINICAL PEARL: The use of bedside/point-of-care ultrasound has dramatically increased in past years and has greatly improved rapid bedside diagnostic capabilities, particularly in life-threatening disease processes. The following section highlights some of the uses of point-of-care ultrasonography in emergency medicine; however, it is important to remember that formal ultrasound studies are useful in confirming bedside findings when appropriate, and are indicated in the evaluation of stable patients for many illnesses.

◼ BEDSIDE (POINT OF CARE) ULTRASOUND

Abdomen

- Indication for focused assessment with sonography in trauma (FAST) scan: Abdominal trauma blunt or penetrating
  - ○ Pertinent findings: Free fluid in the abdominal cavity, collection of blood within the paracolic gutters, evidence of solid organ injury through direct visualization

Cardiac Indications

- Pericardial effusion/cardiac tamponade, trauma patients (in the setting of the FAST exam), cardiac arrest
  - ○ Pertinent findings: Fluid visualized in the pericardial sac in pericardial effusion, right ventricular (RV) collapse visualized in cardiac tamponade, lack of cardiac activity in cardiac arrest
- Aortic dissection: Transthoracic echocardiography (TTE)/transesophageal echocardiography (TEE) for aortic dissection patients who are not stable enough for CTA
  - ○ Pertinent findings: Intimal flap, true and false lumens, thrombosis in the false lumen; associated pericardial effusion, aortic regurgitation, or hemopericardium

Eye Indications

- Suspected retinal detachment
  - Pertinent findings: Hyperechoic line in the floats or undulates within vitreous humor with eye movement

Renal/Bladder Indications

- Suspected bladder stone or renal stone
  - Pertinent findings: Mobile, echogenic calculi can be noted in the bladder, ureters, or urethra with posterior shadowing
  - Pertinent findings: There may be associated bladder wall thickening or, in the case of the kidneys, hydronephrosis or hydroureter

Chest Indications

- Traumatic pneumothorax (as part of the extended FAST exam), hemothorax, rib fracture, congestive heart failure/pulmonary edema.
  - Pertinent findings
    - Sliding lung sign and "comet tail" findings rule out pneumothorax; lung point sign (lung sliding sign with juxtaposed absence of lung sliding in same space) confirms pneumothorax
    - Pleural fluid in hemothorax
    - Cortical discontinuity or buckling in rib fracture
    - B-lines appear as vertical hyperechoic lines extending inferiorly from pleural line in pulmonary edema

Abdominal Indications

- Suspected intra-abdominal trauma with FAST imaging
  - Pertinent findings
    - Intra-abdominal injury: Free fluid (appears as an anechoic collection, clotted blood may appear echogenic) in the hepatorenal space (Morison's pouch), the perisplenic space/splenorenal recess, retrovesicular or rectouterine pouch (Douglas's pouch)
- Suspected abdominal aortic dissection
  - Pertinent findings: Intimal flap, true and false lumens, dilated aorta, thrombosis within the false lumen

> **CLINICAL PEARL:** Care should be taken in measuring the aorta to ensure that the measurement is wall to wall (true lumen) and not of the false lumen.

- Abdominal ultrasound for acute pancreatitis, cholecystitis, or choledocolithiasis and evaluation of the renal system
  - Pertinent findings
    - Pericholecystic fluid, gallbladder wall thickening, evidence of gallstones in cholecystitis; dilatation of the bile duct (>6 mm + 1 mm per decade for patients older than 60 years of age) or intrahepatic biliary tree in choledocholithiasis

- Peripancreatic fluid, pancreatic cysts in pancreatitis
- Echogenic foci or acoustic shadowing, hydronephrosis or ipsilateral decrease/loss of ureteral jet with kidney stones

Pelvis/Genitourinary System Indications

- Bedside ultrasound in a female who has a positive urine pregnancy test to rule out ectopic pregnancy
  - ○ Pertinent findings: Existence of an adnexal mass and an empty uterine cavity are indicative of ectopic pregnancy until proven otherwise
  - ○ Also can be used to assess a threatened abortion under 20 weeks' estimated gestational age
- Scrotal ultrasound to rule out testicular torsion (NOTE: This is a male genitourinary [GU] emergency.)
  - ○ Pertinent findings: Color Doppler ultrasound can reveal scrotal blood flow and there is usually no flow to the affected testis in cases of torsion

Musculoskeletal/Soft-Tissue Indications

- Suspected foreign body
  - ○ Pertinent findings: Location of foreign body prior to retrieval
- Suspected abscess
  - ○ Pertinent findings: Confirmation of hypoechoic collection in subcutaneous space
- Muscle tear, hematoma, or tendon rupture (e.g., biceps, quadriceps, Achilles)
  - ○ Pertinent findings
    - Torn, retracted muscle fibers in muscle tear or strain
    - Intramuscular hematoma
    - Defect or discontinuity in tendon fibers in partial or complete tendon tears

Vascular Indications

- Doppler ultrasonography for lower extremity deep vein thrombosis (DVT)
  - ○ Pertinent findings: Lack of venous compressibility on sonography due to existence of thromboembolism
- Location of vessel lumen for insertion of central or peripheral vascular access

X-RAY

Head/Facial Bones Indication

- Nasal bone fracture (isolated injury)

> **CLINICAL PEARL:** If multiple facial bone injuries are suspected, CT is the preferred imaging modality.

○ Pertinent findings: Defect in nasal bone on lateral view

> **CLINICAL PEARL:** Nasal bone x-rays do NOT need to be obtained in the ED if tenderness and swelling are isolated to the nasal bridge, nares are patent, no significant nasal septal deviation, or no septal hematoma is present.

Neck/Cervical Spine/Thoracic Spine/Lumbar Spine Indication

- Fracture or dislocation suspected
  ○ Pertinent findings: Vertebral fracture pattern or dislocated vertebra

> **CLINICAL PEARL:** If significant spinal trauma or associated traumatic injury is suspected, CT is preferred imaging modality.

> **CLINICAL PEARL:** If a patient has a history of significant head trauma and presents with a distracting injury or associated cervical spine injury, ensure that CT scan of the brain AND the cervical spine are done simultaneously.

Chest Indication

- Chest trauma, pneumothorax, hemothorax/pleural effusion, aortic dissection, chest pain (to rule out noncardiac etiologies/alternative diagnoses)
  ○ Pertinent findings
    - Chest trauma: May demonstrate rib fractures, sternal fracture, scapular fracture, fracture pattern, number and location of affected ribs
    - Pneumothorax/hemothorax: Air (pneumothorax) or blood/fluid (hemothorax, pleural effusion) in the pleural space between the visceral and pleural linings
      - Tracheal deviation may be visualized in tension pneumothorax
    - Aortic dissection: Widened mediastinum
    - PE: Pleural effusion, Hampton's hump, Westermark's sign, Fleischner sign (in cases of large PE)

> **CLINICAL PEARL:** Although previous text indicates possible findings in cases of chest trauma, aortic dissection, and PE, it will likely be necessary to obtain advanced imaging (e.g., CT, CTA) for definitive diagnosis.

Abdomen Indications

- Intra-abdominal trauma
  - ○ Pertinent findings: free air in bowel perforation (traumatic or nontraumatic etiology)
- Small bowel obstruction
  - ○ Pertinent finding: Sentinel bowel loops, dilated bowel loops, evidence of ileus

Pelvis Indication

- Trauma, suspected fracture
  - ○ Pertinent findings: Fracture pattern and location

Musculoskeletal/Soft Tissue Indication

- Fracture or dislocation of specific bone/joint, foreign body
  - ○ Pertinent findings: Fracture pattern and location, joint dislocation, radiopaque foreign body if present (see eChapter 3, Additional Resources to Enhance the Emergency Medicine Rotation, for a sampling of images).

OTHER DIAGNOSTIC TESTING

EKG

- Indication: Chest pain, dyspnea, palpitations, syncope, suspected acute coronary syndrome (ACS), suspected arrhythmia, or electrolyte abnormality
- Pertinent findings: Evaluate for myocardial ischemia and injury (ST segment evaluation, ST segment depression, T wave inversion, Q waves); arrhythmia, QT interval prolongation

LUMBAR PUNCTURE

- Indication: altered mental status, suspected meningitis/encephalitis, SAH (with negative CT results)
- Pertinent findings: Xanthochromia or red blood cells (RBCs) in cerebrospinal fluid (CSF) in SAH; CSF may demonstrate elevated opening pressure, positive Gram stain, elevated white blood cell (WBC) count, abnormal protein and glucose levels in meningitis (see Table 1.13)

TONOMETER

- Indication: Suspected glaucoma
- Pertinent findings: Intraocular pressure (IOP) >20 mmHg (normal range 10–20 mmHg)

SLIT LAMP

- Indication: Ocular trauma, infection, or inflammation; suspected acute angle-closure glaucoma
- Pertinent findings: Conjunctival trauma, inflammation, chemosis; corneal abrasions, ulcers, foreign bodies, lacerations; hypopyon or hyphema in inflammation or trauma; cells and flare in uveitis/iritis; shallow anterior chamber in acute angle-closure glaucoma

ARTERIAL DUPLEX ULTRASOUND/ANKLE–BRACHIAL INDEX (ABI):

- Indication: Suspected arterial occlusion, resting ischemic pain, evidence of arterial compromise on physical exam (diminished pulses, pallor, diminished sensation, etc.)
- Pertinent findings: Reduced velocity at site of stenosis, size and location of plaque/occlusion site, abnormal waveforms, diminished or absent color flow on arterial duplex ultrasound; ABI <0.9 in atherosclerotic vessels/arterial disease

DIRECT COMPARTMENT MANOMETRY

(generally performed by surgery team when indicated)
- Indication: Suspected compartment syndrome
- Pertinent findings: Increased pressure within tissue compartment [3]
  - ○ Normal level: 0 to 8 mmHg
  - ○ Pain develops: 20 to 30 mmHg
  - ○ Capillary blood flow becomes compromised: 25 to 30 mmHg
  - ○ Ischemia occurs when tissue pressures approach diastolic pressure

NUCLEAR MEDICINE STUDIES

Some commonly used nuclear medicine studies in emergency medicine include nuclear stress tests, ventilation/perfusion scans (V/Q scan), and hepatobiliary iminodiacetic acid (HIDA) scans

Nuclear stress test

- Indication: Suspected ACS (radionuclide myocardial perfusion imaging)
- Interpretation: Assessment of myocardial viability and perfusion during rest and physical or pharmacologically induced stress to evaluate for mismatch

Pulmonary V/Q Scan

- Indication: Pulmonary embolus diagnosis
- Interpretation/pertinent findings: computed tomography angiography (CTA) is the modality of choice in diagnosing pulmonary thromboembolism; however, ventilation/perfusion scans are used if CT-PA is not available or if the patient has a contraindication to administration of contrast

dye (such as impaired renal function or allergy to contrast); pulmonary emboli produce a mismatch that is defined as ventilation maintained but perfusion absent; depending on the size of the defect (i.e., how much lung tissue is not being perfused due to a blood clot), the scans are divided into categories of normal, low probability, or high probability for a PE; if a patient has a normal CXR and a low probability for a PE, it is unlikely he or she has a PE; the combination of an abnormal CXR and a high probability V/Q scan makes it more likely the patient has a PE and should be treated with anticoagulants

HIDA Scan

- Indication: Aids in the diagnosis of cholecystitis; in patients with obstruction of the cystic duct by a stone, the tracer applied will not appear in the gallbladder
- Interpretation: In patients with obstruction of the common bile duct, the tracer will not appear in the small intestine; findings indicate an obstructing gallstone

REFERENCES

1. Ferri FF. *Ferri's Best Test: A Practical Guide to Clinical Laboratory Medicine and Diagnostic Imaging.* 4th ed. Philadelphia, PA: Elsevier; 2019.
2. Herring W. *Learning Radiology: Recognizing the Basics.* 3rd ed. Philadelphia, PA: Elsevier; 2016.
3. Stracciolini A, Hammerberg EM. Acute compartment syndrome of the extremities. In: Moreira ME, Bachur RG, eds. *UpToDate.* https://www.uptodate.com/contents/acute-compartment-syndrome-of-the-extremities. Accessed July 2019.

4

Patient Education and Counseling in Emergency Medicine

Introduction

Understanding legal matters, screening patients for safety, and providing appropriate patient education are all important aspects to consider in emergency medicine. This chapter will discuss these issues in further detail. It is important to be familiar with these topics as it will help you to provide comprehensive care for your patient.

AGE-APPROPRIATE SCREENINGS

FALL RISK

- Patients with injuries (e.g., dominant upper extremity fracture) or equipment (e.g., sling, splint, crutches) that affect mobility, ability to perform activities of daily living (ADL), or safety in the home (e.g., stairs) should have proper education and risk assessment prior to discharge from the ED. Inquire about loose carpets and rugs, proper lighting, placement of electrical cords, and slippery surfaces. Encourage the use of a cane or walker for ambulation. Consider recommending hand railings throughout the residence. Fall-risk assessment is particularly important for patients in whom anticoagulation is being considered or implemented.
- Family members or ancillary staff, such as social workers or case managers, should be involved in safety discussion and discharge planning.

- Physical therapy consultation may be helpful in evaluating a patient's ability to ambulate or perform ADL safely and adequately.

Abuse

- Patients with assault-related injuries should be assessed for safety in the home prior to discharge in cases of confirmed or suspected domestic or sexual assault.
- Specific considerations to keep in mind in assessing a victims of abuse are
  - Abusers may be significant others, family members, acquaintances, or other caregivers.
  - Abuse may involve children, intimate partners, family members, or the elderly.
  - Abuse may be emotional, physical, financial, sexual, or take the form of neglect.
- Elder abuse[1]
  - Risk factors: Advanced age; female gender; inability to care for oneself; dementia; social isolation or depression; lower socioeconomic status; external family stressors; caretakers with history of mental illness, substance abuse, or financial dependency on the victim
  - Signs of abuse: Bruising, abrasions/lacerations, bite marks, or burns on skin; suspicious fractures; malnutrition or dehydration; pressure ulcers; indicators of sexual abuse (e.g., trauma to the perineal region, abdomen, or breasts, sexually transmitted infections); indicators of financial abuse (e.g., change in ability to pay for medications, utilities, housing, food)
  - Screening: Providers should interview patients alone to avoid intimidation by abusers; patients should be asked about living arrangements, food preparation, medication administration, finances, and should be asked directly about specific abuse concerns
- Intimate partner abuse[2]
  - Risk factors: Younger age, female gender, lower socioeconomic status, family or personal history of violence, pregnancy, alcohol or substance abuse, history of mental illness
  - Signs of abuse: Injury with inconsistent explanation, particularly of the head, neck, teeth, or genital region; injuries of the forearms (defensive wounds); bruising, abrasions/lacerations, bite marks, or burns on skin; suspicious fractures; indicators of sexual abuse (e.g., trauma to the perineal region, abdomen, or breasts; sexually transmitted infections; unintended pregnancy)
  - Screening: Providers should interview patients alone to avoid intimidation by abusers; providers should assure patients of confidentiality and should question patients in a nonjudgmental way; multiple screening tools exist to aid in screening patients and generally include questions about whether or not a patient feels safe, has been threatened, or has been harmed (physically, emotionally, or sexually)

- Child abuse[3]
  - Risk factors: Learning disabilities, psychiatric disease, or speech and language disorders; congenital anomalies or intellectual disability; failure to thrive; unplanned pregnancy or unwanted child; unrelated adolescent or adult male in the household; intimate partner violence; family stressors (e.g., divorce, illness, job loss); caregiver substance or alcohol abuse
  - Signs of abuse: Unexplained trauma or implausible mechanism of injury; delay in seeking care; abrasions/lacerations, bite marks, or burns on skin; suspicious bruising patterns (e.g., bruising on infants younger than 6 months of age, bruises on torso, ear, neck, or buttocks, bruises with the pattern of a striking object); scald injuries; suspicious fractures (e.g., rib fractures, long bone fractures in nonambulatory infants, multiple fractures in various stages of healing); suspicious parent behaviors
  - Screening: Support for universal screening guidelines for child abuse is lacking; increased provider awareness and careful evaluation of potential abuse victims are key components in evaluation of child abuse cases
- Designated hospital team members, social workers, case managers, or law enforcement may need to be involved in patient care and discharge planning

LEGAL ISSUES IN EMERGENCY MEDICINE

INFORMED CONSENT

- In the acute care setting, patients are required to make critical decisions regarding their care or the care of their loved ones after receiving information that may be difficult to process. It is up to the emergency medicine (EM) provider to explain the risks and benefits of any procedure/intervention. Informed consent is the legal standard under which providers educate patients or their representatives (i.e., power of attorney) about such interventions.[4]
- This process provides the patient the ability to actively participate in his or her care, involves the patient in the medical decision-making process, enhances communication between patient and provider, allows for the patient to ask questions involving alternative therapies, and can reduce medical–legal risk or discontent in cases of complications.
- Patients must have the mental capacity to make decisions regarding their healthcare in order for informed consent to be valid. Patients who lack this capacity may have informed consent provided by a designated healthcare proxy. You should communicate all details of the informed consent in language that a patient understands.

> **CLINICAL PEARL:** It is important to obtain translator services when necessary and to explain details in comprehensive language (e.g., using uncomplicated terms and avoiding medical jargon).

- According to the American College of Emergency Physicians (ACEP), informed consent must include all of the following:[5]
  - Deliver adequate information regarding the nature and purpose of the proposed treatment, which must also include discussing the alternatives, risks, benefits, and whether or not the patient decides to forgo treatment/testing.
  - Be free of coercion.
  - Ensure the patient possesses the capacity to make medical decisions.
- When obtaining informed consent, there should be appropriate written documentation of the consent. This should include a signature from the patient or representative and the provider. Some institutions also require an additional signature by a witness.
- Examples of interventions that require informed consent
  - Administration of pharmacological agents such as tissue plasminogen activator (tPA)
  - Administration of blood or blood products such as platelets, PRBCs (packed red blood cells), or plasma
  - Diagnostic procedures such as lumbar puncture
  - Intubation

LEAVING AGAINST MEDICAL ADVICE

Sometimes patients choose to leave the ED prior to completion of their workup or intervention. Risk factors in patients at higher risk for leaving against medical advice (AMA) include male gender, younger age, psychiatric illness, low income, and dependence on alcohol or an illicit substance.[4]

Patients come into the facility with legitimate, high-acuity complaints such as chest pain, trauma, or a condition requiring surgery. Some of the reasons patients may sign out as AMA include fear of having to pay a high bill, having childcare/parental care or pet care issues at home, hoping to have another facility manage their care, requests for more opiate-dependent management or because they wish to have a cigarette but are not typically allowed to leave the department.[4]

When a patient signs out AMA, this requires a detailed explanation of the consequences of his or her departure. Some may include worsening condition, a debilitating condition, rupture of a viscous (singular form of organs) if not managed, and so on. If you encounter such a situation, make a deliberate effort to explain the risks and benefits of leaving AMA without any judgment. Make an effort to support the patient fully. Suggestions include working collaboratively to address any fears or home-care issues the patient may have. Perhaps encourage the patient to reach out to family or a religious leader to help make a decision.

> **CLINICAL PEARL:** A patient under the influence of alcohol or substances is unable to sign out AMA as his or her decision-making capacity is considered impaired and he or she may be a risk to his or her own safety. Keep in mind that a patient cannot be held against his io her will unless committed.

When a patient signs out AMA, there should be three signatures on the documentation: the provider's, the patient's, and a witness's. There should be two copies made: one for the chart and one for the patient. The interaction between provider and patient should remain collaborative and the patient should be encouraged to return for any concern.

EMERGENCY MEDICAL TREATMENT AND LABOR ACT

The Emergency Medical Treatment and Labor Act (EMTALA) is a federal law that was enacted in 1986 and requires any patient coming to the ED to be screened, stabilized, and treated regardless of ability to pay, insurance status, national origin, or race.[6] This law ensures that any patient presenting to an ED will receive nondiscriminatory care and that the patient must receive a medical screening examination to determine whether a medical emergency is present. EMTALA defines a medical emergency as any condition (including severe pain) that would result in placing an individual's health, bodily function, or organs at risk of serious impairment without immediate medical attention. EDs are required to post signs notifying patients of their right to medication screening examination and treatment. Under EMTALA, examination and treatment cannot be delayed to inquire about payment or insurance coverage.

If a patient is determined to have a medical emergency, treatment must be provided until the emergent condition is resolved or stabilized. If such care cannot be provided (i.e., the hospital does not have the capability or personnel to treat the emergent medical condition), the patient must be transferred in an appropriate manner to another hospital. Hospitals that are capable of receiving specialized transfers must accept transfers from hospitals that lack such capabilities. According to EMTALA, a patient is considered stable if the treating physician determines that no significant deterioration in the patient's condition will occur during the transfer. An unstable patient may be transferred if the physician certifies that the medical benefits outweigh the risk of transfer or if the patient requests a transfer in writing after being informed of the hospital's obligations under EMTALA. According to EMTALA, transfer of an unstable patient may be considered "appropriate" if the following conditions are met:[6]

1. The transferring hospital must provide ongoing care within its capability until transfer.
2. Copies of medical records must be provided.
3. Transferring hospital must confirm that the receiving facility has space, qualified personnel to provide care, and has agree to accept the transfer.
4. The transfer must be made with appropriate medical equipment with qualified personnel.

Violations of EMTALA must be reported to the Centers for Medicare & Medicaid Services (CMS) or another state agency and may be penalized by termination of the hospital or physician Medicare provider agreement, hospital or physician fines, or lawsuits suing for personal injury or to recover damages.

PREVENTIVE MEDICINE GUIDELINES

ALCOHOL, TOBACCO, AND SUBSTANCE USE

- Patients being treated for alcohol, tobacco, or other substance use-related illness or injury should be counseled on drug use and given resources, if available, for help in cessation.

> **CLINICAL PEARL:** It is important to address these issues in a nonthreatening, nonjudgmental manner.

- Assessment of patients with suspected alcohol or other substance abuse should involve asking the patient (and possibly collateral sources of information) about past and present substance use patterns, family history of substance abuse, quantity and frequency of use, and history of related medical and psychiatric conditions.
- Numerous screening tools are available to assess patients for substance abuse (e.g., TAPS [Tobacco, Alcohol, Prescription medications and other Substance use Tool], AUDIT [Alcohol Use Disorders Identification Test], CAGE [cut down, annoyed, guilty, eye-opener], Opioid Risk Tool).

VEHICLE AND RECREATIONAL SAFETY

- Opportunities for education in seatbelt safety, helmet, and other protective gear use may arise for patients involved in motor vehicle, bicycle, or other recreational activity accidents.

SUN/ULTRAVIOLET EXPOSURE SAFETY

- Opportunities for education on sunscreen use and avoidance of ultraviolet (UV) injury to skin or eyes (e.g., welders, skiers) may arise in patients with burn injuries.

WORKPLACE SAFETY

- Opportunities to discuss potential issues with implementing and adhering to workplace safety protocols involving
  - Use of safety equipment
  - Implementing and following safety protocols
  - Heavy-lifting techniques
  - Potentially hazardous chemical or environmental exposures

SELECTED PATIENT EDUCATION TOPICS PERTINENT TO EMERGENCY MEDICINE

FOLLOW-UP INSTRUCTIONS

- All patients being discharged home from the ED should be given clear instructions for follow-up with
  - Primary care provider
    - For routine injuries and illness
    - Newly diagnosed chronic disease (e.g., hypertension, diabetes)
  - Specialist
    - Injuries requiring subacute surgical management (e.g., orthopedics, plastic surgery)
    - Further evaluation after life-threatening disease processes have been ruled out (e.g., cardiology, neurology, gastroenterology)
  - ED
    - Wound check, suture/staple removal for patients unable to obtain follow-up with outside provider
    - ANY recurrent or worsening symptoms related to the initial ED visit
      - Clear education should be provided to the patient and household contacts when possible
- Wound care instructions
  - Patients should be instructed on how to care for wounds:
    - How long wounds should be kept dry
    - Whether or not wounds can get wet or be submerged in water
    - Localized wound care/prophylactic antibiotic use
    - When patients should follow up for suture/staple removal
    - Signs/symptoms of infections, dehiscence, or other reasons to return for reevaluation
- Injury instructions
  - Patients should be given clear instructions on
    - Splint/sling care and usage
    - Range-of-motion exercises when appropriate
    - Crutch use and weight-bearing restrictions

- Red-flag symptoms
  - Patients who are being discharged from the ED in whom life-threatening illness or injury has been ruled out, should be given clear instructions on reasons to return to the ED based on their original chief complaint:
    - Chest pain: New or worsening pain, exertional symptoms, dyspnea, dizziness, or nearsyncope
    - Headache: New or worsening pain, syncope, vomiting, altered mental status, focal neurologic deficit
    - Traumatic injury: New or worsening pain to injured area, numbness/weakness/tingling, changes in skin color
    - Soft-tissue injury/burns: Erythema extending from wound, increased warmth or redness, fever/chills/malaise, purulent discharge, wound dehiscence,numbness/weakness/tingling to injured area, changes in skin color

Vaccinations

Hepatitis B

- Human bites or body fluid exposure
  - Assess risk of potential transmission of hepatitis B, hepatitis C, or HIV and perform baseline testing on patient or counsel patient to have baseline testing done when appropriate.
  - Patients who are unvaccinated or who have negative anti-HBs (hepatitis B surface antibodies) should receive both hepatitis B immune globulin and should begin the hepatitis B vaccination series.

Rabies

- Rabies prophylaxis
  - The rate of rabies in domestic animals in the United States is low, therefore if an animal is healthy and/or vaccinated, quarantine and observation of the animal for 10 days prior to initiating postexposure prophylaxis for rabies is acceptable.
  - If the animal's health or vaccination status cannot be confirmed, consultation with local health agencies (e.g., local health department) or Centers for Disease Control and Prevention (CDC) guidelines may provide helpful resources. Use the rabies hotline at 877-539-4344.
- Dog and cat bites
  - Determine to whom, if anyone, the animal belongs and the animal's vaccination status/rabies risk.

- Other animal bites
  - Animal bites other than dog and cat bites should be treated on a case-by-case basis. CDC (www.nc.cdc.gov/travel/page/be-safe-around-animals) and World Health Organization (www.who.int/news-room/fact-sheets/detail/animal-bites) websites provide helpful resources.
  - Per CDC guidelines, raccoons, skunks, foxes, most carnivorous animals, and bats should be treated as rabid unless the animal is available for testing.
  - Patients with bites from these animals should be given postexposure prophylaxis for rabies unless laboratory testing proves that the animal in question is not rabid.
- Rabies prophylaxis regimen
  - Rabies vaccine: 1 mL intramuscular (IM) injection on day 0, 3, 7, 14 (additional dose given on day 21 if immunocompromised)
  - Rabies immune globulin (if not previously vaccinated against rabies): 20 units/kg as a single dose given in and around wound site if possible, remaining volume should be administered IM at suitable site (e.g., deltoid, buttocks) away from rabies vaccine injection site
  - Note: Further discussion on rabies can be found in Chapter 5, Selected Topics in Emergency Medicine Patient Care: Traumatic Injury

TETANUS

- Tetanus toxoid vaccine (Td or Tdap) should be given if
  - Date of last vaccination was 10 or more years ago for clean, minor wounds
  - Date of last vaccination was more than 5 years ago for all other contaminated or complicated wounds
  - Tetanus *immune globulin* should be given for contaminated or complicated wounds in patients who have unknown tetanus vaccination status or who have received fewer than three doses of tetanus vaccinations/boosters

REFERENCES

1. Halphen JM, Dyer CB. Elder mistreatment: abuse, neglect and financial exploitation. In: Schmader KE, ed. *UpToDate*. https://www.uptodate.com/contents/elder-mistreatment-abuse-neglect-and-financial-exploitation. Updated July 16, 2019.
2. Weil A. Intimate partner violence: diagnosis and screening. *UpToDate*. https://www.uptodate.com/contents/intimate-partner-violence-diagnosis-and-screening
3. Boos SC. Physical child abuse: recognition. *UpToDate*. https://www.uptodate.com/contents/physical-child-abuse-recognition
4. Siff JE. Legal issues in emergency medicine. In: Tintinalli JE, Stapczynski J, Ma O, et al, eds. *Tintinalli's Emergency Medicine: A Comprehensive Study Guide*. 8th ed. New York, NY: McGraw-Hill; 2016:2030–2042.

5. Safa M. Determining decisional capacity. Quality Improvement and Patient Safety Section Newsletter. 2016. https://www.acep.org/how-we-serve/sections/quality-improvement–patient-safety/newsletters/october-2016/determining-decisional-capacity

6. American College of Emergency Physicians. EMTALA fact sheet. https://www.acep.org/life-as-a-physician/ethics–legal/emtala/emtala-fact-sheet

5

Selected Topics in Emergency Medicine Patient Care

Introduction

There are a number of specific scenarios that you may encounter while treating patients in the ED. Although many of these situations are intertwined with a patient's medical complaint, you may find yourself confronted with nonmedical situations regarding your patient's care that must be addressed. This chapter discusses some common scenarios you may face while caring for patients in the ED.

ADVANCED DIRECTIVES/END-OF-LIFE CARE

Less than 50% of American adults have an advanced directive.[1] The ED provider should document whether the patient has an advanced directive or a "do not resuscitate" (DNR) form. This form facilitates cessation of CPR should the patient sustain a cardiac or respiratory arrest. If there is no DNR form, there are other forms to look for (which differ from state to state), including:

- Physician Orders for Life-Sustaining Treatment (POLST)
- Medical Orders for Life-Sustaining Treatment (MOLST)

Many forms detail the patient's treatment wishes, including intravenous (IV) line placement, administration of oxygen, pain medication, IV fluids, any minor surgical interventions, intubations, and antibiotic administration.

For patients who present to the ED with imminent death, life-sustaining measures can be discontinued if there are documents to support this, and/or if the patient's healthcare proxy/power of attorney (POA) decides to do so. The patient should be kept comfortable in the meantime. If life-sustaining treatment is to be discontinued, this should be discussed with the patient and/or healthcare proxy in detail and should include the following components:

- Possible symptoms and outcomes
- Explain to the family that the patient may demonstrate restlessness, shortness of breath, or air hunger in his or her last few moments
- If there is use of a cardiac bedside echocardiogram to view cardiac activity, explain that having a few beats per minute is expected but not consistent with life-sustaining blood flow to the organs
- The availability of a religious provider, such as a chaplain

Ensure there is a quiet, private room for grieving family members that is secluded from noisy, high-traffic areas and that comfortable seating is available. For patients with imminent death and end-of-life care, opiate infusions plus intermittent midazolam should be initiated and titrated to the patient's comfort level.[2] Treating a patient with 0.5 to 5 mg of haloperidol via IV can produce a calming effect on a patient who may develop delirium during this time as well.[2]

CARE OF INCARCERATED PATIENTS AND PATIENTS IN POLICE CUSTODY

Patients in the prison system in the United States have access to medical care within their facilities;however, emergency medical treatment may be sought by incarcerated patients for various reasons. Patients may require treatment for an acute illness, trauma, or for complications of chronic diseases such as cardiovascular disease, hypertension, chronic obstructive pulmonary disease, or diabetes. Studies of prison populations worldwide have revealed high rates of psychiatric disease and increased prevalence of infectious diseases, such as HIV, hepatitis B, hepatitis C, and tuberculosis, and patients may require emergency treatment related to these disease processes.[3]

Patients who arrive to the ED in police custody may require evaluation for traumatic injury sustained prior to or during arrest. Patients may be under the influence of drugs or alcohol or may demonstrate other acute behavioral disturbances. Law enforcement agents may present warrants for obtaining evidence from a patient (e.g., ethanol alcohol level) for legal purposes. It is important for ED staff to use designated specimen containers (e.g., special seals or signatures required) provided by law enforcement agents and to follow all protocols for proper chain-of-custody evidence collection.

Special circumstances must be considered when treating patients in the custody of law enforcement:

- ED staff and patient safety
  - Disruptive or violent patients should be separated from other patients and evaluated efficiently to avoid undue disruption of the ED environment.
  - Patients in custody should remain in designated restraints (except when necessary to remove for thorough evaluation) and with officers at all times to avoid increased risk to staff or other patients.
- Restraints
  - State and local legislation varies with regard to restraint of prisoners.
  - All patients should be managed on a case-by-case basis depending on presenting complaint and level of security required for the patient.
  - Patients may require removal of restraints, under supervision of the accompanying officers, to facilitate evaluation and treatment of the patient *keeping in mind the safety of the patient and ED staff during such interactions.*
- Confidentiality of medication information
  - Presence of officers during evaluation and treatment of a patient can raise issues of confidentiality of health information.
  - To ensure privacy, law enforcement officers may step out of the room when treating nonviolent or minor offenders; however, public safety overrides medical confidentiality for patients involved in more serious criminal activity.[4]
- Ingestion of foreign bodies or foreign substances
  - Patients may sometimes admit to having swallowed or concealed drugs or other foreign bodies.
  - Patients who admit to ingestion of foreign bodies should be evaluated for signs/symptoms of obstruction (x-ray can help determine location of item) and should be carefully observed until item has passed.
  - Appropriate surgical consultation should be obtained if concern for obstruction exists or if patient is at high risk of systemic toxicity (e.g., from ingested drugs).

Patients in custody of law enforcement should be treated with the same compassion and respect as shown to any other patient in the ED. It is important to keep in mind the safety of your patient, the staff, and other patients in the ED, as well as your own personal safety during the evaluation of these patients.

DRUG-SEEKING BEHAVIOR

Some patients will seek medical care in the ED with the intent of obtaining medication or prescriptions for controlled substances (e.g., opioid analgesics, benzodiazepines, sedatives, stimulants) for misuse or illicit sale. Although it is important to evaluate all patients in the ED in a thorough, nonjudgmental way to ensure that life-threatening illness or injury can safely be ruled out, it is also important to be aware of such behaviors. Indiscriminate administration and prescription of controlled substances can have catastrophic consequences for the patient and has led to significant morbidity and mortality in the United States.

Other factors to consider when evaluating a patient exhibiting potential drug-seeking behaviors include:

- Inconsistent history
  - Patient may relay inconsistent details about his or her history to different members of the ED staff.
  - Reported medical history does not match patient's previous records.
  - Use of false identification; prior medical record names/patient identifiers do not match.
  - Exaggerated or false symptoms are reported.
  - Multiple visits are made to multiple facilities that the patient does not disclose.
  - Patient reports numerous drug allergies.
- Inconsistent physical exam
  - Patient may appear comfortable when ED staff are not at the bedside or may be easily distracted from his or her distress.
  - Reexamination by other providers or on reevaluation does not produce consistent findings.
  - Signs or symptoms fail to correspond with expected physiologic or anatomic manifestations of disease (e.g., neurologic symptoms do not correspond to an expected dermatome).
  - Signs or symptoms do not correspond with objective laboratory or radiologic findings.
- Multiple prior ED visits for similar or other pain-related complaint
- Drug-monitoring program data suggesting controlled substance misuse
  - Early refills, multiple prescribers, prescriptions filled at multiple pharmacies
- Documentation from previous ED visits by providers regarding concern for drug-seeking behavior

Additional risk factors for the misuse of controlled substances include a history of conduct disorder, psychiatric symptoms, and a personal or family history of substance use disorder.[5]

> **CLINICAL PEARL:** Patients with suspected drug-seeking behavior should be addressed by your preceptor and/or attending physician. Although these behaviors are important to keep in mind and you may suspect this behavior after your evaluation of the patient, this is always a diagnosis of exclusion. These clinical situations require careful discussion and clear communication between provider(s) and the patient.

Patients with suspected drug-seeking behavior should be treated with the same compassion and respect you would demonstrate in treating any other patient in your care. Many of these patients have a history of chronic pain syndromes or other psychosocial factors that should be considered and can further complicate their care. It is important to develop and implement your treatment and disposition plan with the patient, keeping the following things in mind:

- Clear communication between provider and patient is important.
  - Patients should feel like their concerns have been acknowledged and addressed.
  - Providers should discuss why they may or may not be administering or prescribing requested medications, keeping patient safety in mind.
- For patients with chronic pain, discussing alternative treatment managements can be beneficial (e.g., physical therapy, pain management, non-pharmacologic therapies).
- Ensure the patient has adequate follow-up with a primary care provider or specialist.
- Direct patients to substance abuse resources when appropriate.
- Develop future treatment plans.
- Clearly document concerns and discussions with the patient so future providers may access this information.

MALINGERING AND FACTITIOUS DISORDERS

Both malingering and factitious disorders involve deceptive behavior that exaggerates or simulates physical or psychological illness. The intent of malingering is secondary gain, typically in the form of work avoidance, avoidance of other obligations, to obtain drugs, or to receive financial compensation. For example, a malingering patient may feign a back injury or tamper with a laboratory specimen (e.g., pricking one's finger to create fictitious hematuria) for the purpose of obtaining opiate pain medication. Patients with factitious disorders simulate illness in order to assume a sick role without the intent of secondary gain. Some examples of such behavior are deceptive use of self-harm (without suicidal intent) for the purpose of playing the role of an injured patient or inappropriate self-administration of medication to induce illness.

All patients with suspected malingering or factitious disorder warrant a thorough evaluation as this is a diagnosis of exclusion. Patients may exhibit similar inconsistencies in their presentation and exam as discussed in the drug-seeking behavior section. Evidence of factitious behavior may be directly observed by the provider or other ED staff members or may be gathered via medical records, video evidence, or other collateral contacts. Other behaviors that are suspicious for malingering or factitious disorder are:

- High rates of healthcare utilization
- Use of multiple healthcare facilities, providers, or pharmacies
- Evasion or refusal to providehealth history information
- Evaluation of the patient reveals extensive history of illness or injuries (e.g., numerous surgical scars) or extensive prior testing and procedures (including those that are high risk)
- Disease follows unusual course (e.g., rapid resolution of symptoms upon administration of therapy or admission to the hospital, new symptoms emerging as others resolve, inconsistent response to standard treatments)

Management of patients with malingering or factitious disorder can be challenging. Some strategies for effectively managing are:

- One provider should oversee patient's care.
- Consultation by or referral to psychiatry should be considered.
- Assess suicide risk and monitor patient for self-injurious behavior.
- Guide diagnostic and treatment plans with objective clinical findings.
- Consider and treat other comorbid psychiatric conditions.

Of utmost importance is treating all patients, including those with suspected malingering or factitious disorder in a fair, nonjudgmental, and supportive manner. It is important to avoid overlooking or ignoring true illness or injury in the evaluation of these patients as this can lead to negative outcomes for both the patient and the provider.

MANAGEMENT OF THE VIOLENT PATIENT

Recent data indicate that hospital workers are at high risk for experiencing violence in the workplace.[6] Clinicians who work in the ED experience the highest level of patient violence because high-risk patients are frequently evaluated and treated in this setting.[7] Risk factors for violence include:

- External influences: Overcrowded waiting rooms, inadequate security, poor lighting
- Patient influences: Ingestion of drugs or alcohol, history of violent behavior, access to firearms

Pay special attention to the following groups, which are at risk of becoming chronically violent, meaning they have exhibited four or more episodes of this behavior:[7]

- Older men with a diagnosis of schizophrenia, history of violence toward others, and substance use disorder
- Borderline personality/antisocial personality disorder with history of violence toward others and substance use disorder
- Antisocial personality disorder occurring with major mental disorders

Signs of imminent violence include

- Clenching jaw/fists
- Profane or overtly sexual language
- Throwing inanimate objects
- Speaking loudly

The initial management of this patient population centers on deescalating the situation. When obtaining a history, maintain a line of questioning that is empathetic and nonthreatening. If there is suspicion of violence or aggression, perhaps interview the patient with the accompaniment of other ED staff and security. If a patient does require restraint, medications may help initially. Some options include benzodiazepines and diphenhydramine. If a patient seems cooperative despite agitation, the medications can be administered by mouth. Administration using an intramuscular approach is typically reserved as a last resort but may be required for the safety of both the patient and staff. In the ED, it is common to use a polypharmacy approach of an antipsychotic, such as haloperidol, and diazepam with diphenhydramine. Although physical restraints of all kinds are a last resort, clinicians must make every effort to defuse the situation without them. Patients should always receive continuous one-to-one attention if they are physically restrained so as not to injure themselves (i.e., they should never be left alone).

PATIENTS WITH HEALTHCARE PROXIES

Patients who lack the mental capacity to make healthcare decisions on their own behalf may have a designated healthcare proxy (or healthcare POA). Such cases may include patients with dementia, developmental delay, or other congenital or acquired cognitive disability. A healthcare proxy may be a relative or may be a court-appointed individual or institution. A common scenario you may encounter in the ED is a patient who is a ward of the state under the care of a group home or other residential/healthcare institution.

When providing care to patients who lack the capacity to make decisions on their own behalf, it is important to review the documentation designating the POA (this documentation often accompanies the patient). Once the healthcare proxy is identified, you should maintain open communication with the proxy regarding all aspects of the patient's evaluation and treatment during his or her ED stay. Any procedures requiring informed consent (e.g., procedural sedation, lumbar puncture, blood transfusion) should be reviewed with the healthcare proxy and appropriate signatures obtained. If patients are being discharged home, you should clearly review the patient's diagnosis, treatment plan, and follow-up instructions with the healthcare proxy. The central focus of the relationship between the provider and the healthcare proxy should be to provide ethical care that is in the best interest of the patient.

PATIENTS WITH LIMITED ENGLISH PROFICIENCY

Medicine itself is a language distinct from any other. The vernacular used can be confusing for novice healthcare students, let alone the layperson. In addition, the languages a patient uses and the culture he or she is a part of can be barriers to understanding and obtaining appropriate care. As a student, seek the services provided by your institution for patients with limited English proficiency. Translated material and interpreter lines may be accessible. Document in the chart what services are used in the event that this may be helpful during future visits. Keep in mind that not all languages have words for something that exists in other languages/cultures.

The Centers for Disease Control and Prevention (CDC) website has several resources to allow for access to translator services:[8]

- CDC.gov in Spanish: www.cdc.gov/spanish/index.html
- Easy to Understand Medicine Instructions in 6 Languages: www.ahrq.gov/professionals/quality-patientsafety/pharmhealthlit/prescriptionmed-instr.html
- Healthy Roads Media: www.store.healthyroadsmedia.org
- HealthReach: healthreach.nlm.nih.gov

REFERENCES

1. Weaver L, Hobgood C. Death notification and advance directives. In: Tintinalli JE, Stapczynski J, Ma O, et al, eds. *Tintinalli's Emergency Medicine: A Comprehensive Study Guide*. 8th ed. New York, NY: McGraw-Hill; 2016:2017–2019.
2. Zalenski RJ, Zimny E. Palliative care. In: Tintinalli JE, Stapczynski J, Ma O, et al, eds. *Tintinalli's Emergency Medicine: A Comprehensive Study Guide*. 8th ed. New York, NY: McGraw-Hill; 2016:2013–2016.
3. Fazel S, Baillargeon J. The health of prisoners. *Lancet*. 2011;377(9769):956–965. doi:10.1016/S0140-6736(10)61053-7
4. Boyce SH, Stevenson RJ. Prison medicine. In: Tintinalli JE, Stapczynski J, Ma O, et al, eds. *Tintinalli's Emergency Medicine: A Comprehensive Study Guide*. 8th ed. New York, NY: McGraw-Hill; 2016.

5. Becker WC, Starrels JL. Prescription drug misuse: epidemiology, prevention, identification, and management. In: Saxon AJ, ed. *UpToDate*. https://www.uptodate.com/contents/prescription-drug-misuse-epidemiology-prevention-identification-and-management?search=prescription-drug-misuseepidemiology-prevention-identification-and-management&source=search_result&selectedTitle=1~150&usage_type=default&display_rank=1. Updated August 13, 2019.

6. Violence occupational hazards in hospitals. National Institute for Occupational Safety and Health website. https://www.cdc.gov/niosh/docs/2002-101/default.html

7. Tishler CL, Reiss NS, Dundas J. The assessment and management of the violent patient in critical hospital settings. *Gen Hosp Psychiatry*. 2013; 35(2):181–185. doi:10.1016/j.genhosppsych.2012.10.012

8. Culture & health literacy. Centers for Disease Control website. https://www.cdc.gov/healthliteracy/culture.html

9. Betancourt JR, Renfrew MR, Green AR, et al. *Improving Patient Safety Systems for Patients with Limited English Proficiency*. Rockville, MD: Agency for Healthcare Research and Quality; 2012. http://www.ahrq.gov/professionals/systems/hospital/lepguide/index.html.

6

Common Procedures in Emergency Medicine

Introduction

One of the many reasons why Physician assistants (PAs) may choose to go into Emergency Medicine is the capability to perform procedures. The variety of hands-on experience can include everything from a small tetanus injection to putting a chest tube in a trauma patient. Although the procedures required by institutions vary from site to site depending on the capability and geographic location, this chapter will review many of the more common procedures PAs in the emergency department may be called upon to execute.

DIGITAL BLOCK

Indication

Wound repair of a digit or other procedure involving digit/nail structures for which local anesthesia is required for pain control. For fingers and toes other than the great toe, block options include traditional digital block, transthecal block, or subcutaneous block. Thumb and great toe block techniques include three- and four-sided ring block methods.

Equipment

- PPE (gloves, gown, mask with eye shield)
- 5-mL syringe for lidocaine
- 18-gauge needle or blunt-tip needle (to draw up anesthetic)

- 25-gauge needle (may attempt to use 27-gauze needle to minimize pain at injection site for fingers; thickened skin and most toe blocks will require 25-guage needle)
- Local anesthetic (1%–2% lidocaine with *without* epinephrine)
- Sterile drape

Procedure

1. Put on PPE.
2. Cleanse skin with alcohol swab.
3. Draw up anesthetic with 18-guage or blunt-tip needle, avoid using more than 3 to 4 mL.
4. For traditional digital block, place hand palm side down (or foot plantar side down) on a sterile drape.
   a. Hold syringe perpendicular to the finger/toe and insert the needle at the base of the finger into the subcutaneous tissue just distal to the metacarpophalangeal (MCP/metatarsophalangeal (MTP) joint.
   b. Advance the needle through the web space toward the palmar/plantar surface without pushing the needle through the skin (approximately 1 cm).
   c. Withdraw plunger slightly to ensure you are not in a vessel and begin injecting anesthetic into palmar/plantar web space while simultaneously withdrawing needle along web space, infiltrating the tissues as you go until you infiltrate area surrounding subcutaneous dorsal nerve space before withdrawing needle completely (1–2 mL of anesthetic should be sufficient).
   d. Repeat same procedure on opposite side of digit you are anesthetizing.
5. For transthecal block (or flexor tendon sheath digital block), place the patient's hand palm side up on a sterile drape, locate the flexor tendon along the distal palmar crease of the affected digit (palpating while having patient flex the digit can help to identify the tendon).
   a. Repeat steps 1 to 3, then, using a 25-gauge needle, hold the syringe at a 45° angle just distal to the palmar crease.
   b. Advance the needle into the flexor tendon sheath and slowly inject 1 to 2 mL of anesthetic. If you meet resistance, withdraw slightly and attempt to inject again.
6. For subcutaneous block, place the patient's hand palm side up on a sterile drape, locate the palmar skin crease at the base of the affected digit.
   a. Repeat steps 1 to 3, then, using a sterile glove, pinch soft tissue just distal to the proximal skin crease with one hand and insert syringe into the midpoint of the skin crease with the other.
   b. Slowly inject 1 to 2 mL of anesthetic solution into subcutaneous space and massage solution into the tissues.
7. For the three-sided thumb/toe block, place the patient's hand palmar side down (foot plantar side down) on a sterile drape.

   a. Repeat steps 1 to 3, hold the syringe perpendicular to the lateral aspect of the thumb/toe and insert the needle just distal to MCP/MTP.

   b. Advance the needle through the web space toward the palmar/plantar surface without pushing the needle through the skin (approximately 1 cm/1.5–2 cm for great toe).

   c. Withdraw plunger slightly to ensure you are not in a vessel and begin injecting anesthetic into palmar/plantar web space while simultaneously withdrawing needle along web space, infiltrating the tissues as you go (1–2mL should be sufficient).

   d. Inject over the dorsal area of the thumb/great toe by partially withdrawing needle and redirecting it medially, across the dorsal aspect of the thumb/toe, injecting anesthetic from the lateral to medial aspect (0.5–1 mL) until you infiltrate the entire dorsal area.

   e. Inject the medial aspect of the thumb/toe just distal to the MCP/MTP, entering in the area previously anesthetized.

   f. Advance the needle through the medial web space toward the palmar/plantar surface without pushing the needle through the skin (approximately 1 cm/1.5–2 cm for great toe).

   g. Withdraw plunger slightly to ensure you are not in a vessel and begin injecting anesthetic into palmar/plantar web space while simultaneously withdrawing needle along medical web space, infiltrating the tissues as you go (1–2 mL should be sufficient).

8. The four-sided block method can be applied if complete anesthesia of the thumb or great toe is not achieved with the three-block method.

   a. Perform the three-sided block described in step 7.

   b. Inject an additional 1 mL of anesthetic across the palmar/plantar surface by entering a previously anesthetized area and advancing the needle medially to laterally or laterally to medially, infiltrating the tissues as you go.

9. Allow up to 10 to 15 minutes for anesthesia to take effect. Check sensation of the distal digit or affected area with a needle prick prior to beginning procedure to ensure area is completely anesthetized.

FOREIGN-BODY REMOVAL: EARS

Indication

Indications for FB removal from the ears include history of placement by the patient, foul-smelling discharge from the ear, visualization, or recurrent bleeding.[1]

Equipment

- Ear speculum
- Universal precautions/face mask with shield for provider

- Alligator forceps
- Otoscope
- Cerumen spoon
- Irrigation material (tray, ear syringe from 20 to 60 mL with 20-guage angio-cath attached, room temperature tap water, towels)

Procedure

1. Set up station and explain the procedure to the patient.
2. Have the patient sitting upright to facilitate visualization.
3. Inspect both ears to document physical exam findings.
4. Attempt to grasp the FB with alligator forceps or cerumen spoon depending on the type of object noted.
   a. Cerumen hook or spoon works well for cerumen.
   b. Hook works well for spherical objects, which are more proximal.

> **CLINICAL PEARL:** A small suction tube attached to wall suction can be used for objects as well but do so with caution so as not to puncture the tympanic membrane (TM).

5. After removal, ensure complete removal and document physical exam.

FOR CERUMEN REMOVAL

1. Use similar setup as indicated previously.
2. Consider inserting 1 to 2 mL of liquid docusate into the ear to break up the cerumen.
3. Wait approximately 10 to 20 minutes and attempt cerumen removal with the use of the cerumen hook or irrigation with the use of an irrigation tray.

There is risk of pushing the object deeper into the canal or even puncturing the tympanic membrane (TM). If the object cannot be directly visualized or removed, or if the TM becomes ruptured, the patient should receive antibiotics and a consult toENT should be made.

REFERENCE

1. Desai BK. Ear foreign body removal. In: Ganti L, ed. *Atlas of Emergency Medicine Procedures*. New York, NY: Springer Science+Business Media; 2016.

FOREIGN-BODY REMOVAL: EYES

Indication

There is often a discussion as to whether foreign-body (FB) removal from the eye requires immediate consultation with ophthalmology. For patients who have the following, ophthalmology should be consulted sooner rather than later:

- High-velocity FB[1]
- Deeply embedded FB
- Any sign of globe compromise such as loss of extraocular movement, changes in the contour of the globe, or a positive Seidel sign
- Evidence of intraocular bleeding such as hyphema
- Evidence of associated iritis
- Chemical alkaline burns

Equipment
- Slit lamp for exam
- Topical tetracaine ophthalmic analgesic solution
- Cotton-tip applicator or spud/burr for removal (alternatively, a 22-guage angiocatheter catheter tip can be used for removal, but do so with caution)
- Gloves
- Opthalmoscope
- Snellen chart to document visual acuities (with and without corrective lenses, if patient uses)
- Fluorescein stain for the cornea
- Eyewash sink station for irrigation

> **CLINICAL PEARL:** If an eyewash sink is unavailable: An alternative solution is to attach IV tubing to a bag of normal saline with a 22- or 20-guage catheter at the tip. Once tetracaine has been administered to the eye, irrigate with normal saline using the catheter tip. Ensure the patient has towels on a pillow and change patient into a hospital gown so as not to get his or her clothes wet.

Procedure
1. Obtain informed consent from the patient if required by your institution.
2. Obtain and document formal visual acuity along with a detailed physical exam.
3. The physical exam should include lid eversion. Lid eversion can be done using the wooden handle of a sterile cotton swab. Once the eyelid is everted, it can be removed and the cotton swab can be utilized to swab away an FB trapped under the eyelid, if it is readily visible and accessible.

> **CLINICAL PEARL:** This is especially important with contact wearers as the contact lenses tend to migrate in an upward fashion.

4. Apply anesthetic topically.
5. Use a moistened cotton swab for FB removal under slit lamp guidance. If the FB can be visualized with the naked eye, removal is possible without slit lamp.

> **CLINICAL PEARL:** For metallic FB, care should be taken so as not to leave a rust stain on the cornea, and ophthalmology consult should be obtained immediately. The advantage of using an FB removal needle is that the rust ring can be removed simultaneously.

6. Tetanus should be administered as needed.
7. Consider application of topical antibiotics and appropriate follow-up with opthalmology.[1]

REFERENCE

1. Desai BK. Corneal foreign body removal. In: Ganti L, ed. *Atlas of Emergency Medicine Procedures.* New York, NY: Springer Science+Business Media; 2016.

FOREIGN-BODY REMOVAL: SKIN/SOFT TISSUE

Indication

A skin or soft-tissue FB is a substance that is not naturally part of the body.[1] An FB in the skin/soft tissue should be suspected with any history in which the skin is broken. Any time the skin is breached, consider a retained FB. Common materials include glass, wood, and metallic objects. On occasion, a skin/soft-tissue FB may occur in a patient who is under the influence of alcohol or other substances, so this must be addressed first as the risk of further injury increases if a patient is uncooperative.

Physical Exam

The approach to skin/soft-tissue FB assessment should begin with an appropriate physical exam, including wound exploration and documentation of neurovascular status. Document whether the patient has appropriate peripheral pulses intact along with appropriate sensation intact. Document whether the findings are new or chronic.

Imaging

X-RAY

Clinicians evaluating the skin/soft tissue for FB should have a low threshold for ordering/performing imaging studies. There are many options, including ultrasound, CT, and plain x-rays. Being able to see an FB on plain x-ray depends on the FB material, size, and orientation.[1] Metallic objects are easily visualized. Almost all glass objects in soft tissue, including bottles, windshield glass, and light bulbs, are at least somewhat radiopaque and can be detected by plain x-rays unless obscured by bone.[1] Plastics may not be visible on imaging due to their varying density. Depending on the type of injury, other FB types to look for are included in Table 6.1 with the corresponding possible history.

> **CLINICAL PEARL:** In order to identify the size, depth, and further composition of an FB, sometimes it is helpful to place an inanimate object, such as a paper clip or penny, next to the anatomical site in question for comparison.

Similar to plain film, CT can provide evidence of FB in the skin/soft tissue with a more three-dimensional view. However, it can be costly, takes more time, and exposes the patient to more radiation.

ULTRASOUND

Sonography is becoming more prevalent in the use of FB detection in the ED. It is particularly useful in evaluating vegetative matter that is radiolucent (wood, cactus needles, thorns).[1]

> **CLINICAL PEARL:** Never probe the depth of a wound with your fingers (even if gloved) as it may increase the risk of exposure to bloodborne pathogens, especially if the potential FB is sharp.

TABLE 6.1 Foreign Body With Associated History

Foreign Body	Associated History
Glass	MVA involving windshield, punching a window, bottle used as a weapon
Asphalt	Asphalt: Motor vehicle or motorcycle crash, pedestrian struck, fall off a bicycle
Teeth	Common during a fight

MVA, motor vehicle accident.

> **CLINICAL PEARL:** Teeth are associated with Boxer's fracture of the hand (4th/5th metacarpal head fracture).

Equipment

It is important to have appropriate equipment and lighting to perform an assessment of skin/soft tissue FB. If you do not have adequate lighting, it may be helpful to use a gooseneck lamp or move to a room with improved lighting. Wound exploration should be performed wearing gloves. If there is potential for bleeding or vascular injury, wear a mask and gown.

FB REMOVAL

A decision to remove an FB is one that should occur in conversation with the collaborating ED provider. If removal of the FB may cause more undue injury to the patient and is not located adjacent to vital structures, the decision can be made to electively hold removal.

There is no one technique for FB removal. It depends on the location. Take caution with areas, such as the face, distal extremities, or neck, where there are many structures in small spaces. The following equipment may be needed:

- Consent obtained from the patient with risks and benefits noted
- Sterile drapes
- Hemostat or needle driver
- Forceps
- Scalpel
- Tourniquet
- Small 3- or 5-mL syringe with 22- or 24-guage needle for local anesthesia
- Lidocaine without epinephrine (Note: Epinephrine should not be used on fingers/toes/ear lobes/tip of nose/genital region.)
- Betadine or wound-cleansing agent
- Saline for irrigation

Procedure

Once confirmation of the FB has been performed using direct visualization or via imaging, the procedure can begin.

1. If applicable, place a tourniquet/inflated BP cuff on an extremity to avoid blood loss and to facilitate viewing of the region.
2. Administer local anesthesia if required for FB removal.
3. Ensure proper irrigation of the area to clean any debris, but do not use high velocity so as to avoid damaging tissue.
4. If the FB is through a puncture wound, make a proper skin incision to allow for wound exploration and removal of FB. At times, it helps to pinch the surrounding skin and allow for the FB to become exposed and extract with a hemostat.
5. After removal, irrigate the wound again prior to bandaging.
6. If an incision is made in an area that is not cosmetic, leave the incision open and properly bandaged. If a large incision is made, as long as there is no contraindication, sutures can be placed. In areas with gross contamination, leave the wound open and insert sterile packing with a mandatory 48-hour follow-up.[1]

SPECIAL SITUATIONS

- Subungual FB: This may require a digital block before manipulation of the nail or nail bed. The tip of a sterile needle can be used to extract an FB under the nail (such as a wooden splinter). Alternatively, using a scalpel to lift a small wedge-shaped part of the nail where the splinter ends allows for removal.[1]

- Metallic FB: Regarding high-velocity FBs such as bullets: If they are not adjacent to vital structures or vascular structures, and are deep within tissue, they can remain. These objects tend to become encysted and rarely cause infection.[1] For superficial metallic FB, a sterile magnet can be used for removal. Follow the directions noted previously in making an incision or place the magnet over the entry site to facilitate removal.

- Pencil/graphite: It is relevant to remove pencil/graphite objects as they can cause permanent tattooing and there is a risk of melanoma over time if not removed.[1]

- Fishhooks: As in any case, document the patient's neurovascular status. If barbs are involved, they should be cut with the appropriate tool.

> **CLINICAL PEARL:** Due to the presence of tendons and the rich neurovascular circulation in the palm of the hand, an FB that is deep or requires incision for removal may best be performed by a hand surgeon.

FISHHOOK REMOVAL

There are several techniques for fishhook removal.

- The advance-and-cut technique is used for a fishhook embedded when a digital block has been performed. Force the point of the fishhook through the anesthetized skin. Clip off the barb using surgical shears. Then remove the rest of the fishhook by reversing the direction of entry.

- The needle-cover technique can be used when the hook is large and not deep in the skin. Insert a short-bevel 18-guage needle through the entry wound of the hook and sheath the barb of the hook within the needle. If done correctly, the hook and the needle can then be removed together.

- The retrograde technique starts with downward pressure on the shank to disengage the barb, followed by a swift pull off the hook in reverse direction of entry.

TETANUS AND ANTIBIOTIC ADMINISTRATION

- All patients who undergo FB insertion should have their tetanus status updated. Depending on your institution, patients will either receive Tdap. Patients who are immunocompromised, have a wound with high potential for infection/inflammation due to high degree of debridement, or have evidence of FB that could not be removed may be candidates for prophylactic antibiotic administration.

- Excess time from injury to resection of the FB may also require antibiotic administration. There is no data to support prophylactic antibiotic administration for wounds in which the FB was completely resected and wounds remain clean.[1] First-generation cephalosporin is first-line treatment. For patients who may be at risk for MRSA infection (methicillin-resistant *S. aureus*), more broad-spectrum coverage with clindamycin, trimethoprim–sulfamethoxazole or tetracycline may be required.

<small>DISCHARGE INSTRUCTIONS</small>

- Tetanus vaccine should be administered in the nondominant arm. Patients may be instructed to take over-the counter antipyretics as needed for pain or fever.
- In the setting of FB removal, patients should be instructed to keep the extremity elevated, keep the area clean and dry, and have the wound evaluated by a provider (either the ED or primary care provider) in 48 to 72 hours. The patients should be told not to let the wound become waterlogged.
- Should they develop increased redness/swelling to the area, purulent drainage, fever, or red streaks up an extremity indicative of lymphangitis, they are to return to the ED for subsequent evaluation.

REFERENCE

1. Stone DB, Scordino DJ. Foreign body removal. In: Roberts JR, Custalow CB, Thomsen TW, eds. *Roberts and Hedges' Clinical Procedures in Emergency Medicine and Acute Care.* 7th ed. Philadelphia, PA: Elsevier; 2018:708–737.

INCISION AND DRAINAGE OF ABSCESS

Indication

Incision and drainage of an abscess are indicated for patients with soft-tissue infections that involve

- Purulent discharge, fluctuance, or those that contain a subcutaneous collection of pus that can be palpated on physical exam or visualized by ultrasonography

Although cellulitis is treated with warm compresses and oral antibiotics alone, an uncomplicated abscess is treated with incision and drainage. Some abscesses will require incision and drainage along with oral antibiotic therapy, particularly patients with the following:

- Abscesses larger than 2 cm, multiple lesions, extensive surrounding cellulitis,immunocompromise, risk of endocarditis or other comorbid conditions, high risk of transmission of infection to others

Equipment

- Personal protective equipment (PPE; gloves, gown, mask with eye shield)
- 1- to 10-mL syringe (depending on size of abscess)
- 18-gauge needle or blunt-tip needle
- 25-gauge needle

- Local anesthetic (1%–2% lidocaine)
- Antiseptic scrub for skin (e.g., povidone iodine, chlorhexidine)
- 11-blade scalpel
- Swab and culture container (*only if sending wound culture)
- Hemostat
- 10- to 30-mL irrigation syringe; alternatively, anesthetic syringe can be used to irrigate
- Normal saline solution
- Forceps
- Scissors
- ¼-inch or ½-inch packing
- 4×4-inch gauze pads
- Tape

Procedure

1. Put on personal protective equipment.
2. Cleanse skin with antiseptic scrub.
3. Draw up appropriate amount of lidocaine (most commonly 1%–2% solution without epinephrine) into syringe with 18-gauge needle.

> **CLINICAL PEARL:** Lidocaine with epinephrine can also be used to minimize bleeding.

4. Inject lidocaine into area of greatest fluctuance (making sure to direct lidocaine to dermal layer above purulent collection), central pustule, or in location of spontaneous drainage if drainage has already occurred.

> **CLINICAL PEARL:** Although skin anesthesia is usually possible, it can be difficult to provide complete anesthesia to the affected area given the degree of tissue inflammation and diminished efficacy of local anesthetic in the low pH of the infected tissue. Regional nerve blocks can be effective alternatives when possible.[1]

5. Create incision with an 11-blade scalpel along the natural skin crease or fold of affected area across the length of the abscess area.

> **CLINICAL PEARL:** Take care not to incise too deeply to avoid injuring underlying nerve, muscle, or vascular structures. Use the smallest, effective incision size in cosmetic areas, such as the face or neck, to avoid excessive scarring.

6. Swab purulent drainage if sending a culture.

7. Apply gentle pressure to express purulent drainage; insert hemostat to break up loculations (may require additional anesthesia for this step).
8. Irrigate abscess cavity with normal saline to remove further drainage or debris.
9. Cut appropriate length of packing with forceps and scissors and insert loosely (avoid overpacking) into cavity leaving short tail outside wound for ease of removal.

> **CLINICAL PEARL:** As an alternative, a catheter or rubber drain can be placed instead of packing the wound.

10. Place 4×4-inch gauze dressing with tape over wound.
11. Instruct patient in proper wound care and give follow-up instructions for changing or removal of packing in 24 to 72 hours.

> **CLINICAL PEARL:** Repacking is often unnecessary unless significant drainage is still present at follow-up visit, or if the initial abscess was large.

REFERENCE

1. Ambrose G, Berlin D. Incision and drainage. In: Roberts JR, Custalow CB, Thomsen TW, eds. *Roberts and Hedges' Clinical Procedures in Emergency Medicine and Acute Care.* 7th ed. Philadephia, PA: Elsevier; 2019:738–773.

LUMBAR PUNCTURE

Indication

Indications for obtaining cerebrospinal fluid (CSF) can vary. Because it is an invasive procedure commonly done in the ED, this procedure is part of your education. Indications for lumbar puncture include the following:

- Persistent headache despite intervention and a negative brain CT to rule out subarachnoid bleed
- Meningitis (viral/bacterial/fungal) or any other systemic central nervous system (CNS) infection
- Measure intracranial opening pressure (ICP) to rule out intracranial hypertension
- Rule out syphilis of the CNS

Contraindications

The presence of an already-existing infection near the puncture site is a contraindication to performing a lumbar puncture. Relative contraindications include coagulopathy, presence of a space-occupying lesion confirmed via brain imaging, and severe thrombocytopenia. Therefore, obtain coagulation studies, including PT/iINR, partial thromboplastin time (PTT), and platelets, before beginning the procedure.

> **CLINICAL PEARL:** Even for patients who return to the ED with a headache that was recently imaged, repeat imaging prior to the lumbar puncture should be performed.

Equipment
The equipment is found in a prepackaged kit and includes
- Antiseptic and applicator
- Three-way stopcock
- Spinal needles
- Sterile drape
- Manometer
- Syringe
- Lidocaine
- Needles for anesthetic
- 6-inch extension tubing
- Collection tubes

> **CLINICAL PEARL:** The spinal needles included in a lumbar puncture kit tend to be larger bore to allow for expedited removal of CSF; however, there is also risk of a postspinal tap headache. As a result, it may be helpful to use a smaller gauge spinal needle when doing a lumbar puncture. This can take longer; however, there is minimal opportunity for a spinal headache, and the smaller needle may be less painful for the patient. Keep in mind, thinner needles make it more difficult to pass through adult skin and deeper structures, which could result in bending the needle, or the needle veering off the desired course.

Procedure
- Before beginning, be sure to set up the room and your procedure station, and obtain informed consent.[1]
- Obtain the lumbar puncture tray from your facility store room.
- Most lumbar puncture kits come with the medications required for the procedure, including betadine and lidocaine (without epinephrine).
- Obtain consent for the procedure. Written consent should include the indication and potential complications and there should be a verbal conversation as to how the procedure will be carried out. Complications from this procedure include local pain, postspinal headache, infection, bleeding, nerve damage, and paralysis.

> **CLINICAL PEARL:** Explain to the patient that the needle insertion site is well below the level of spinal cord termination.

- If performing the lumbar puncture with the patient sitting upright, you will require assistance from a medical assistant/patient care technician and several pillows for the patient to hug along with a tray table to place the pillows on.
- Lumbar puncture is typically done with the patient in the lateral recumbent position with the goal of creating an imaginary line from the posterior superior iliac crest to the L4 spinous process. The patient should have a pillow to keep the head in line with the vertebral axis. Ensure the shoulders and hips are perpendicular to the table/stretcher.
- Alternatively, patients may require sitting in an upright position because the midline is easier to identify. If performing the procedure with the patient sitting up, be cautious of orthostatic blood pressure (BP) changes and frequently ask the patient he or she is doing to ensure the airway is patent.
    1. Position the patient properly, either seated or in left lateral decubitus position.
    2. Identify the appropriate landmarks, including L4 spinous process and posterior–superior iliac crests.
    3. Prepare the skin with an antiseptic solution using appropriate technique.
    4. Apply the sterile drape.
    5. Create a wheal with anesthetic over the insertion site and infiltrate and anesthetize the deeper layers.
    6. Insert needle in midline, with needle parallel to bed while advancing forward. Check for CSF during needle advancement by removing stylet. Subarachnoid space is infiltrated once CSF appears.
    7. Measure opening pressure with manometer.
    8. Collect CSF samples as needed.
    9. Replace stylet and remove needle.

PROCEDURAL TIPS

- When holding the spinal needle, the bevel of the needle should be facing the ceiling and the spinal needle should be held between the thumbs and index fingers of both hands. Some providers prefer to have the bevel facing toward the patient's left or right side to prevent trauma of the dural fibers.
- The paraspinal ligaments can cause resistance to the needle, but once the needle penetrates the space, a "pop" or noticeable lack of resistance may be felt.

> **CLINICAL PEARL:** In patients who are obese, it is not uncommon for the needle to be inserted all the way down to the hub.

- Sometimes it is easier to remove the stylet of the needle in small increments to see whether the subarachnoid space has been entered and check for initiation of CSF flow. However, the stylet should always be in place when advancing the needle.
- If bone is hit during the procedure, partially withdraw the needle, check for spinal alignment while maintaining sterility, and reenter, ensuring the needle remains midline.
- Once CSF is noted, have the four tubes ready to be filled. It may help to replace the stylet in between tubes to avoid loss of CSF, and therefore, avoid a spinal headache.
- Only fill each tube up to the designated line (which is typically consistent with 1 mL of fluid per tube).
  These tubes should be labeled according to your institution's laboratory standards; the following may be a possible order for the tubes and they should be hand-delivered to ensure there is no error in labeling or potential for loss, considering how invasive the procedure is. It is important to mark the tubes in the appropriate filling order using the numbers 1 to 4:
  Tube 1: Cell count
  Tube 2: Glucose/protein
  Tube 3: Cultures
  Tube 4: Cell count
- After a spinal tap, the patient should be instructed to lay flat for at least 1 hour and intravenous (IV) fluid administration initiated unless there is a contraindication. For a headache, patients can receive caffeine administered as 500 mg in 1-L bag of normal saline over 1 to 2 hours. (Note: A cup of coffee contains 50 to 100 mg of caffeine). If a severe headache persists for several weeks when upright and subsides when supine, consider anesthesia consult for a blood patch.

REFERENCE

1. Euerle B. Spinal puncture and cerebrospinal fluid examination. In: Roberts JR, ed. *Roberts and Hedges' Clinical Procedures in Emergency Medicine and Acute Care.* 7th ed. Philadelphia, PA: Elsevier; 2018:1258–1280.

NASAL PACKING (ANTERIOR)

Indication

Anterior sources of epistaxis are the most common (1). Anterior nasal packing should be considered for epistaxis that is not controlled with direct pressure or silver nitrate cautery . Although accordion petroleum gauze packing is an accepted method for management of anterior epistaxis, newer packing materials, such as nasal tampons and nasal balloon devices, are widely and effectively used.

Ask about any trauma, insertion of a foreign body, or use of anticoagulants (i.e., warfarin, aspirin, etc.) and consider dry air during the winter as an etiology for nosebleed. Consider inquiring about hematological conditions such as Von Willebrand coagulopathy.

If the epistaxis appears to be of posterior etiology or is refractory from recent intervention, an ear, nose, and throat (ENT) consult should be obtained. For patients who are bleeding secondary to anticoagulant use, blood work should be sent, including complete blood count (CBC) and prothrombin time (PT)/international normalized ratio (INR). If a patient has evidence of massive facial trauma or recent surgery involving the area, nasal packing is contraindicated and either oromaxillary facial surgery (OMFS) or plastic surgery should be called.

Equipment
- PPE (gloves, gown, mask with eye shield)
- Wall suction (if available)
- Topical anesthetic (1%–2% lidocaine)
- 10-mL syringe
- Saline (if using nasal tampon)

> **CLINICAL PEARL:** The use of lidocaine with epinephrine is an effective method of achieving simultaneous anesthesia and vasoconstriction.

- Topical vasoconstrictor (intranasal oxymetazoline)
- Nasal speculum with light source or otoscope
- Tongue depressor
- Bayonet forceps (if using petroleum gauze)
- Scissors (for trimming nasal tampon to size)
- Kidney basin (for soaking nasal balloon device in sterile water)
- 2×2-inch and 4×4-inch gauze (cotton balls or dental rolls will also work if available)
- Topical antibiotic ointment (if using nasal tampon)
- Silver nitrate stick
- Packing materials
  - ○ Petroleum gauze
  - ○ Nasal tampon
  - ○ Nasal balloon device (e.g., *Rapid Rhino, Rhino Rocket*)

Procedure
1. Put on PPE.
2. Attempt to identify bleeding site with nasal speculum.
   a. May use intranasal oxymetazoline to slow bleeding enough to identify site.
3. Instruct patient to blow nose to dislodge any clots or carefully suction nares.

4. Soak 2×2-inch gauze (may also use cotton balls or dental rolls) in 1% to 2% lidocaine with epinephrine (or 1%–2% lidocaine without epinephrine followed by intranasal oxymetazoline), roll gauze and apply to each naris.
   a. Have patient sit forward and apply firm, external pressure to nares with fingers to achieve anesthesia and hemostasis (approximately 10–15 minutes).
5. Reassess bleeding site and reconsider silver nitrate cautery if bleeding controlled or only scant oozing. Confirm that a septal hematoma is not present.
6. Insert packing device.
   a. Petroleum gauze*: Advance gauze with bayonet forceps in accordion fashion until several layers are placed to create tamponade effect.
      *Note: This method is rarely used given ease of use and efficacy of currently available packing devices discussed in the following text.
   b. Nasal tampon
      i. Trim tampon to proper length and width to fit nose.
      ii. Lubricate with antibiotic ointment.
      iii. Insert gently advancing posteriorly and parallel to the nasal floor.
      iv. After tampon is inserted, inject 5- to 10-mL saline to expand tampon.
      v. Tie tampon drawstring to a 4 × 4-piece of gauze to anchor tampon in place.
   c. Nasal balloon device
      i. Soak in sterile water for 30 seconds (do not use saline as this can deactivate fibers that promote thrombosis in device).
      ii. Insert gently advancing posteriorly and parallel to the nasal floor until the ring at the base is within the naris.
      iii. Insert air using a syringe to expand cuff until it becomes round and firm.
7. Monitor patient for 10 to 15 minutes, ambulate patient, and check for signs of inadequate hemostasis and recheck placement of tampon or nasal balloon device.
8. Use tongue depressor to adequately visualize posterior pharynx for bleeding or clots.
9. Instruct patient to lean forward and apply firm pressure for 15 minutes for any recurrent bleeding. Patient should return to the ED for any recurrent bleeding that is not controlled with these measures.
10. Patients should be instructed to follow up with otolaryngology specialist within 24 to 48 hours for packing removal and further evaluation.
11. Prescribe prophylactic antibiotics (with coverage against *Staphylococcus aureus*) for patients at risk of developing infection, such as elderly, diabetic, or immunosuppressed patients. Options for prophylaxis include
    a. Amoxicillin–clavulanate
    b. Second-generation cephalosporin (e.g., cefuroxime)
    c. Topical mupirocin 2% ointment

> **CLINICAL PEARL:** The topic of prophylactic antibiotics is somewhat controversial. Although rates of toxic shock syndrome are low and risk of unnecessary use of antibiotic prophylaxis may outweigh any benefit, they are still widely recommended by most otolaryngologists.

REFERENCE

1. Schlosser RJ. Epistaxis. *N Engl J Med*. 2009;360(8):784–789. doi:10.1056/NEJMcp 0807078

WOUND REPAIR

Indication

Wound-repair techniques are used for the purpose of keeping wounds closed to avoid contamination, facilitate healing, and to maximize cosmetic outcomes. Ideally, wounds should be closed within 4 to 6 hours to decrease risk of wound infection. This time may increase to 18 hours for clean, uninfected wounds in any location and up to 48 to 72 hours for low-risk facial wounds.[1,2]

- Staples
  - Scalp wounds
  - Large, linear wounds where cosmetic outcomes are less important (e.g., extremity, trunk)
- Sutures
  - Most widely used wound-repair technique
  - Irregular or deep wounds, wounds requiring layered repair
  - Facial wounds too deep to repair with tissue adhesive
  - Wounds with persistent bleeding
- Tissue adhesives (glue or tape)
  - Linear wounds under little tension, areas of cosmetic concern
  - Wounds with no active bleeding
  - Superficial wounds under low tension
  - Wounds in areas *without* excessive hair (e.g., eyebrows, scalp)
  - Skin tear/superficial avulsion injuries (if avulsed skin is still attached)
  - Wounds with low risk of contamination/infection as adhesive glue effectively seals wound

Equipment

- PPE (gloves, gown, mask with eye shield)
- 1- to 10-mL syringe for lidocaine (depending on size of wound)
- 18-gauge needle or blunt-tip needle

- 25-gauge needle (27- or 30-gauge needle may be used for small lacerations); length of needle should be chosen based on length of wound
- Local anesthetic (1%–2% lidocaine with or without epinephrine)
- Tap water or normal saline solution for irrigation
- 10- to 60-mL irrigation syringe with or without an irrigation shield
- Suture kit or
  - Sterile scissors
  - Forceps
  - Drapes
  - Needle driver
  - Hemostat (if active bleeding/vessel tie needed)
- Wound-closure material
  - Tissue adhesive (glue or tape)
  - Suture material
    - Nonabsorbable (nylon or polypropylene) sutures are generally used for skin closure; absorbable sutures (catgut, polyglactin) are generally used for closure of intraoral lacerations and deeper layers of skin/tissue in layered repairs
    - Most commonly used sizes of suture material between 1-0 (largest) to 10-0 (smallest) are
      - Face/neck: 6-0, may use 5-0 for higher tension areas (under chin)
      - Distal/volar upper extremities and hands: 5-0, 4-0
      - Trunk/extremities with low wound tension: 4-0, 3-0
      - Extremities with higher wound tension: 3-0, 2-0
      - Deep lacerations will involve approximation of deeper tissues (muscle, fascia) with absorbable suture material prior to closure of superficial/skin layer with nonabsorbable suture material
  - Staple device
- 4×4-inch gauze pads
- Tape
- Antibiotic ointment

Procedure

1. Put on PPE.
2. Thoroughly irrigate wound with normal saline or tap water.

> **CLINICAL PEARL:** When possible, it is often more comfortable for patients receiving staples or sutures to administer local anesthesia (see step 7a) to the wound prior to irrigation or debridement.

3. Debride nonviable tissue and contaminants/debris as needed.
4. Dry skin along wound edge after irrigation/debridement.
5. For tissue adhesive tape
   a. Apply benzoin tincture to intact skin along wound edge to improve adhesion. Take caution to keep this out of the wound itself.

    b. Cut ¼-inch to ½-inch wide adhesive tape strips to desired length (allow for approximately 2–3 cm of overlap with skin on either side of the wound) with backing still attached.

    c. Starting at the center of the wound, remove backing to one side of tape and apply to one side of wound while gently approximating other side.

    d. Remove remainder of backing and attach second half of adhesive tape to other side of wound. Repeat until entire wound is approximated, leaving adequate space in between strips to approximate wound without completely occluding it.

    e. Instruct patient to keep clean and dry for 24 to 48 hours and then cleanse with damp cloth;avoid submersion in water. Maintain in place for 1 to 2 weeks, trimming curled edges of the tape as needed.

6. For tissue adhesive glue

    a. Follow steps 1 to 4 as indicated.

    b. Squeeze adhesive tube with fingers to liquefy for use.

    c. Hold wound edges together with forceps or fingers and apply along wound edge. Apply in three to four layers, extending 5 to 10 mm from each end of wound. Amount of adhesive layers applied may vary depending on the type used.

    d. Continue to approximate wound edges for at least 1 minute until adhesive dries.

> **CLINICAL PEARL:** Be careful not to glue your gloved fingers to any part of the patient's skin or wound. Wipe away excessive glue with gauze. You may use antibiotic ointment to create a "dam" effect and prevent glue from adhering to places other than the wound. This is particularly helpful for avoiding contact with eyebrows, eyelids, and eyelashes when repairing facial wounds.

    e. Leave adhesive glue and wound open.

    f. Instruct patients not to apply occlusive bandages or ointments to wound, to avoid submersion in water, and that glue will slough off in 5 to 10 days. Patients may trim dried and curled edges of glue as wound heals.

7. For staples, follow steps 1 to 4 as indicated:

    a. Anesthetize wound.

       i. Draw up lidocaine with 18-gauge needle.

       ii. Switch to 25-gauge needle; insert needle at one end of wound edge (from within the wound, not through intact skin) and advance subcutaneously, paralleling the wound border until you reach the other end of the wound edge.

      iii. Aspirate to ensure you are not in a vessel; if clear, inject lidocaine as you withdraw the needle along the wound border. You should see a small wheal of anesthetic being raised as you inject along wound edge.

Note: Multiple injections along the wound edge as indicated previously may be necessary for longer wounds. As an alternative, ring or digital blocks may be used for lacerations to digits (see "Digital Block" section); regional nerve blocks may be helpful for larger, more complex wounds.

CLINICAL PEARL: Lidocaine with epinephrine should be avoided in distal areas and areas with poor blood supply (digits, cartilaginous areas of ears or nose). Avoid lidocaine toxicity in larger wounds or with smaller patients. Maximum dose of lidocaine is 4.5 mg/kg (up to 300 mg); maximum dose of lidocaine with epinephrine is 7 mg/kg (up to 500 mg).

  b. Drape wound area with sterile drape.
  c. Approximate wound edges so that edges are everted (may require assistance by another person). Starting from the center of the wound, align the middle of the staple device (usually marked with a hash or line) with the center of the wound and squeeze trigger to place staple. Do not apply too much pressure while placing staple to avoid placing the staple too deep, which can cause ischemia; there should be 1 to 2 mm of space between the crossbar of the staple and the wound/skin surface.

CLINICAL PEARL: Deep wounds may require absorbable sutures to close fascial injuries or within superficial fascial and dermal layers to reduce wound tension (see step 9c).

  d. Continue to place staples along wound until entire wound is well-approximated.
  e. May leave wound open to air or dress with sterile dressing. Patients should be instructed to gently clean the wound in 24 to 48 hours.
8. For staple removal
  a. Scalp wounds may have staples removed in 7 days; trunk and upper extremity wounds may have staples removed in 7 to 10 days; lower extremity wounds/wounds over joints/high-tension wounds may have staples removed in 10 to 14 days.
  b. Staple removal device is placed with dual prongs under the staple crossbar facing upward with single prong facing down. Squeeze handles together, this creates an "M" shape in the staple as it is bent upward from the wound, gently remove each staple end from wound.
9. For suture placement, follow steps 1 to 4, 7a as indicated:
  a. Drape wound area with sterile drape.
  b. If wound is deep and requires layered closure, place subcutaneous sutures with absorbable suture material prior to skin closure.
  c. Subcutaneous suture repair

    i. Starting from within the wound, place the first suture through the subcutaneous level at the bottom of the wound/base of the flap, exit in the dermis and draw suture across wound, enter at same level on opposite side of wound at the dermal layer and exit at the subcutaneous level.

> **CLINICAL PEARL:** Grasp the needle with the needle driver at a 90° angle to needle at flat surface just below attached suture material.

    ii. Pull edges together to approximate and tie with a double throw (surgeon's knot) for the first knot, followed by three single throws, alternating the direction of each throw to ensure knot is secure and lies flat. Trim tails as close to knot as possible without cutting knot and leave stitch buried.

    iii. Continue in similar fashion until deeper layers have been approximated or superficial wound tension has been relieved.

  d. Simple interrupted suture repair

    i. Simple interrupted sutures are the most common type of wound repair and work well with wounds under little tension.

    ii. Approximate wound edges: Holding one edge of the wound with forceps, place the first suture approximately 2 to 4 mm (depending on depth of wound) from wound edge, bisecting the laceration into two equal parts.

> **CLINICAL PEARL:** It is preferable to use forceps with teeth to gently lift and evert skin edges rather than grasping or crushing skin; forceps without teeth can crush tissues increasing damage and scarring.

    iii. Grab needle with forceps from inside wound (for wounds under greater tension or with wound edges that are far apart) and reload needle driver, or place first suture through both wound edges in one movement. Pull suture material through wound until 2 to 4 cm remain and tie with a double throw (surgeon's knot) for the first knot, followed by three to five single throws, alternating the direction of each throw to ensure knot is secure and lies flat.

    iv. Slide knot to one side of wound (keep this side uniform for all subsequent sutures) and cut, leaving 1-cm tails (shorter if suturing on face or intraorally).

    v. Continue to bisect each segment of wound with new sutures until wound is well approximated.

  e. Horizontal mattress suture repair

    i. Horizontal mattress sutures are useful for longer wounds and when everted wound edges are desired but there is little subcutaneous tissue underneath.

    ii. Approximate wound edges: Holding one edge of the wound with forceps, place the first suture in the same manner as the simple interrupted suture (see step 9d), reinsert the needle approximately 5 mm from the exit site on the same side of the wound. Exit on the opposite side of the wound, approximately 5 mm from original suture, parallel to the wound edge.

    iii. Pull the suture material through until 2 to 3 cm of suture remains and use this end to tie off the suture in the manner described previouly (see step 9diii) and cut tails to 1 to 2 cm. Take care not to overtighten the knot, as this may strangulate the tissue at the wound's edge.

    iv. Continue until wound is well approximated.

  f. Vertical mattress suture repair

    i. Vertical mattress suture repair is used for wounds under high tension without the need for layered suture repair.

    ii. Approximate wound edges: Holding one edge of the wound with forceps, place the first suture taking a larger, deeper bite for the first pass, exiting at the same depth and distance from wound border on opposite side of the wound. Using the needle driver, grasp the needle facing the opposite direction so as to go back toward the side first entered and reinsert needle on the same side of the wound, closer to the wound border than the original bite, passing through at a more superficial layer to the opposite side of the wound.

    iii. Pull suture material through until 2 to 3 cm remain and tie ends together on the same side of the wound using steps described in 9diii; cut 1- to 2-cm tails.

    iv. Continue until wound is well approximated.

10. Clean wound; apply antibiotic ointment and sterile dressing. Instruct patients to keep wound area clean and dry for 24 hours followed by gentle washing and daily to twice daily bandage changes with topical antibiotic ointment.

11. Suture removal is as follows
   - Face/neck: 3 to 5 days
   - Scalp: 7 days
   - Trunk/upper extremities: 7 days
   - Lower extremities: 8 to 10 days
   - Hand/joint/high-tension wounds: 10 to 14 days

12. To remove sutures, grab suture knot with forceps and cut *one* side of the loop of suture pulling knot end until loop is completely removed from wound.

CLINICAL PEARL: Be sure not to cut suture knot or more than one side of the suture loop as this can allow for sections of suture material to be left within a wound. Thick scabs may be softened with topical antibiotic ointment for 5 to 10 minutes and gently removed with forceps for ease of suture removal.

REFERENCES

1. Hollander JE, Singer AJ. Laceration management. *Ann Emerg Med.* 1999;l34(3): 356–367. doi:10.1016/s0196-0644(99)70131-9.
2. deLemos DM. Closure of minor skin wounds with sutures. In: Stack AM, Wolfson AB, eds. *UpToDate.* https://www-uptodate-com/contents/closure-of -minor-skin-wounds-with-sutures. Updated June 28, 2018.

7

Common Abbreviations in Emergency Medicine

AAA: abdominal aortic aneurysm
ABC: airway, breathing, circulation
ABG: arterial blood gas
ABI: ankle–brachial index
AC: acromioclavicular
ACEP: American College of Emergency Physicians
ACOG: American College of Obstetricians and Gynecologists
ACS: acute coronary syndrome
AF/A fib: atrial fibrillation
AHA: American Heart Association
AKA: above the knee amputation
AKI: acute kidney injury
ALP: alkaline phosphatase
ALT: alanine aminotransferase
AMA: against medical advice
AMS: altered mental status
AP: anteroposterior
aPTT: activated partial thromboplastin time
ARDS: acute respiratory distress syndrome
ARF: acute renal failure
AS: aortic stenosis
ASA: aspirin
AST: aspartate aminotransferase
AVM: arteriovenous malformation
β**-HCG:** beta-human chorionic gonadotropin
BiPAP: bilevel positive airway pressure
BKA: below the knee amputation
B/L: bilateral
BMP: basic metabolic panel
BNP: B-type natriuretic peptide
BP: blood pressure

BRAT: banana, rice, applesauce, toast
BSA: body surface area
BUN: blood urea nitrogen
CA: carcinoma
CABG: coronary artery bypass graft
CAD: coronary artery disease
CAP: community-acquired pneumonia
CBC: complete blood count
C/C: chief complaint
C-collar: cervical collar
CCU: cardiac/coronary care unit
CDC: Centers for Disease Control and Prevention
CKD: chronic kidney disease
CMP: comprehensive metabolic panel
CMS: Centers for Medicare & Medicaid Services
CN: cranial nerve
CNS: central nervous system
COPD: chronic obstructive pulmonary disease
CPAP: continuous positive airway pressure
CPK: creatine phosphokinase
Cr: creatinine
CRP: C-reactive protein
CSF: cerebrospinal fluid
CSLR: crossed straight leg raise
CTA: computed tomography angiography
CTPA: CT pulmonary angiography
CURB-65 score: confusion, blood urea nitrogen, respiratory rate, blood pressure, age >65 score
CVA: cerebrovascular accident/costovertebral angle
CVT: central venous thrombosis
CXR: chest x-ray
D/C: discontinue
DIP: distal interphalangeal joint
DJD: degenerative joint disease (osteoarthritis)
DKA: diabetic ketoacidosis
DM: diabetes mellitus
DNR: do not resuscitate
DOE: dyspnea on exertion
DP: dorsalis pedis
DRE: digital rectal exam
DTR: deep tendon reflexes
DVT: deep vein thrombosis
ECT: ecarin clotting time
EF: ejection fraction
eFAST: extended focused assessment with sonography in trauma

EMS: emergency medical services
EMTALA: Emergency Medical Treatment and Labor Act
ENT: ear, nose, and throat
EOM: extraocular muscles
ESR: erythrocyte sedimentation rate
ETOH: ethanol/alcohol
Ex-fix: external fixation
FAST: focused assessment with sonography in trauma
FB: foreign body
F/U: follow up
FX: fracture
GCS: Glasgow Coma Scale
GERD: gastroesophageal reflux disease
GFR: glomerular filtration rate
GI: gastrointestinal
GSW: gunshot wound
GU: genitourinar
HA: headache
HAP: hospital/healthcare-associated pneumonia
HCO$_3$: bicarbonate
HCT: hematocrit
HEART: history, EKG, age, risk factors, and troponin score
HEENT: head, eyes, ears, nose, and throat
HF: heart failure
HGB: hemoglobin
H/H: hemoglobin/hematocrit
HHNS: hyperosmolar hyperglycemia nonketotic syndrome
HIDA: hepatobiliary iminodiacetic acid
HLD: hyperlipidemia
H/O: history of
HSV: herpes simplex virus
HTN: hypertension
HZO: herpes zoster ophthalmicu
ICD: implantable cardioverter defibrillator
ICH: intracerebral hemorrhage/intracranial hemorrhage
ICP: intracranial pressure
I&D incision and draingle
IJ: internal jugular
INR: international normalized ratio
IOP: intraocular pressure
IR: interventional radiology
IV: intravenous
IVC: inferior vena cava
IVDU: intravenous drug use
JVD: jugular venous distention

Lac: laceration
LBBB: left bundle branch block
LBP: low-back pain
LES: lower esophageal sphincter
LFT: liver function test
LLQ: left lower quadrant (abdomen)
LMWH: low-molecular-weight heparin
LNMP: last known menstrual periods
LP: lumbar puncture
LUQ: left upper quadrant (abdomen)
LV: left ventricle
LVEF: left ventricular ejection fraction
LVH: left ventricular hypertrophy
MAP: mean arterial pressure
MCP: metacarpophalangeal
MCV: mean corpuscular volume
MI: myocardial infarction
MRA: magnetic resonance angiography
MRCP: magnetic resonance cholangiopancreatography
MRSA: methicillin-resistant *Staphylococcus aureus*
MRV: magnetic resonance venography
MSDS: material safety data sheet
MTP: metatarsophalangeal
MVA: motor vehicle accident
MVC: motor vehicle collision
MVP: mitral valve prolapse
NIHSS: National Institutes of Health Stroke Scale
NPH: normal pressure hydrocephalus
NPO: nil per os (nothing by mouth)
NSAIDs: nonsteroidal anti-inflammatory drugs
NSR: normal sinus rhythm
NSTEMI: non–ST-elevation myocardial infarction
N/V: nausea/vomiting
NYHA: New York Heart Association
OCP: oral contraceptive pill
OD: oculus dexter (right eye)
OMFS: oral and maxillofacial surgery
ORIF: open reduction and internal fixation
OS: oculus sinister (left eye)
OU: oculus uterque (both eyes)
PaCO$_2$: partial pressure of carbon dioxide
PaO$_2$: partial pressure of oxygen
PCC: prothrombin complex concentrate
PCI: percutaneous coronary intervention
PCL: posterior cruciate ligament

PCP: phencyclidine
PCR: polymerase chain reaction
PE: pulmonary embolism/physical exam
PEFR: peak expiratory flow rate
PERC score: pulmonary embolism rule-out criteria score
PESI: Pulmonary Embolism Severity Index
PID: pelvic inflammatory disease
PIP: proximal interphalangeal
Plt: platelets
PMH: past medical history
PNA: pneumonia
PO: per os (by mouth)
POA: power of attorney
POLST: Physician Orders for Life-Sustaining Treatment
PPI: proton-pump inhibitor
PRBC: packed red blood cell
PRN: pro re nata (as needed)
PSI/PORT score: Pneumonia Severity Index/Pneumonia Patient Outcomes
    Research Team score
PT: posterior tibialis/prothrombin time
PTT: partial thromboplastin time
PTX: pneumothorax
PUD: peptic ulcer disease
PVC: pulmonary vascular congestion
PVD: peripheral vascular disease
RBBB: right bundle branch block
RBC: red blood cell
Rh: Rhesus D
RICE: rest, ice, compression, elevation
RLQ: right lower quadrant (abdomen)
R/O: rule out
ROM: range of motion
ROS: review of systems
RSI: rapid sequence intubation
RUQ: right upper quadrant (abdomen)
RV: right ventricle
RVH: right ventricular hypertrophy
SAH: subarachnoid hemorrhage
SaO$_2$: oxygen saturation
SB: sinus bradycardia
SBO: small bowel obstruction
SBP: spontaneous bacterial peritonitis
SC: subcutaneous
SDH: subdural hematoma
SIADH: syndrome of inappropriate antidiuretic hormone

SL: sublingual
SLE: systemic lupus erythematosus
SLR: straight leg raise
SOB: shortness of breath
S/P: status post
SPO$_2$: peripheral capillaryoxygen saturation (capillary)/pulse oximetry
SR: sinus rhythm
ST: sinus tachycardia
STEMI: ST-elevation myocardial infarction
STI: sexually transmitted infection
SW: stab wound
TBI: traumatic brain injury
TdAP: tetanus, diptheria, acellular pertussis (vaccine)
TEE: transesophageal echocardiography
THR: total hip replacement
TIA: transient ischemic attack
TIMI score: Thrombolysis in Myocardial Infarction score
TKR: total knee replacement
TLSO: thoracic lumbar sacral orthosis
TM: tympanic membrane
TMP/SMX: trimethoprim–sulfamethoxazole
tPA: tissue plasminogen activator
TTE: transthoracic echocardiography
UA: urinalysis
UCL: ulnar collateral ligament
UH: unfractionated heparin
URI: upper respiratory infection
US: ultrasound
USPSTF: U.S. Preventive Services Task Force
URI: upper respiratory infection
UTI: urinary tract infection
UV: ultraviole
VBG: venous blood gas
VF: ventricular fibrillation
V/Q scan: ventilation/perfusion scan
VT: ventricular tachycardia
WBC: white blood cell
ZES: Zollinger–Ellison syndrome

Index